AMERICAN ACADEMY
OF OPHTHALMOLOGY®
Protecting Sight. Empowering Lives.

MW01702000

1 | Update on General Medicine

Last major revision 2019–2020

2022–2023

BCSC

Basic and Clinical Science Course™

EBO
Published after collaborative review with the European Board of Ophthalmology subcommittee

The American Academy of Ophthalmology is accredited by the Accreditation Council for Continuing Medical Education (ACCME) to provide continuing medical education for physicians.

The American Academy of Ophthalmology designates this enduring material for a maximum of 10 *AMA PRA Category 1 Credits*™. Physicians should claim only the credit commensurate with the extent of their participation in the activity.

Originally released June 2019; reviewed for currency August 2021; CME expiration date: June 1, 2023. *AMA PRA Category 1 Credits*™ may be claimed only once between June 1, 2019, and the expiration date.

BCSC® volumes are designed to increase the physician's ophthalmic knowledge through study and review. Users of this activity are encouraged to read the text and then answer the study questions provided at the back of the book.

To claim *AMA PRA Category 1 Credits*™ upon completion of this activity, learners must demonstrate appropriate knowledge and participation in the activity by taking the posttest for Section 1 and achieving a score of 80% or higher. For further details, please see the instructions for requesting CME credit at the back of the book.

The Academy provides this material for educational purposes only. It is not intended to represent the only or best method or procedure in every case, nor to replace a physician's own judgment or give specific advice for case management. Including all indications, contraindications, side effects, and alternative agents for each drug or treatment is beyond the scope of this material. All information and recommendations should be verified, prior to use, with current information included in the manufacturers' package inserts or other independent sources, and considered in light of the patient's condition and history. Reference to certain drugs, instruments, and other products in this course is made for illustrative purposes only and is not intended to constitute an endorsement of such. Some material may include information on applications that are not considered community standard, that reflect indications not included in approved FDA labeling, or that are approved for use only in restricted research settings. **The FDA has stated that it is the responsibility of the physician to determine the FDA status of each drug or device he or she wishes to use, and to use them with appropriate, informed patient consent in compliance with applicable law.** The Academy specifically disclaims any and all liability for injury or other damages of any kind, from negligence or otherwise, for any and all claims that may arise from the use of any recommendations or other information contained herein.

Cover image: From BCSC Section 12, *Retina and Vitreous.* Confocal scanning laser ophthalmoscopy multicolor fundus image (30° field of view) of a healthy eye. *(Courtesy of Lucia Sobrin, MD.)*

FSC www.fsc.org MIX Paper from responsible sources FSC® C001701

Printed in China.

Basic and Clinical Science Course

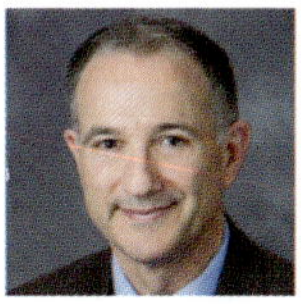

Christopher J. Rapuano, MD, Philadelphia, Pennsylvania
Senior Secretary for Clinical Education

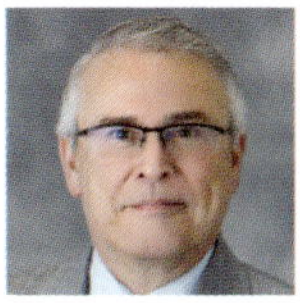

J. Timothy Stout, MD, PhD, MBA, Houston, Texas
Secretary for Lifelong Learning and Assessment

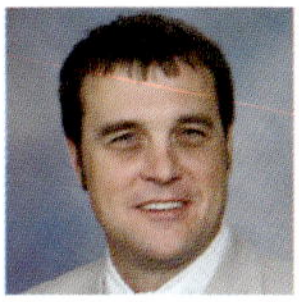

Colin A. McCannel, MD, Los Angeles, California
BCSC Course Chair

Section 1

Faculty for the Major Revision

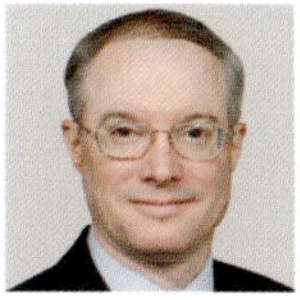

Herbert J. Ingraham, MD
Chair
Danville, Pennsylvania

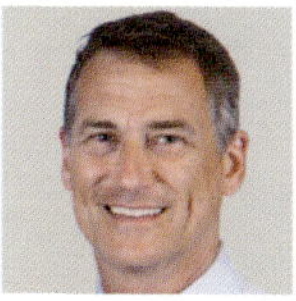

Darin K. Bowers, MD
Lynchburg, Virginia

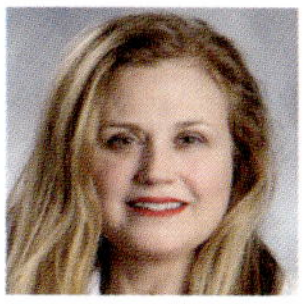

A. Luisa Di Lorenzo, MD
Troy, Michigan

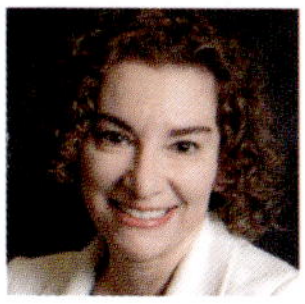

Peggy H. Gramates, MD
Pineville, Louisiana

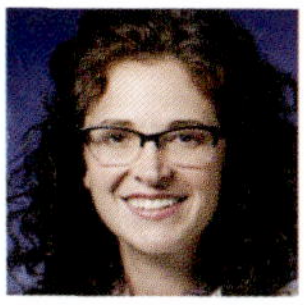

Ariane D. Kaplan, MD
Ann Arbor, Michigan

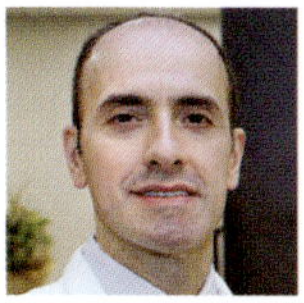

Paul J. Lama, MD
Rochelle Park, New Jersey

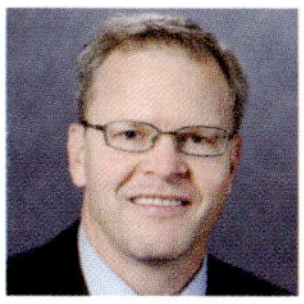

Steven L. Mansberger, MD, MPH
Portland, Oregon

The Academy wishes to acknowledge the following committees for review of this edition:

Committee on Aging: Andrew G. Lee, MD, Houston, Texas

Vision Rehabilitation Committee: Joseph L. Fontenot, MD, Mobile, Alabama

Practicing Ophthalmologists Advisory Committee for Education: Steven J. Grosser, MD, *Primary Reviewer,* Golden Valley, Minnesota; Bradley D. Fouraker, MD, *Chair,* Tampa, Florida; Alice Bashinsky, MD, Asheville, North Carolina; David J. Browning, MD, PhD, Charlotte, North Carolina; Cynthia S. Chiu, MD, Oakland, California; Stephen R. Klapper, MD, Carmel, Indiana; Troy M. Tanji, MD, Waipahu, Hawaii; Michelle S. Ying, MD, MSPH, Ladson, South Carolina

The Academy also wishes to acknowledge the following committee for assistance in developing Study Questions and Answers for this BCSC Section:

Self-Assessment Committee: Deepa Abraham, MD, Seattle, Washington; William R. Barlow, MD, Salt Lake City, Utah; William L. Becker, MD, St Louis, Missouri; Michele M. Bloomer, MD, San Francisco, California; John J. Chen, MD, PhD, Rochester, Minnesota; Zelia M. Correa, MD, Baltimore, Maryland; Deborah M. Costakos, MD, Milwaukee, Wisconsin; Theodore Curtis, MD, Mount Kisco, New York; Laura C. Fine, MD, Boston, Massachusetts; Robert E. Fintelmann, MD, Phoenix, Arizona; Mark Greiner, MD, Iowa City, Iowa; Jeffrey M. Goshe, MD, Cleveland, Ohio; Paul B. Griggs, MD, Seattle, Washington; David R. Hardten, MD, Minnetonka, Minnesota; Rachel M. Huckfeldt, MD, Boston, Massachusetts; Sarah S. Khodadadeh, MD, Vero Beach, Florida; Douglas R. Lazzaro, MD, Brooklyn, New York; Amanda C. Maltry, MD, Minneapolis, Minnesota; Brian Privett, MD, Cedar Rapids, Iowa; Sunita Radhakrishnan, MD, San Mateo, California; Jordan J. Rixen, MD, Lincoln, Nebraska; Mark I. Salevitz, MD, Scottsdale, Arizona; Ravi S. J. Singh, MD, Shawnee Mission, Kansas; Mitchell B. Strominger, MD, Reno, Nevada; Janet Y. Tsui, MD, Santa Clara, California; Ari L. Weitzner, MD, New York, New York; Zoë R. Williams, MD, Rochester, NY; Kimberly M. Winges, MD, Portland, Oregon

In addition, the Academy wishes to recognize the important contributions of Jerry A. Dancik, MD, in the development of Chapter 3, and Lisa Henderson, MD, Linda Gadioli, and Brett Wheat in the development of Chapter 16.

Finally, the Academy acknowledges the following consultants for their important work on Chapter 17: Angela R. Elam, MD, Kristen Nwanyanwu, MD, MHS, and Fasika A. Woreta, MD, MPH.

EB

European Board of Ophthalmology: Peter J. Ringens, MD, PhD, *EBO-BCSC Program Liaison,* Maastricht, Netherlands; Christina N. Grupcheva, MD, PhD, FEBO, *EBO Chair for BCSC Section 1,* Dijon, France

Financial Disclosures

Academy staff members who contributed to the development of this product state that within the 24 months prior to their contributions to this CME activity and for the duration of development, they have had no financial interest in or other relationship with any entity that produces, markets, resells, or distributes health care goods or services consumed by or used in patients, or with any competing commercial product or service.

The authors and reviewers state that within the 24 months prior to their contributions to this CME activity and for the duration of development, they have had the following financial relationships:*

Dr Bowers: Allergan (S)

Dr Browning: Aerpio Therapeutics (S), Alcon Laboratories (S), Alimera Sciences (C), Emmes (S), Genentech (S), Novartis Pharmaceuticals (S), Ohr Pharmaceutical (S), Pfizer (S), Regeneron Pharmaceuticals (S), Springer (P), ZEISS (O)

Dr Correa: Castle Biosciences (C)

Dr Fintelmann: ALPHAEON CREDIT (O), Strathspey Crown (O)

Dr Fouraker: Addition Technology (C, L), Alcon Laboratories (C, L), OASIS Medical (C, L)

Dr Goshe: Carl Zeiss Meditec (L)

Dr Grosser: InjectSense (O), Ivantis (O)

Dr Grupcheva: Allergan (L), Théa (C, L), Johnson & Johnson (L, S)

Dr Hardten: Allergan (C, L, S), Avedro (C), Eye Surgical Instruments (C, O), Johnson & Johnson (C), Oculus (L), Optical Systems Design (C, O), TLC Vision (C)

Dr Huckfeldt: AGTC (S), MeiraGTx (S), Spark Therapeutics (S)

Dr Klapper: AdOM Advanced Optical Technologies (O)

Dr Mansberger: Aerie Pharmaceuticals (C), Allergan (S), Bausch + Lomb (C), Envisia Therapeutics (C, S), Gore Medical (C), National Eye Institute (S), Nicox (C)

Dr Nwanyanwu: Eyeful LLC (O)

Dr Privett: Omeros (O)

Dr Radhakrishnan: Netra Systems (C, O)

The other authors and reviewers state that within the 24 months prior to their contributions to this CME activity and for the duration of development, they have had no financial interest in or other relationship with any entity that produces, markets, resells, or distributes health care goods or services consumed by or used in patients, or with any competing commercial product or service.

* C = consultant fee, paid advisory boards, or fees for attending a meeting; E = employed by or received a W2 from a commercial company; L = lecture fees or honoraria, travel fees or reimbursements when speaking at the invitation of a commercial company; O = equity ownership/stock options in publicly or privately traded firms, excluding mutual funds; P = patents and/or royalties for intellectual property; S = grant support or other financial support to the investigator from all sources, including research support from government agencies, foundations, device manufacturers, and/or pharmaceutical companies

Recent Past Faculty

A. Jan Berlin, MD
Maria Jancevski, MD
Jaclyn L. Kovach, MD
Maria A. Woodward, MD

In addition, the Academy gratefully acknowledges the contributions of numerous past faculty and advisory committee members who have played an important role in the development of previous editions of the Basic and Clinical Science Course.

American Academy of Ophthalmology Staff

Dale E. Fajardo, EdD, MBA, *Vice President, Education*
Beth Wilson, *Director, Continuing Professional Development*
Denise Evenson, *Director, Brand & Creative*
Ann McGuire, *Acquisitions and Development Manager*
Stephanie Tanaka, *Publications Manager*
Susan Malloy, *Acquisitions Editor and Program Manager*
Jasmine Chen, *Manager of E-Learning*
Lana Ip, *Senior Designer*
Beth Collins, *Medical Editor*
Eric Gerdes, *Interactive Designer*
Lynda Hanwella, *Publications Specialist*
Debra Marchi, *Permissions Assistant*

American Academy of Ophthalmology
655 Beach Street
Box 7424
San Francisco, CA 94120-7424

Contents

Introduction to the BCSC

The Basic and Clinical Science Course (BCSC) is designed to meet the needs of residents and practitioners for a comprehensive yet concise curriculum of the field of ophthalmology. The BCSC has developed from its original brief outline format, which relied heavily on outside readings, to a more convenient and educationally useful self-contained text. The Academy updates and revises the course annually, with the goals of integrating the basic science and clinical practice of ophthalmology and of keeping ophthalmologists current with new developments in the various subspecialties. To address a particularly important and timely issue, Chapter 17, Social Determinants of Health, has been added to Section 1. This is a preview of the chapter on this topic that will appear in the 2023–2024 major revision.

The BCSC incorporates the effort and expertise of more than 100 ophthalmologists, organized into 13 Section faculties, working with Academy editorial staff. In addition, the course continues to benefit from many lasting contributions made by the faculties of previous editions. Members of the Academy Practicing Ophthalmologists Advisory Committee for Education, Committee on Aging, and Vision Rehabilitation Committee review every volume before major revisions. Members of the European Board of Ophthalmology, organized into Section faculties, also review each volume before major revisions, focusing primarily on differences between American and European ophthalmology practice.

Organization of the Course

The Basic and Clinical Science Course comprises 13 volumes, incorporating fundamental ophthalmic knowledge, subspecialty areas, and special topics:

1. Update on General Medicine
2. Fundamentals and Principles of Ophthalmology
3. Clinical Optics and Vision Rehabilitation
4. Ophthalmic Pathology and Intraocular Tumors
5. Neuro-Ophthalmology
6. Pediatric Ophthalmology and Strabismus
7. Oculofacial Plastic and Orbital Surgery
8. External Disease and Cornea
9. Uveitis and Ocular Inflammation
10. Glaucoma
11. Lens and Cataract
12. Retina and Vitreous
13. Refractive Surgery

References

Readers who wish to explore specific topics in greater detail may consult the references cited within each chapter and listed in the Basic Texts section at the back of the book.

These references are intended to be selective rather than exhaustive, chosen by the BCSC faculty as being important, current, and readily available to residents and practitioners.

Multimedia

This edition of Section 1, *Update on General Medicine,* includes videos related to topics covered in the book. Selected by members of the BCSC faculty to present important topics that are best delivered visually, the videos are available to readers of the print and electronic versions of Section 1 (www.aao.org/bcscvideo_section01). Mobile-device users can scan the QR code below (a QR-code reader may need to be installed on the device) to access the video content.

Self-Assessment and CME Credit

Each volume of the BCSC is designed as an independent study activity for ophthalmology residents and practitioners. The learning objectives for this volume are given on page 1. The text, illustrations, and references provide the information necessary to achieve the objectives; the study questions allow readers to test their understanding of the material and their mastery of the objectives. Physicians who wish to claim CME credit for this educational activity may do so online by following the instructions at the end of the book.*

Conclusion

The Basic and Clinical Science Course has expanded greatly over the years, with the addition of much new text, numerous illustrations, and video content. Recent editions have sought to place greater emphasis on clinical applicability while maintaining a solid foundation in basic science. As with any educational program, it reflects the experience of its authors. As its faculties change and medicine progresses, new viewpoints emerge on controversial subjects and techniques. Not all alternate approaches can be included in this series; as with any educational endeavor, the learner should seek additional sources, including Academy Preferred Practice Pattern Guidelines.

The BCSC faculty and staff continually strive to improve the educational usefulness of the course; you, the reader, can contribute to this ongoing process. If you have any suggestions or questions about the series, please do not hesitate to contact the faculty or the editors.

The authors, editors, and reviewers hope that your study of the BCSC will be of lasting value and that each Section will serve as a practical resource for quality patient care.

* This activity meets the Self-Assessment CME requirements defined by the American Board of Ophthalmology (ABO). Please be advised that the ABO is not an accrediting body for purposes of any CME program. ABO does not sponsor this or any outside activity, and ABO does not endorse any particular CME activity. Complete information regarding the ABO Self-Assessment CME Maintenance of Certification requirements is available at https://abop.org/maintain-certification/cme-self-assessment/.

Objectives

Upon completion of BCSC Section 1, *Update on General Medicine,* the reader should be able to

- describe the various factors to consider in critically reviewing clinical research
- explain the importance of the randomized, controlled clinical study in evaluating the effects of new treatments
- describe the classification, pathophysiology, and presentation of diabetes mellitus, as well as the diagnostic criteria for this disease
- describe the various therapeutic approaches for diabetes mellitus
- classify the levels of hypertension based on blood pressure measurements
- list the major classes of antihypertensive medications, their characteristics, and their adverse effects
- discuss the indications for dietary and pharmacologic treatment of hyperlipidemia
- describe the various diagnostic procedures used in the evaluation of patients with coronary heart disease
- state the current treatment options for ischemic heart disease, heart failure, and cardiac arrhythmias
- list the common causes of stroke
- distinguish between obstructive and restrictive, reversible and irreversible, pulmonary diseases, and give examples of each type
- discuss the major behavioral disorders and possible therapeutic modalities for these conditions (including the ocular adverse effects of psychoactive medications)
- list some of the factors associated with a patient's adherence or nonadherence to medical regimens

- explain the rationale for and value of screening programs for various systemic diseases
- discuss the major disease processes affecting most of the adult population, and briefly explain how preventive measures may reduce the morbidity and mortality that these diseases cause
- list the most prevalent types of cancer for men and for women together with the appropriate screening methods for detecting them
- describe current concepts about the etiologies of most malignancies
- describe traditional as well as more novel approaches to the treatment of various types of cancer
- describe the ophthalmic manifestations of the major systemic diseases covered in this volume
- list the most common human pathogens and their manifestations
- discuss the epidemiology, clinical features, and treatment of HIV infection
- list the newer antiviral, antifungal, and antibacterial agents and their benefits and adverse effects
- describe the early manifestations and treatment of malignant hyperthermia
- describe the current American Heart Association guidelines for performing cardiopulmonary resuscitation
- discuss the impact of social determinants of health on patient wellness

CHAPTER 1

Using Research to Improve Clinical Practice

Highlights

- Research can help answer important clinical questions such as the utility of diagnostic and screening tests or the benefits, risks, probabilities, and expected outcomes of surgeries.
- It is important for clinicians to understand how to measure and compare their clinical practice and how to present data to demonstrate improved clinical practice.
- The use of big data (eg, the IRIS program) or the lean technique can improve clinical outcomes, efficiency, and patient satisfaction.

Ophthalmologists use clinical research to establish best practices for patient care. This chapter will help the clinician understand how to critically review research and apply the results to the clinical practice of ophthalmology.

Researching Answers to Clinical Questions

Formulating the clinical question is the first step in resolving a diagnostic or management issue. Examples of clinical questions in ophthalmology include: What are the results of minimally invasive glaucoma surgeries in patients with low-pressure glaucoma versus higher-pressure glaucoma? Do racial and ethnic minority populations in the United States have a higher risk of proliferative vitreoretinopathy after pars plana vitrectomy? What is the expected survival of an endothelial graft in a patient with Fuchs dystrophy?

Clinicians can use various sources of information to research their answers to questions, including general textbooks on ophthalmology, review journals on specific subjects (eg, *Survey of Ophthalmology* [www.surveyophthalmol.com]), and educational material from the American Academy of Ophthalmology ([AAO]; www.aao.org/clinical-education) (eg, Preferred Practice Pattern guidelines, *Focal Points* modules). In addition, clinicians can use the Cochrane Library (www.cochranelibrary.com) to access high-quality meta-analyses regarding specific management issues (eg, surgery for nonarteritic ischemic optic neuropathy, intervention for involutional lower-eyelid ectropion).

PubMed (https://pubmed.ncbi.nlm.nih.gov) is another great resource for primary sources of information. Clinicians with more specific questions or who are looking for specific data can narrow their search to the most applicable articles. PubMed provides detailed instructions on using appropriate keywords such as type of study: from laboratory-based studies of basic science (eg, cell culture, molecular biology) to animal studies (eg, testing of new drugs or specific surgical techniques) to clinical studies (eg, case reports, case series, randomized controlled trials).

Critical Reading of Studies

Before committing time to reading a published study, the clinician should review its abstract to ascertain whether the study addresses the question of interest. After reviewing the abstract, the clinician should read the rest of the study critically to determine the characteristics of the study population, recruitment strategy, sample size, intervention, outcomes of interest, and statistical methods used, and thus evaluate whether the study is valid and applicable to the clinical question.

Are the study population and recruitment strategy applicable to my patients?

Understanding a study's population and its recruitment strategy is key to understanding the setting of the study. Was the trial clinic-based, multicenter, or community-based? In therapeutic trials, the inclusion and exclusion criteria describe the characteristics of those who were or were not treated with an intervention. Specific patient groups may have been excluded because they were considered a vulnerable population. For example, most trials of ocular hypotensive drugs exclude children and pregnant women; as a result, there are minimal data on the safety and efficacy of most ocular hypotensive agents in these 2 groups of patients. Thus, if a clinician wants to do research before deciding whether to use a specific ocular hypotensive agent in a pregnant woman or in a child, most of the evidence can be found only in individual case reports or retrospective case series.

The next step in evaluating a study is exploring whether the study created selection bias by assigning the intervention to certain participants. Was the intervention randomly assigned? Was the treated group comparable to the control group? The purpose of randomly assigning an intervention to participants is to minimize bias on the part of the investigators and the patient. For example, an investigator may create selection bias by inadvertently enrolling less complex patients for a new surgery, potentially biasing their outcomes toward better results.

Whether the selection was biased or random can be determined by examining whether the participants assigned to each group are similar in the characteristics that may affect the outcome of interest. For example, when evaluating a study assessing the effect of laser treatment versus anti–vascular endothelial growth factor (anti-VEGF) treatment on diabetic retinopathy, the clinician should examine whether patients' hemoglobin A_{1c} levels, blood pressure, and severity of disease are similar between study groups, because these factors may alter the progression of retinopathy. Use of a control group is also important because it indicates whether the results of the intervention are above and beyond beneficial effects of participants' enrollment in a trial, which usually includes selected, motivated patients.

Clinical trials may study a narrow subset of a disease, making the results applicable and generalizable only to similar patients. A common error is extrapolating such data to apply to all patients or varying degrees of disease severity. For example, if a treatment is successful only in patients with mild glaucomatous damage who underwent trabeculectomy but not in those with advanced glaucomatous damage, the study results should be applied only to similar patients—in this case, patients with mild glaucomatous damage.

Was the sample large enough to detect a difference?

The sample size must have enough power to reject the *null hypothesis,* which states that there is no difference (in the outcome of interest) in the group that received the intervention compared with the group that did not receive the intervention. A study must have enough power to reject the null hypothesis. When this occurs, it suggests support for the "alternative hypothesis," which states that a true difference exists between the groups. *Power* depends on the sample size (number of participants), the expected difference in the outcome of interest in the intervention group compared with the control group (eg, improvement in visual acuity, resolution of macular edema), and the variability (eg, standard deviation) of the outcome of interest. In general, an intervention with a larger treatment effect and smaller variability requires a smaller sample size. These characteristics should be reported in the Methods section of the study.

Are the treatments and outcomes clinically relevant?

The clinician should ascertain whether the study's results can be applied to his or her patients. Questions to consider include the following:

- Is the intervention available and applicable to the current practice environment?
- Are the outcomes clinically important?
- Are all clinically important outcomes evaluated?
- Is the treatment difference clinically significant?

It is important to consider whether the intervention is useful in practice. It may be too expensive, too difficult to perform, or no longer in general use. If so, the study may pose little benefit to current clinical care.

Is the intervention reproducible?

The study should describe the intervention in enough detail to allow the experiment to be replicated. For example, a surgical study should explain all the steps of the procedure so that different surgeons are able to perform the procedure in the same manner in each case. Did all surgeons involved in the study perform it similarly, and were their results similar? Did the study include a training session before the start of the study, monitor specific aspects of the surgical procedure, and standardize postoperative care? In general, a study should avoid differences in study procedures except for the intervention of interest. In addition, to decrease the risk of investigator bias, the study should try to mask the observer to the intervention. *Investigator bias* may occur when the investigator expects a different result in the intervention group and adjusts his or her measurement of the outcome of interest to satisfy this expectation.

Is the outcome clearly defined and reliable?

The study should clearly state the primary and secondary outcomes of interest as well as the expected change for these outcomes. For example, if the primary outcome is improvement in visual acuity, the study should indicate the logMAR value that represents improvement, the range, the distribution of results (eg, normal, skewed to the right or left), and the variability. These statements allow the reader to determine whether the study was able to prove or disprove the null hypothesis.

Many outcomes (eg, visual acuity, intraocular pressure [IOP], macular thickness as measured with optical coherence tomography [OCT]) will have measurement error. This measurement error will increase the variability of the outcome of interest or create a difference in results when no true difference in outcomes exists. Therefore, a study should standardize measurement of the outcome of interest for all investigators. For example, the Ocular Hypertension Treatment Study created a standardized method to check IOP. The "recorder" placed the tonometry dial at 20 mm Hg while an "observer" measured the IOP and adjusted the dial to the intersection of the tonometry mires without viewing the dial. Finally, the recorder recorded the IOP measurement and changed the dial back to 20 mm Hg, then repeated the measurement sequence. The sequence was repeated a third time if the measurements differed by 2 mm Hg. By using a masked recorder and observer, and repeating the testing, the study created a standardized method intended to decrease measurement error and the variability of IOP measurement.

Was the follow-up time and reporting long enough?

The validity of a study is anchored on (1) adequate duration of follow-up and (2) follow-up of all participants. Thus, in evaluating a study, the clinician should look for how many of the participants completed follow-up and whether the study reported outcomes for all participants. For example, in a study assessing the use of atropine eyedrops versus patching for treatment of amblyopia, a follow-up of 3–6 months may be adequate; similar follow-up periods may be appropriate for tracking macular edema resolution after laser or drug therapy or monitoring visual acuity improvement after cataract extraction. Conversely, glaucoma progresses over long periods; therefore, trials assessing visual field loss in glaucoma would require longer follow-up, such as 5 years. Consequently, the typical rate of disease progression is an important guide in establishing the duration of follow-up required.

Finally, the study should report the results for all participants, which is called an "intention to treat" analysis. The study should state the reasons for loss to follow-up, and any differences in reasons between the study groups. For example, participants in the intervention group of a drug trial may be more likely to drop out than those in the placebo group if they experience ocular adverse effects from the drug, such as burning or stinging.

Is the analysis appropriate for the outcome?

Statistical tests depend on the type of data used to determine the difference between 2 treatment groups. For example, if the data are normally distributed (ie, parametric, conforming more or less to a bell-shaped curve) and are continuous (eg, age), then a *t* test comparing the intervention and control groups can be performed. For continuous data that are not normally distributed, researchers can use nonparametric tests such as the

Mann-Whitney U test or the Wilcoxon signed rank test. For categorical data (present or absent; small, medium, or large), the study may use a chi-square test. All of these tests provide a *P* value, which is a number that indicates the likelihood that a difference between the 2 groups is due to chance alone. For example, a *P* value of $<.05$ suggests that the likelihood that the difference between the 2 groups is due to chance alone is less than 5%. The lower the *P* value, the less likely it is that the difference is due to chance and the more likely it is that the difference represents a true difference. Figure 1-1 shows a flow chart for various types of data and study designs.

Is the difference between the groups clinically significant?

Even though a statistical test may suggest a statistically significant difference in the results between 2 groups, the clinician should consider whether the magnitude and nature of the difference are clinically meaningful. For example, a statistically significant difference in visual acuity may only be 2 letters on a Snellen chart, but this difference may not be clinically noticeable to patients and may be within the margin of measurement error for visual acuity. In addition to evaluating primary outcome variables, the study should evaluate secondary clinically important variables related to the safety of the intervention. These variables include dropout rates, pain, and allergic reactions.

Is there a conflict of interest?

A conflict of interest (COI) occurs when a person or organization receives financial or other interests in an entity (eg, a device company) that could consciously or unconsciously

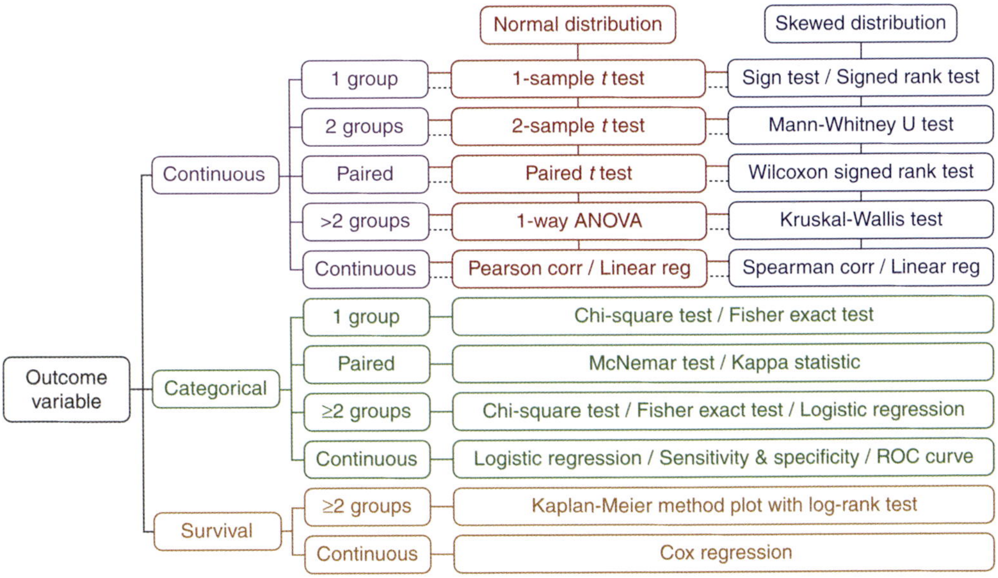

Figure 1-1 Flow chart of commonly used statistical tests. ANOVA = analysis of variance; Cox regression = Cox proportional hazards regression model; Linear reg = linear regression; Pearson corr = Pearson product moment correlation; ROC = receiver operating characteristic; Spearman corr = Spearman rank correlation. See also Figure 1-8, which shows examples of histograms with normal and skewed data distributions.

motivate them to make decisions that benefit the entity. An example of a COI would be if a person who was a paid speaker for an entity wrote and published a paper describing that entity's new device and its benefits. Because of the relationship between the author and the entity, there is a risk that the COI could positively influence the author's decision-making in the entity's favor. If the author of the paper biases the study results to describe large benefits for the device with minimal risk, the author may secondarily benefit by receiving more paid speaking engagements from the entity.

Although this COI and the author's role in the paper may not represent an impropriety, such an impropriety is one reason that medical journals require authors and other decision makers to disclose any COIs. Secondarily and most importantly, medical journals also require the author and other individuals with COIs to present an *accurate* and *balanced* assessment of the benefits and *all of the risks* of the drug or new device. Even if their motivations do not include a direct financial benefit in the form of COI, all authors are motivated to publish their findings in research journals, for reasons that may include academic promotion, future research grants, and their national reputation. Overall, any research should include an accurate and balanced assessment of the results regardless of whether the authors have COI, and readers should use their best judgment about whether the research includes a balanced presentation of the results.

Understanding Study Design

Clinical research uses a wide array of study designs. In *observational studies,* also known as *nonexperimental studies,* investigators evaluate characteristics, behaviors, and exposures in participants with a particular disease, condition, or complication. An observational study reports only the characteristics of the study population; it does not directly manipulate behaviors (eg, cigarette smoking) or exposures (eg, use of a medication, laser treatment). In *experimental studies,* typically clinical trials, subjects are assigned to a particular treatment, such as a prescribed behavior (eg, eating a diet high in antioxidant foods), or a therapeutic or preventive intervention (eg, use of an oral neuroprotective agent for patients with glaucoma, antioxidant vitamin supplementation for patients with early age-related macular degeneration [AMD]).

When conducted and interpreted appropriately, each type of study design may provide valuable information. Researchers employ observational studies when describing the presentation and progression of disease, generating hypotheses, and efficiently assessing data that may already exist for testing a hypothesis about an intervention. Examples of observational studies include case reports, case series, case-control studies, cross-sectional studies, and cohort studies. In contrast, prospective randomized controlled trials provide the best evidence regarding the effects of an intervention. Finally, meta-analyses provide a methodology to summarize the results of multiple clinical trials addressing similar research questions. Figure 1-2 depicts the levels of evidence that can be obtained from different study designs; note that meta-analyses and controlled trials offer the highest levels of evidence.

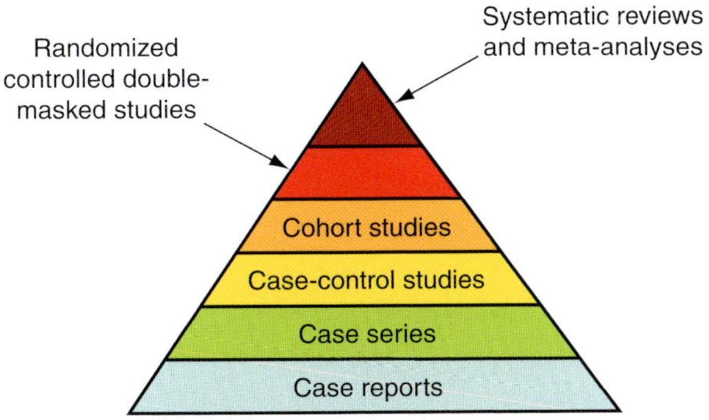

Figure 1-2 The pyramid of evidence, which illustrates the relative strength of different study designs. *(Adapted with permission from Medical Research Library of Brooklyn.* Guide to Research Methods: The Evidence Pyramid. EBM Tutorial. *https://library.downstate.edu/evidence-based-medicine.html.)*

Case Reports

A case report describes a finding in regard to a single patient to alert readers to a rare condition or unusual treatment result. For example, in 2005, Friedman reported retinal vasculitis in an apparently healthy patient with none of the common causes of vasculitis, such as toxoplasmosis, syphilis, Behçet disease, sarcoidosis, lupus, or herpes. A magnetic resonance imaging (MRI) scan of the patient's brain revealed findings typical of multiple sclerosis (MS). Although clinicians recognize that retinal vasculitis develops in MS patients, this study was the first to report retinal vasculitis as the initial presentation of MS. This case report demonstrated that clinicians should consider MS when they have tested for more common causes of vasculitis, but the etiology remains unclear.

Case reports cannot provide information on treatment efficacy or assert whether a disease is caused by an exposure. At most, they can suggest a previously unsuspected finding or mechanism of disease.

Friedman SM. Retinal vasculitis as the initial presentation of multiple sclerosis. *Retina.* 2005;25(2):218–219.

Case Series

Case series investigate the presentation, history, and/or follow-up of a group of patients and provide valuable information on the natural history or prognosis of a disease. Case series may differ from clinical trials in regard to patient selection, patient characteristics, and length and completeness of follow-up; these characteristics may establish the quality and applicability of a case series. The case series provides preliminary information for a larger study with a comparison group.

Case series can include bias if they only include patients with severe disease from tertiary referral centers such as university-based clinics, or patients with only mild cases of a disease. For example, a study examining a new minimally invasive glaucoma surgery in patients with glaucoma may show incremental lowering of IOP and the need for fewer medications 6 months after the surgery. However, in the Methods section of the study, the reader discovers that the study population came from a tertiary glaucoma center that specialized in a new procedure to reduce patient dependence on drops. Also, the study only included patients with stable glaucoma. In other words, the study was biased toward patients with mild disease and was therefore not generalizable to patients with other severities of glaucoma; it was also biased to decrease the number of medications because the providers and patients involved in the study were motivated to decrease or stop their glaucoma drops after the procedure.

Case series might not standardize the collection of patient information, measurements, tests, and other evaluations. This may result in underreporting or overreporting of results. For example, the technicians, examination rooms, lighting, and charts used to measure visual acuity may differ within the various clinics. Or study personnel may record visual acuity differently; for example, some may record the nearest whole line (20/25) while others record to the letter (20/25 + 2).

Lengths of follow-up intervals may vary within a single case series. If there are differences in follow-up time, the study should report what the specific follow-up times were, such as 1, 2, and 3 years after the initiation of treatment. When the outcome being measured is an event, such as corneal graft failure, a *survival analysis* can account for the varying lengths of follow-up. If the study does not follow all of its participants for the full length of the possible follow-up period, these losses to follow-up may cause the reported outlook for the case series to be biased. For example, in a case series of patients with macular edema from branch retinal vein occlusion, some patients may choose not to return because their macular edema has resolved, and their vision has improved; some patients may experience further loss of vision and seek care from another ophthalmologist; and some patients may move to another location. Overall, if a large percentage of patients do not return for complete follow-up, the study results may not be valid; the remaining subjects may have had an unusually good or unusually bad course compared with the subjects lost to follow-up.

Case-Control Studies

Figure 1-3 illustrates the structure of case-control studies. Case-control studies investigate a hypothesis about an association between exposures or potential risk factors (eg, smoking, medical conditions, therapies) and outcomes of interest (eg, loss of visual acuity, development of glaucoma, corneal graft failure, complications of cataract surgery). Case-control studies select a group of participants with the disease of interest (cases) and a group of comparable individuals who are free of disease (controls). Each study compares the past exposures and characteristics of the 2 groups to determine whether differences exist between the groups. If so, the study will conclude that the exposures or characteristics that differ are associated with the disease.

Researchers select cases and controls from a current database and obtain the history of exposures through patient surveys and/or review of medical records. Thus, researchers can perform case-control studies more quickly and inexpensively than cohort studies (discussed later in the chapter), because cohort studies require extra time and money to

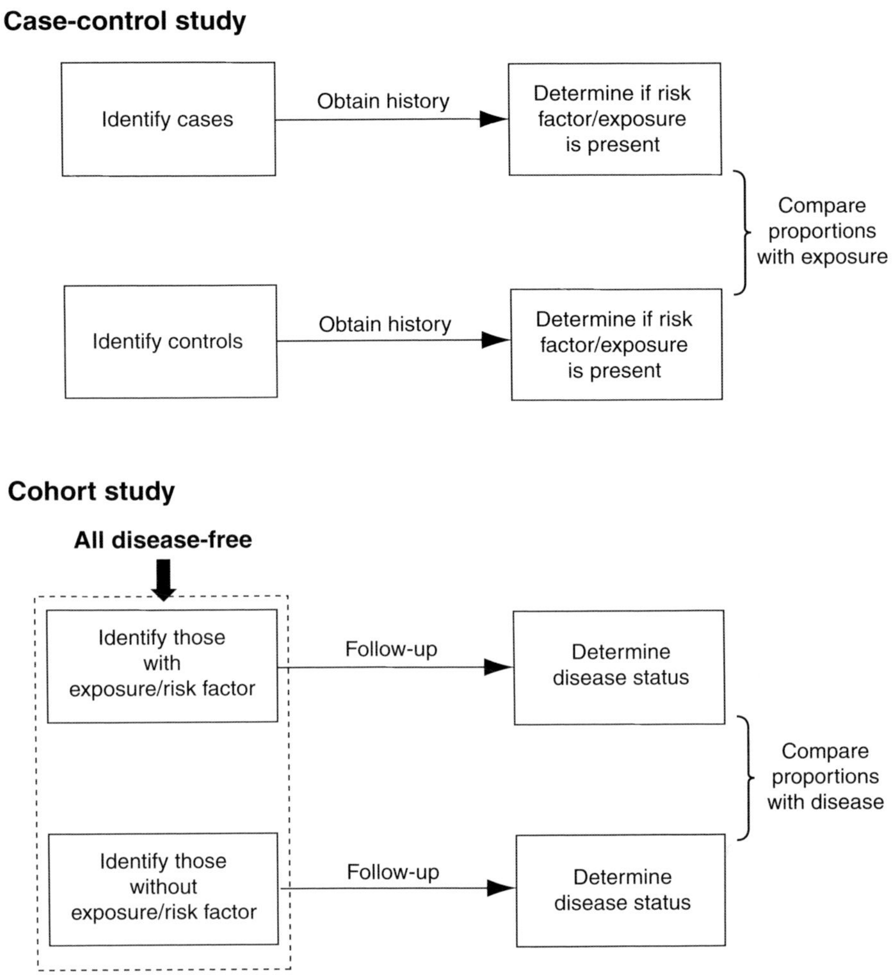

Figure 1-3 Simplified schematics of observational study designs.

follow participants. During record reviews or patient interviews, case-control studies can collect data on many potential risk factors simultaneously.

However, exposure data may be less accurate in case-control studies than in cohort studies. For example, patients with retinal vein occlusion (cases) may be more likely than control patients to recall taking medications (eg, aspirin) in the past because control patients, who do not have the disease, may be less motivated to scrutinize their past behavior. Therefore, a higher proportion of cases than controls might report use of aspirin in the past 6 months, even if in truth the proportion of aspirin users was the same in both cases and controls. This *recall bias* in cases may strengthen the association between aspirin use and vein occlusion.

Case-control studies may be subject to selection bias if they do not have an appropriate control group. For example, a study may show that myopia offers a protective effect on retinal vein occlusion if the study collects its cases from a retinal group but collects its controls from a general ophthalmology practice that offers refractive surgery for myopia. The proportion of individuals with myopia would be smaller among the cases (from the retinal group) than among the controls (from the general practice). The study may conclude that myopia is protective against retinal vein occlusion, but the apparent association would actually be attributable to selection bias. To learn more about other sources of bias, an interested reader may consult general epidemiology textbooks, such as the following.

Rothman KJ, Greenland S, Lash TL. *Modern Epidemiology.* 3rd, mid-cycle revision ed. Philadelphia: Lippincott Williams & Wilkins; 2012.

Cross-Sectional Studies

Cross-sectional studies correlate exposures and risk factors with the presence of disease without the benefit of knowing the timing or sequence of exposure and disease development. An example of a cross-sectional study is one in which a researcher collects a blood sample from patients and records their lens status (phakic, pseudophakic, or aphakic) at the same time. The study could evaluate the association between a history of cataract surgery (case status) and cholesterol level and gender (potential risk factors). However, if the mean cholesterol level is higher in cases than in those without a history of cataract surgery, the researcher would not know whether the elevated cholesterol level occurred before cataract surgery. With this study design, it is also important to consider whether a *confounding factor* may be affecting the association. For this study, age could be a confounding factor, because cholesterol levels increase with age, as does the likelihood of cataract surgery. The researcher could use data analysis tools such as stratification and/or regression analysis to adjust for age and then determine whether the cholesterol–cataract surgery association is still present in each of the age strata.

Cohort Studies

Researchers may use cohort, or follow-up, studies to investigate the association between exposures or potential risk factors and patient outcomes. These studies identify subjects who are free of the disease of interest and classify them by the presence or absence of potential risk factors. Then the study follows these subjects for subsequent development of the disease of interest (see Fig 1-3).

The Los Angeles Latino Eye Study (LALES) is an example of a population-based cohort study with prospective data collection. This study examined and interviewed approximately 6000 residents of Los Angeles, California, and followed them longitudinally for the incidence of ocular disease. Researchers explored potential risk factors for diseases such as AMD, diabetic retinopathy, glaucoma, and cataract using the residents' exposures at the beginning of the study and the incidence of the diseases years later. For example, the investigators discovered new cases of macular degeneration over a 4-year period in Latino individuals. The study found that older age and pulse pressure (difference between systolic and diastolic pressure) were independently associated with new onset early AMD, soft indistinct drusen, and retinal pigmentary abnormalities. This is an example of prospectively assessing the risk factor (blood pressure and age) for an outcome of interest (incidence of AMD).

Cohort studies can provide associations between risk factors and disease. The primary weakness of this study design is that participants with the risk factor of interest may differ in many ways from those without the risk factor, and those other characteristics may affect the incidence of the disease. One example relates to the higher incidence of graft failure among patients with interrupted sutures. It would be inaccurate to conclude that use of interrupted sutures increases the risk of graft failure, because ophthalmologists use interrupted sutures in patients with a preexisting risk of graft failure, such as stromal vascularization. In this example, stromal vascularization is a confounding factor. Statistical analysis techniques, such as stratified analysis and regression analysis, can adjust for the effect of known confounding factors. However, quite often investigators do not understand all the factors that affect the incidence of a disease. For this reason, cohort studies may identify associations and disease incidence, but these associations are not considered causal.

Choudhury F, Varma R, McKean-Cowdin R, Klein R, Azen SP; Los Angeles Latino Eye Study Group. Risk factors for four-year incidence and progression of age-related macular degeneration: the Los Angeles Latino Eye Study. *Am J Ophthalmol.* 2011;152(3):385–395.

Clinical Trials

Figure 1-4 demonstrates the major difference between clinical trials and cohort studies: clinical trials randomly assign patients to different treatment groups (exposure groups). Random assignment yields treatment groups with similar characteristics in regard to variables that may alter outcomes or the risk of complications from the treatment. This control of confounding factors is a major advantage of clinical trials over other study designs.

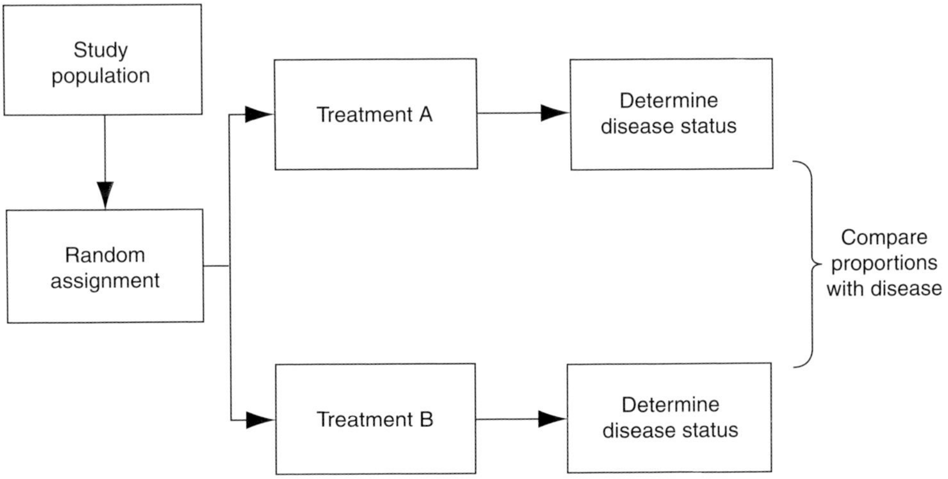

Figure 1-4 Simplified schematic of a randomized controlled trial.

All the previously mentioned features of high-quality observational studies, such as the following, should also be applied to randomized controlled trials:

- a well-defined research question and objectives
- explicit inclusion and exclusion criteria
- an adequate sample size
- standardized procedures
- predefined, objective primary and secondary outcomes
- masking of patients, treating clinicians, and evaluators to the assigned treatment
- complete follow-up of all patients

The CONSORT (Consolidated Standards of Reporting Trials) Statement, an evidence-based set of recommendations, includes a checklist of features that should be included in the design and reporting of clinical trials.

When evaluating a clinical trial, the clinician should consider 2 issues in addition to the other features of high-quality studies. The first is whether the study excluded patients from data analysis because they did not meet all of the eligibility criteria, experienced adverse effects and stopped treatment, or did not adhere to the treatment regimen. Exclusion of these types of patients creates biased results because the excluded patients' results may differ from those of the patients included in the analysis. For this reason, clinical trials should include an intention-to-treat analysis, which includes the data from all enrolled participants, and separate analyses of those who completed the trial and those who did not.

Results from subgroups of patients (eg, young vs old, hypertensive vs nonhypertensive) should be regarded with suspicion. By statistical chance alone, a study can identify a subgroup of patients for whom the benefit of treatment is statistically significant. A subgroup evaluation may be considered valid if the investigators identified the subgroup a priori in the study design, treatment results vary similarly across subgroups (eg, success steadily decreases in each age stratum as the participants become younger), and a biologically plausible explanation exists for the finding.

Systematic Reviews and Meta-analyses of Clinical Trials

Because they combine evidence from 2 or more clinical trials, systematic reviews and meta-analyses provide the strongest evidence for assessing interventions for a particular condition (see Fig 1-2). For example, to compare the safety and efficacy of intracameral cefuroxime, moxifloxacin, and vancomycin at the end of cataract surgery, Bowen and colleagues reviewed the results of 17 studies with over 900,000 eyes. They showed an 80% decrease ($P < .001$) in risk of endophthalmitis when using intracameral antibiotics. They also reported minimal toxicity for moxifloxacin; dosing errors related to toxicity for cefuroxime; and rare toxic retinal events with vancomycin use. Overall, this meta-analysis strongly supports intracameral antibiotics after cataract surgery to prevent endophthalmitis.

Bowen RC, Zhou AX, Bondalapati S, et al. Comparative analysis of the safety and efficacy of intracameral cefuroxime, moxifloxacin and vancomycin at the end of cataract surgery: a meta-analysis. *Br J Ophthalmol.* 2018;102(9):1268–1276.

Interpreting Diagnostic and Screening Tests

The goal of this section is to help the reader interpret diagnostic and screening tests. The first example presents a relatively straightforward case; it involves a screening test with a binary (yes/no) outcome, a disease that the patient either has or does not have, and a patient about whom nothing is known at the time of screening. The subsequent discussions examine complicating features that often occur in ophthalmic practice and in research. The reader should consider these complicating features when evaluating results of diagnostic and screening tests.

The Straightforward Case

A fictitious study evaluates use of a simple, quick strabismus test in 100 children, comparing it to a longer, more expensive full examination with a pediatric ophthalmologist as the *gold standard.* The study finds that 30 children have strabismus and 70 do not. However, after undergoing the quick screening test, 60 children have abnormal results and 40 children have normal results. Table 1-1 shows the screening test result data. The screening test performance is described as follows:

- *Sensitivity:* The test correctly identifies 20 of every 30 children who have strabismus (67%). The equation is a/(a + c). The denominator, (a + c), represents all of the test subjects who have the disease (strabismus).
- *Specificity:* The test correctly identifies 30 of every 70 children who do not have strabismus (43%). The equation is d/(b + d). The denominator (b + d), represents all of the test subjects who do not have the disease (normal).
- *Positive predictive value (PPV):* If a child's test results are abnormal, there is only a 1 in 3 chance (20/60) that the child actually has strabismus (33%). The equation is a/(a + b). The denominator, (a + b), represents all of the subjects with abnormal test results.
- *Negative predictive value (NPV):* If a child's test results are normal, there is a 3 in 4 chance (30/40) that the child is actually disease-free (75%). The equation is d/(d + c). The denominator, (d + c), represents all the test subjects with normal test results.
- *Accuracy:* The screening test is correct in 50 of 100 cases (50%). The equation to determine accuracy is (a + d)/(a + b +c + d).

Table 1-1 Results for Strabismus Screening Test in Clinic

Screening Test Result	Strabismus	No Strabismus	Totals
Abnormal	a. Truly abnormal (20)	b. Falsely abnormal (40)	60
Normal	c. Falsely normal (10)	d. Truly normal (30)	40
Totals	30	70	100

Sensitivity is 20/30 (67%); specificity is 30/70 (43%); positive predictive value is 20/60 (33%); negative predictive value is 30/40 (75%); accuracy is 50%.

Table 1-2 Results for Strabismus Screening Test in Shopping Center

Screening Test Result	Strabismus	No Strabismus	Totals
Abnormal	a. Truly abnormal (2)	b. Falsely abnormal (58)	60
Normal	c. Falsely normal (1)	d. Truly normal (39)	40
Totals	3	97	100

Sensitivity is 2/3 (67%); specificity is 39/97 (40%); positive predictive value is 2/60 (3%); negative predictive value is 39/40 (98%).

Sensitivity is the percentage of test subjects who both have the disease of interest and have abnormal test results, and *specificity* is the percentage of disease-free people who have normal results. However, it is also important to remember that neither sensitivity nor specificity takes into account the prevalence of disease in the study population.

Table 1-2 illustrates the performance of the hypothetical strabismus test if it yields the same results (60 children with abnormal test results and 40 children with normal test results) when performed in a shopping center where the prevalence of strabismus is only 3% (much lower than in the situation previously discussed). The sensitivity is still 67%, and the specificity is about the same, at 40%. However, because of the high number of falsely abnormal results, 58 children without disease and only 2 children who truly have strabismus would be referred for complete examinations. In this example, the PPV is only 3% (2/60). The NPV is 98% (39/40). Because of the low prevalence of strabismus in this setting, most children whose test results were abnormal would actually be disease-free. This increases the costs of unnecessary follow-up testing and increases anxiety for the parents. Clearly, the prevalence of disease in the population of interest and the screening test's PPV and NPV should be considered before the test is used for screening a population.

Choosing a gold standard is a key aspect of conducting a diagnostic testing study. The reader of such a study should ascertain whether the gold standard (in this case a pediatric ophthalmologist) was *masked* to the results of the strabismus test; if not, this may have created confirmatory bias, potentially artificially increasing the diagnostic precision of the screening test. The gold standard should also have been previously published and accepted by contemporaneous experts. Finally, the gold standard should be repeatable under the same conditions; for example, would the pediatric ophthalmologist come to the same diagnosis (strabismus vs. no strabismus) if they examined the child a second time? In conclusion, the gold standard should be scrutinized for its applicability to the clinical situation.

Complicating Features

Using ROC curves to compare different screening thresholds with a continuous predictive variable

When the screening test measures a continuous value, such as IOP, it becomes more complicated to evaluate the screening test. Figure 1-5 uses data from the Baltimore Eye Survey to graphically display sensitivity and specificity for each value of IOP. The usual cutoff for normal IOP, 21 mm Hg, has a sensitivity of 49% and a specificity of 90%. The intersection of sensitivity and specificity is the optimal threshold for maximum sensitivity and specificity in a screening test. This intersection occurs at 18 mm Hg, where the sensitivity is 65%

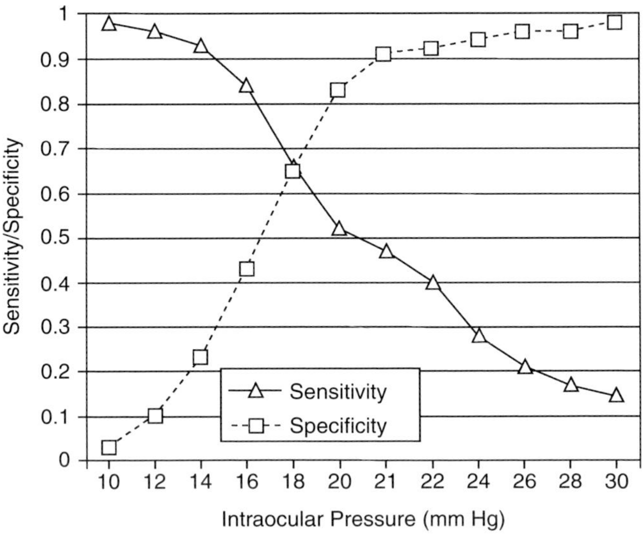

Figure 1-5 Sensitivity and specificity of an intraocular pressure (IOP) cutoff as a screening tool for glaucoma. For each IOP level (along the x-axis), the values for sensitivity and specificity are plotted. This demonstrates that with a higher level of IOP as a screening cutoff for glaucoma (for example, IOP >30 mm Hg), the sensitivity decreases and the specificity increases. *(Used with permission from Tielsch JM, Katz J, Singh K, et al. A population-based evaluation of glaucoma screening: the Baltimore Eye Survey.* Am J Epidemiol. *1991;134[10]:1102–1110.)*

and the specificity is 66%. With continuous variables, like IOP, there is a trade-off between sensitivity and specificity: a higher sensitivity results in a lower specificity, and vice versa.

Figure 1-6 depicts another graphical representation of sensitivity and specificity called a *receiver operating characteristic (ROC) curve*. By convention, an ROC curve plots sensitivity on the y-axis and (1 – specificity) on the x-axis. The larger the area under the curve, the more diagnostically precise is the screening test. The line with the diamond-shaped symbols represents a hypothetical screening test with optimal results; the line with the triangles represents a poor screening test with an ROC area of only 50%; and the line with the circles—the middle curve—represents the Baltimore Eye Survey data used in Figure 1-5. An ROC curve can inform selection of an optimal cutoff point for a screening test by identifying the sensitivity–specificity pair located closest to the upper left of the ROC plot.

Overall, these figures demonstrate that IOP measurement is not a very good screening tool for glaucoma because no cut-off reaches the ideal sensitivity/specificity (upper left of diamond line). Other significant factors in choosing a cutoff point for a screening test are the population to be screened and the relative importance of sensitivity and specificity. If the consequence of missing a diagnosis is very important such as blindness, an investigator may choose a test with high sensitivity but poor specificity. For example, a low cutoff for erythrocyte sedimentation rate might be chosen for a person who has recent vision loss and who is suspected of having giant cell arteritis.

Tielsch JM, Katz J, Singh K, et al. A population-based evaluation of glaucoma screening: the Baltimore Eye Survey. *Am J Epidemiol.* 1991;134(10):1102–1110.

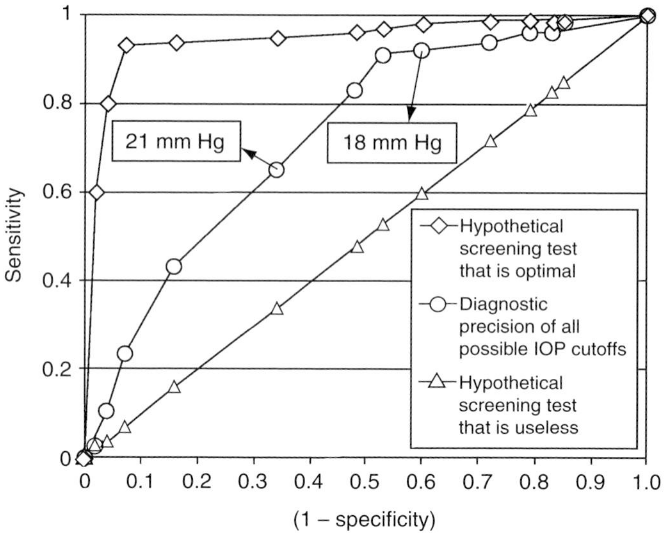

Figure 1-6 ROC curve of IOP as a screening tool for glaucoma with sensitivity on the y-axis and (1 – specificity) on the x-axis. The middle line replots the data from Figure 1-5, showing all combinations of IOP. Two boxes identify the diagnostic precision of IOP ≥18 mm Hg and IOP ≥21 mm Hg. The other lines represent an optimal (upper line) and a useless (lower line) screening test, respectively. *(Produced with data from Tielsch JM, Katz J, Singh K, et al. A population-based evaluation of glaucoma screening: the Baltimore Eye Survey.* Am J Epidemiol. *1991;134[10]:1102–1110.)*

Using ROC curves to compare different screening devices

Studies can use ROC curves to compare new diagnostic tests. ROC curves can be used to compare tests that use different units or different scales. Figure 1-7 shows 3 ROC curves illustrating the ability of 3 glaucoma imaging devices to discriminate between healthy eyes and eyes with glaucomatous visual field loss via imaging of the optic nerve head and nerve fiber layer. The area under each ROC curve represents a summary measure of the relative efficacy of the screening test. The ROC curves appear similar for inferior average nerve fiber layer thickness as measured with OCT and for scanning laser polarimetry with variable corneal compensation (GDx VCC nerve fiber index), while the ROC curve for confocal scanning laser ophthalmoscopy (HRT linear discriminant function) is lower. In other words, the figure suggests a higher diagnostic precision for scanning laser polarimetry and OCT than confocal scanning laser ophthalmoscopy.

Medeiros FA, Zangwill LM, Bowd C, Weinreb RN. Comparison of the GDx VCC scanning laser polarimeter, HRT II confocal scanning laser ophthalmoscope, and Stratus OCT optical coherence tomograph for the detection of glaucoma. *Arch Ophthalmol.* 2004;122(6):827–837.

The effect of pretest probability of disease

Pretest probability of disease uses knowledge of the patient before any screening or diagnostic tests are performed. For example, the investigator may know that the patient has a first-degree relative with glaucoma as well as a thinner-than-average central corneal thickness (both are risk factors for glaucoma). This information suggests a pretest probability

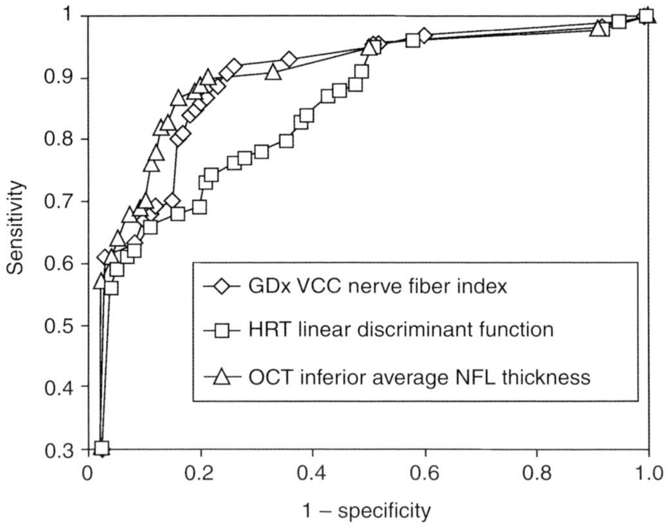

Figure 1-7 ROC curve of 3 glaucoma imaging devices. The single parameter chosen for display for each instrument was the one that performed the best in the authors' study. There was no statistically significant difference in the area under the ROC curves for these 3 parameters. *(The HRT linear discriminant function is from a paper by Bathija et al, referenced by Medeiros et al; the GDx and OCT parameters are standard test outputs provided by the manufacturers. Graph drawn with data from Medeiros FA, Zangwill LM, Bowd C, Weinreb RN. Comparison of the GDx VCC scanning laser polarimeter, HRT II confocal scanning laser ophthalmoscope, and Stratus OCT optical coherence tomograph for the detection of glaucoma.* Arch Ophthalmol. *2004;122[6]:827–837.)*

of glaucoma about 3 times higher than that of a person picked at random from the general population. How much does a diagnostic test improve the ability to diagnose glaucoma in this patient with a higher pretest probability? How much higher is the relative risk of glaucoma if the test result is positive?

Bayes theorem allows the pretest probability of disease to be combined with the diagnostic precision of a screening test to produce a posttest probability of disease. To use this theorem, the *likelihood ratio* must be calculated. The likelihood ratio of a positive test is the sensitivity divided by (1 – specificity). For a sample test with 80% sensitivity and 90% specificity (0.8/[1 – 0.9]), the positive likelihood ratio is 8. The likelihood ratio of a negative test is (1 – sensitivity) divided by the specificity. For the same sample test, the negative likelihood ratio is (1 – 0.8)/0.9, or 0.22. Positive likelihood ratios start at 1 and continue to infinity—the bigger, the better. Negative likelihood ratios range from 0 to 1—the smaller, the better. If the goal is to diagnose disease, the test with the larger positive likelihood ratio is the better test; conversely, if the goal is to rule out disease, the test with the smaller negative likelihood ratio is better.

If the positive likelihood ratio is multiplied by the pretest probability of disease, the result is the *posttest probability of disease*. Thus, for the example patient with the positive family history, thin cornea, and pretest probability of 3, a positive test with a positive likelihood ratio of 8 will result in a posttest probability of glaucoma that is 24 times that of a person drawn at random from the population.

Table 1-3 Changes in PPV and NPV Depending on Pretest Probability in a Test With 80% Sensitivity, 90% Specificity

Pretest Probability of Disease, %	Positive Predictive Value (PPV), %	Negative Predictive Value (NPV), %
1	7.5	99.8
10	47.1	97.6
50	88.9	81.8
90	98.6	33.3

Table 1-3 demonstrates another important consideration regarding pretest probability of disease. Consider the case of a 65-year-old woman with no risk factors for glaucoma and a pretest probability of disease of 1.0%. A positive test result for glaucoma would raise her probability of disease to 7.5%. Most patients with a positive test result would not actually have the disease! Similarly, an 85-year-old man with a strong positive family history, thin central corneal thickness, and an IOP of 30 mm Hg might have a pretest probability of disease of 50.0%. If his test result were negative, he would still have a posttest probability of disease of 18.2%, greater than that of the 65-year-old woman! This example illustrates the importance of considering the pretest probability of disease in deciding whether to employ a diagnostic test. In general, screening tests do not perform well when the prevalence of disease is low.

Intermediate diagnostic categories, such as "glaucoma suspect," are often encountered in clinical practice. Sensitivity–specificity and ROC curves cannot account for such categories, because they require borderline subjects to be categorized as either having the disease (eg, glaucoma) or not having it (eg, no glaucoma). However, a likelihood ratio can be calculated for a borderline category, which reflects the risk of patients exhibiting that characteristic (eg, "glaucoma suspect").

Use of tests in combination

Studies can combine tests in series or in parallel. An example of combining 2 tests *in series* is when a clinician performs the second test only if the first is positive. The correlation between the 2 tests must be considered when they are used in series. Consider the following case: a study uses cup–disc ratio, determined via optic nerve head photography, as a diagnostic test. If the result is positive, the peripapillary retinal nerve fiber layer thickness observed on OCT imaging is used to confirm the diagnosis. The study provides likelihood ratios for each test. Although it may be tempting to use the product of the 2 likelihood ratios and the pretest probability to calculate a posttest probability, if the screening tests are correlated with one another the predictive ability will appear artificially higher. Because cup–disc ratio and retinal nerve fiber layer thickness both examine tissues of the optic nerve head, albeit using different technologies, they are highly correlated. Thus, because the 2 tests are not independent, the results from the performance of the 2-test strategy are likely to be different from the posttest probability calculated from the product of the 2 likelihood ratios and the pretest probability.

Other studies have combined tests *in parallel*, considering the result positive if either test result is positive. This strategy works best when the tests have good specificity (combining tests this way makes overall specificity deteriorate) and address different aspects of a disease. Kopplin and colleagues found that a visual acuity of less than 20/40, abnormal/poor-quality nonmydriatic imaging, abnormal frequency doubling perimetry, or abnormal/poor-quality confocal scanning laser ophthalmoscopy resulted in an ROC curve area of 0.827 for detection of visually significant eye disease (eg, cataract, macular degeneration, glaucoma).

Kopplin LJ, Mansberger SL. Predictive value of screening tests for visually significant eye disease. *Am J Ophthalmol.* 2015;160(3):538–546.e3.

Clinical acceptance and ethics of testing

Clinicians should avoid tests that provide a small increment in the likelihood ratio of detecting disease or that are expensive or painful. Also, all tests carry some burden, including the potential for adverse effects (eg, corneal abrasion from tonometry), psychological fear of a disease (eg, related to a screening test for glaucoma), and additional testing and follow-up examinations for abnormal or unusual results. A clinician should avoid a test if it will not change patient management. Similarly, screening for eye disease should include a process for follow-up of those who have abnormal results, regardless of their insurance status. Screening provides little value to participants who are told they might have a disease but are given no method of obtaining a follow-up evaluation or treatment.

Generalizability

Most studies investigate new screening or diagnostic tests in a clinical setting before evaluating them in a population-based sample (largely because of the high cost of performing population-based research). Clinicians should consider whether the data for a new test will apply to their screening population. Even a clinic-based study may not have patients like those in another practice. For example, a study may include only young glaucoma patients without other eye diseases, such as macular degeneration. This leads to excellent sensitivity and specificity, but the results may differ in a sample of patients who have borderline glaucoma and are older.

Summary

Researchers use a variety of measures to evaluate the diagnostic precision of screening and diagnostic tests. Sensitivity and specificity are the simplest and easiest to understand, but their disadvantage is that they do not account for the prevalence of disease in the target population. PPV and NPV are more useful in that regard. ROC curves provide a comprehensive view of the relationship between the sensitivity and specificity of a continuous test result (eg, IOP) and can be used to compare diagnostic tests. Clinicians can use likelihood ratios and pretest probability of disease to critically evaluate screening and diagnostic tests in their clinical setting.

Riegelman RK. *Studying a Study and Testing a Test: Reading Evidence-based Health Research.* 6th ed. Philadelphia: Lippincott Williams & Wilkins; 2012.

Discussing Benefits, Risks, Probabilities, and Expected Outcomes With Patients

Physicians and their clinical team members need to educate patients regarding their disease, including potential preventive measures, treatments, and outcomes.

Clinical research defines *risk* as the conditional probability of an event, usually an adverse event. *Risk difference* is the absolute difference in the risk between 2 groups of individuals. *Relative risk* is the ratio of 2 risk measures. The risk difference depends on the unit of measure, whereas relative risk is dimensionless because it involves division of 2 risk measurements. In the Ocular Hypertension Treatment Study (OHTS), the risk difference of glaucoma development for subjects who were not treated compared with those who were treated was 5% (9.5%–4.5%) across 5 years. The relative risk of not being treated compared with receiving treatment was 211% (9.5%/4.5%). Both measures are consistent with the data, but clinicians or patients may interpret them very differently. Numerically, a 5% increased risk of glaucoma (if ocular hypertension is not treated) might seem small to a patient, while a 211% increased risk might seem large. A key piece of information that may help in the interpretation of such results is the *baseline probability of the outcome.* For example, the baseline probability of developing glaucoma with untreated ocular hypertension is 9.5%. In most cases, baseline probabilities or expected outcomes can help patients understand risk and make an informed decision about a procedure.

The *number needed to treat (NNT)* can also be helpful when describing how likely a treatment or medication will improve an outcome for an individual patient. In the above example, the study shows a 5% absolute risk reduction (ARR) in the proportion of patients without glaucoma if they use ocular hypotensive medications. The ARR is 5%, and the number needed to treat is 20 (100/5). In other words, a clinician could tell the patient that in order to prevent 1 patient from developing glaucoma over 5 years, 20 patients would need to be treated with ocular hypotensive medications. Armed with this information, the patient can decide whether to use an ocular hypotensive medication.

For those providers with capitated payments, it may be useful to consider the impact of the new procedure or treatment on societal cost. This cost can be determined by calculating the added cost using the NNT. For example, if the retail cost of a generic glaucoma medication for 1 patient is $70/month, or $4200 over 5 years, the excess cost of using ocular hypotensive medications calculated with the NNT would be $84,000 ($4200 × 20) for 1 patient to see the benefits from using these ocular hypotensive medications.

The advantage of the NNT is that it only uses absolute risk reduction and is less likely to exaggerate the impact of a new procedure or medication. However, the NNT does not take other important factors into consideration, such as the negative effects on quality of life related to eyedrop use, nor other possible factors such as systemic adverse effects resulting from the use of ocular medications. The NNT does provide a straightforward attempt to describe the likelihood that a patient will be helped, harmed, or unaffected by a treatment.

In observational studies, investigators may also present their results as *odds ratios.* In an odds ratio, the odds of a subject with the disease (case) having an exposure (eg, smoking) are compared with the odds of a subject without the disease (control) having the exposure. When the disease is rare, the odds ratio approximates the relative risk of the exposure, because the denominators for both the odds under comparison are close to 1. For example, in the meta-analyses on potential risk factors for late AMD, which occurs relatively infrequently, the odds ratio for smoking is 2.35, meaning smokers have a 235% risk for development of late AMD compared with nonsmokers. As previously stated, the baseline risk is key; if it is low (ie, less than 1%), then an odds ratio of 2.0 still results in a low risk for an individual patient.

Exposure to specific factors may or may not be clinically significant, and it may not be *causal*, or one of the root causes of the disease. Because it is difficult to distinguish causal risk factors from noncausal risk factors in observational studies, researchers often use causal criteria to identify which risk factors are causal and which are not.

Medical providers use *risk calculators* in a number of ways, for example, to predict an individual patient's risk of cardiovascular disease, risk of having a child with Down syndrome, likelihood of survival from an intensive care unit, and likelihood of experiencing other medical conditions. Ophthalmologists have used risk calculators to help simplify complex study results and apply these results to individual patients. For example, the OHTS regression equation used 5 variables (cup–disc ratio, central corneal thickness, untreated IOP, pattern standard deviation from the visual field, and age) to predict the risk of a patient developing glaucoma as a result of ocular hypertension. The OHTS risk calculator is available for free online (https://ohts.wustl.edu/risk/). Other available risk calculators include those for macular degeneration, keratoconus, and glaucoma progression. Many risk calculators can be downloaded onto a mobile device. Overall, the advantage of risk calculators is that they simplify complex results to provide an estimate of the mean baseline probability of disease development or surgery complications in individual patients. Risk calculators can also identify those patients at high risk of developing disease and select them for a lower NNT and lower societal costs.

De Moraes CG, Sehi M, Greenfield DS, Chung YS, Ritch R, Liebmann JM. A validated risk calculator to assess risk and rate of visual field progression in treated glaucoma patients. *Invest Ophthalmol Vis Sci.* 2012;53(6):2702–2707.

Kass MA, Heuer DK, Higginbotham EJ, et al. The Ocular Hypertension Treatment Study: a randomized trial determines that topical ocular hypotensive medication delays or prevents the onset of primary open-angle glaucoma. *Arch Ophthalmol.* 2002;120(6):701–713.

Mansberger SL. A risk calculator to determine the probability of glaucoma. *J Glaucoma.* 2004;13(4):345–347.

How to Measure and Improve Clinical Practice

Using Big Data to Improve Clinical Practice

Large studies using claims data have demonstrated considerable regional differences in practice and in the quality of eye care in the United States and worldwide. For example, Stein and colleagues showed a large difference in the use of laser trabeculoplasty between ophthalmologists and optometrists in Oklahoma. Were these high usage rates standards of care, or did they represent overusage, particularly when compared to other treatments?

An analysis of the Medicare database revealed that some ophthalmologists had large Medicare expenditures when compared with those of the average ophthalmologist. This big data analysis, among others, prompted investigators to discover fraud in our health care system. Big data can also be used to evaluate how individual ophthalmologists compare to their peers for an outcome of interest, such as the proportion of patients who need to return to the operating room after cataract surgery. If an ophthalmologist has a higher complication rate than that of his or her peers, this information may prompt that ophthalmologist to begin a quality improvement project to lower their patient complication rate via education and further training. Big data offer clinicians many opportunities to measure and improve eye care, particularly when accompanied by an organizing framework to understand the data and develop improvement activities (see the following sections).

Medicare Provider Utilization and Payment Data: Physician and Other Supplier Look-up Tool Database. Baltimore, MD: Centers for Medicare & Medicaid Services. https://www.cms.gov/Research-Statistics-Data-and-Systems/Statistics-Trends-and-Reports/Medicare-Provider-Charge-Data/Physician-and-Other-Supplier. Accessed September 10, 2021.

Stein JD, Zhao PY, Andrews C, Skuta GL. Comparison of outcomes of laser trabeculoplasty performed by optometrists vs ophthalmologists in Oklahoma. *JAMA Ophthalmol.* 2016; 134(10):1095–1101.

Issues in Designing a Measurement System

A useful measurement system may include quality indicators. For example, one question ophthalmologists commonly face is whether they have dilated a diabetic patient's eyes at least once every 2 years. How might one validate that a dilated eye examination was performed? One cumbersome validation method would be to video record ophthalmologists while they perform patient examinations and then review that recording to confirm the completion of the dilated eye examination. Other validation options may include (1) written documentation indicating that dilating drops were placed in the eye; (2) notations in the medical record indicating that a peripheral dilated eye examination was performed, such as noting whether it was normal or abnormal; and (3) a diagram or drawing of the retina periphery. All of these would be valid measures.

Once a valid measure has been chosen, *reliability* needs to be determined. First, the analysis should yield the same results if performed by the same clinician at a different time. For example, are the same results obtained when a measure is made with the same instrument the second time and the third? Measures that minimize errors when repeated have good *test–retest reliability,* or reproducibility. Second, the analysis should yield the same results if performed on the same subject multiple times. If the person doing the measurement gets the same results on the same subject, after multiple attempts, there is good *intrarater reliability.* Third, the analysis should yield the same results if performed by different clinicians. Organizations should design measures (as well as a training system for the staff and a support system that will capture and analyze the data) to allow different people to use the same measure and obtain similar results. Measures that have this characteristic are said to have good *interrater reliability.*

In research, 2 statistical techniques are commonly used to determine the degree of agreement between 2 different tests that detect a particular disease in a group of patients.

One method is to simply tally the number of times that the results of the 2 tests agree (ie, both tests indicate disease present, both tests indicate no disease) and then divide that number by the total number of items being assessed, thereby yielding the *percent agreement.* Another method, the κ (kappa) statistic, measures the agreement between 2 or more individuals or entities while taking into account the potential for agreement via chance alone. Kappas greater than 0.75 represent excellent agreement; those from 0.40 to 0.75, fair to good agreement; and those below 0.40, poor agreement. However, not all experts agree on these kappa cutoff points; and other cutoffs for agreement may be recommended.

Once a valid and reliable measure has been established, the organization should first consider the population of interest and the inclusion and exclusion criteria. For example, a study of the quality of cataract surgery might exclude retina specialists (exclusion criterion) and include only comprehensive ophthalmologists who spend at least 50% of their time seeing patients (inclusion criterion).

Second, the organization needs to determine whether the studied event occurs at a frequency that will allow meaningful differences to be found. Are the events so rare ("floor effect") or so common ("ceiling effect") that little value is to be gained in using such a measurement system? Organizations should consider conducting a pilot study to investigate these issues before implementing a system.

Third, whenever possible, organizations should use measures that are easily obtained, yet are valid and reliable. Systems that do not require much additional work are more practical for the purpose of monitoring practices. Thus, billing files may provide sufficient information on the completion of specific process quality steps, such as the performance of regular visual field testing in patients with glaucoma, and outcomes, such as incidence of suprachoroidal hemorrhage after intraocular surgery.

Implementation of a Monitoring System

An ideal monitoring system would capture data regarding every patient of interest for a given practitioner. Doing so would collect the maximum number of cases for statistical analyses and provide maximum statistical power for reliable estimates of uncommon or rare events. In addition, a 100% analysis would minimize bias due to missing patients. For example, electronic billing data could identify every patient who had intraocular surgery (identified by specific Current Procedural Terminology [CPT] codes) in a practice during a specified period and any subsequent surgeries (again identified by CPT codes) within the next 30 or 90 days to determine a specific complication (identified by its International Classification of Diseases code), such as retinal detachment or endophthalmitis. This would reflect *outcome quality.*

In contrast, questions about *process quality*—such as whether a target pressure range was set for every patient with glaucoma—are not amenable to a 100% analysis because that type of data may not be entered in current administrative databases; instead, it may need to be extracted from medical records by a trained reviewer. Information obtained from billing databases may allow assessment of other process quality measures, such as gonioscopy.

An organization's next step is to review its records. What standards should be used for such a review? What criteria should be used? *Explicit* criteria, which have a yes/no outcome or limited categories (eg, optic nerve documentation could include a statement regarding the nerve's condition, the vertical cup–disc ratio, or a drawing or photograph), have higher reliability than *implicit* criteria (the reviewer's judgment that overall quality was good or not good), particularly for interrater reliability. For ophthalmology practices, the American Academy of Ophthalmology (AAO) provides Preferred Practice Pattern guidelines and a summary benchmarks series, both of which can be used to obtain explicit criteria. Similarly, the American Board of Ophthalmology includes explicit criteria in its Practice Improvement Modules for maintenance of board certification. These are available at www.aao.org/ppp and at https://abop.org, respectively.

Record reviews may reveal that some medical records are unavailable or are missing data or information on visits. Every effort should be made to obtain unavailable records. If these records remain unavailable, the number of unavailable records should be recorded, and replacement records from the randomization should be reviewed. A high proportion of missing medical records may suggest bias. For records with missing visits, it may be possible to capture important data from other available visits. If the review criteria require that every visit is checked, the options are to (1) exclude that patient, (2) exclude that patient only for analyses needing that missing-visit data, (3) impute the missing values through statistical modeling of available data, or (4) treat the missing visit as either meeting or not meeting the criteria (generally the latter). The key steps are to decide what to do and then apply that decision consistently over time (and report the decision with the data and results).

An important element of establishing a system for monitoring quality of care is performing power calculations to determine sample sizes, because these calculations provide confidence that a nonsignificant difference is truly nonsignificant (and is not due to having an insufficient sample size). See the section "Was the sample large enough to detect a difference?" earlier in this chapter.

One final consideration is the external validity of the method used to determine whether a quality measure was met. Using chart review, McGlynn and colleagues determined that the rate of annual dilated eye examination among patients with diabetes mellitus was only 19%. But when they used billing codes, they found that the rate was 50%. Was the discrepancy due to poor documentation of the procedure or inaccurate billing practices? The data may have been recorded incorrectly, by either the observer or the person abstracting the data from the data source. Other errors could be related to coding issues, data entry problems, and incorrect diagnoses. In summary, each discrepancy needs to be examined further, and the whole monitoring system may need to be redesigned. As stated previously, conducting a pilot study with a handful of participants can help with study design, increase validity, and save time when developing a monitoring system.

In 2013, AAO introduced its IRIS (Intelligent Research in Sight) Registry, a centralized system for collecting electronic eye care data from ophthalmology practices. This registry automatically abstracts data from modern electronic medical record systems. In comparison to large claims-based registries, which collect data about electronic billing, IRIS contains specific information related to the medical treatment of eye disease (eg, visual acuity, IOP) and is agnostic to insurance status. This allows ophthalmologists to examine results of medical treatment of eye disease and develop improvement activities.

AAO's other goals for the registry include the provision of benchmark reports for quality of care and identify opportunities for improvement. The registry can also create large data sets for diseases such as AMD, cataract, and glaucoma, facilitating exploration of trends in treatment, costs, and other factors. It also allows collection of data regarding rare diseases, such as retinitis pigmentosa. For example, Rao and colleagues compared the visual acuity after 1 year in patients undergoing treatment for neovascular age-related macular degeneration (nAMD). The researchers found no difference in visual acuity results when comparing 3 common medications for nAMD (bevacizumab, ranibizumab, and aflibercept). This result suggested that all tested medications could be used, and providers may consider other distinguishing characteristics of the treatments such as cost when deciding which medication to recommend. This may be an important tool to help ophthalmologists continually monitor and improve their performance quality.

McGlynn EA, Asch SM, Adams J, et al. The quality of health care delivered to adults in the United States. *N Engl J Med.* 2003;348(26):2635–2645.

Rao P, Lum F, Wood K, et al. Real-world vision in age-related macular degeneration patients treated with single anti-VEGF drug type for 1 year in the IRIS Registry. *Ophthalmology.* 2018;125(4):522–528.

Analysis of the Results

Once the results have been compiled, organizations must interpret the data correctly. For projects designed to detect important deviations from expected performance, it is important to use tests that determine statistical significance. For many measures, comparisons of mean performance are satisfactory—for example, the percentage of AAO benchmark process indicators for cataract that providers have achieved. However, for others, the best way to compare performance may be to analyze the number of patients whose care meets a given threshold. For example, investigators may want to know the percentage of patients who have at least a 90% quality score. Once that measure is obtained, researchers can compare it among providers.

In addition, when evaluating quality results investigators should consider clinical significance and difference, and factors beyond the provider's control. Patients could refuse the cost of additional tests or refuse to be dilated because they need to be able to drive. Outcomes of chronic diseases are even more difficult to evaluate than process measures such as dilation of a patient with diabetes mellitus. For example, the rate of blindness from glaucoma over 20 years is subject to the severity at presentation and the risk for progression among the pool of patients. Quality of care for chronic diseases like glaucoma may be affected by patients' ability to return for regular care and use their recommended treatments regularly, as well as their socioeconomic status. Thus, measuring whether the provider performs specific examination steps, such as examining the optic nerve (*process*), is appropriate, whereas looking at rates of blindness over 20 years (*outcomes*) may not be appropriate.

Organizations can use statistical analyses to evaluate potential differences in quality between providers. They can control for patients' socioeconomic status and demographic characteristics, as well as other factors that may be related to the outcome of interest.

These analyses may show that a factor that cannot be "treated" by the provider (eg, socioeconomic status) is the issue and is outside the provider's control. Even with these caveats, quality improvement is critical to medicine. In addition, the purpose is not to be punitive but to encourage improvement in all providers and improvement in individual providers from year to year.

Methods of Presenting Data to Facilitate Continuous Improvement

After the results have been analyzed, the next step is to graphically display and disseminate them. There are many ways to present data. First, the data can be displayed using a frequency distribution such as a histogram (Fig 1-8) or using a scatter diagram (Fig 1-9). Are the data *normally distributed* (ie, distributed in a bell-shaped curve), or are they skewed? The answer to this question affects the selection of statistical tools and analyses, and it can provide important insights into potential underlying factors. Alternately, 2 distinct subgroups may be found in the data and need to be defined. For example, care in solo practices may differ from care in large single-specialty groups for a particular disease area.

Second, a Pareto chart (Fig 1-10) can provide insights into the cumulative distribution of key factors of interest. The chart combines a histogram with a cumulative frequency line, making it possible to assess performance across the range of values for the variable of interest.

Third, run charts or control charts (Fig 1-11) can help organizations understand changes that have occurred over time. Rates of events, especially uncommon ones, can fluctuate. Are the fluctuations significant, both statistically and clinically, compared with those during prior periods or from other institutions or practices? In run charts and control charts, event rates are plotted over time with both upper and lower control limits and averages. This presentation enables reviewers to determine (1) whether an aberrant data point is really a meaningful finding or is due to random error and (2) how the organization is faring compared with peer organizations, if data from peers are available.

The purpose of these data analyses is to identify variation in the factor of interest. Factors that are due to the way the system is established and that are inherent in its current state of operations are called *common cause factors.* To improve performance in this area, the organization will have to redesign and reengineer the system. For example, there may be a known rate of "unreliable" visual fields in glaucoma, despite the best training of technicians and screening of patients. In contrast, there are "special causes" of variation that are due to a specific, identifiable factor, often a specific provider or person. Rapid identification of "special cause" variance allows for quick correction of variation that exceeds normal rates. However, improving the performance of the overall system and reducing the common cause variation will improve care and affect the most patients. By "shifting the curve," the organization can improve care for every patient, as opposed to just identifying the outlier providers and assisting in their rehabilitation.

Other Features of Continuous Quality Improvement

Studies suggest that just measuring and reporting results improves performance indicators by up to 6%. However, organizations that continually incorporate quality improvement

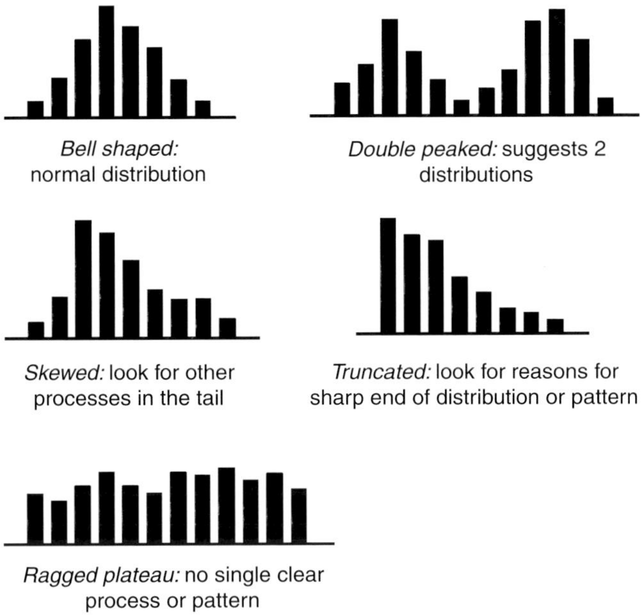

Figure 1-8 Types of histograms with different data distributions. *(Reproduced from the Quality Assurance Project.)*

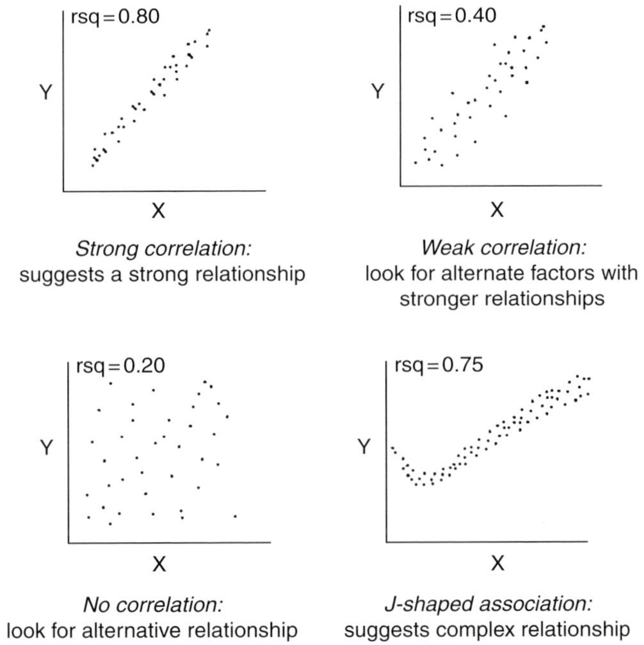

Figure 1-9 Scatter diagram interpretation. An rsq value of 0.80 means that 80% of the variation can be explained by the relationship between x and y. An rsq of more than 0.50 is respectable and results close to 0 mean that the variables are unrelated. *(Reproduced from the Quality Assurance Project.)*

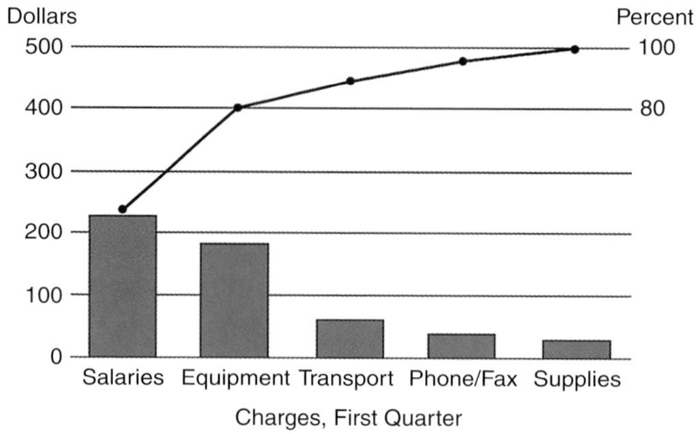

Figure 1-10 Pareto chart. *(Reproduced from the Quality Assurance Project.)*

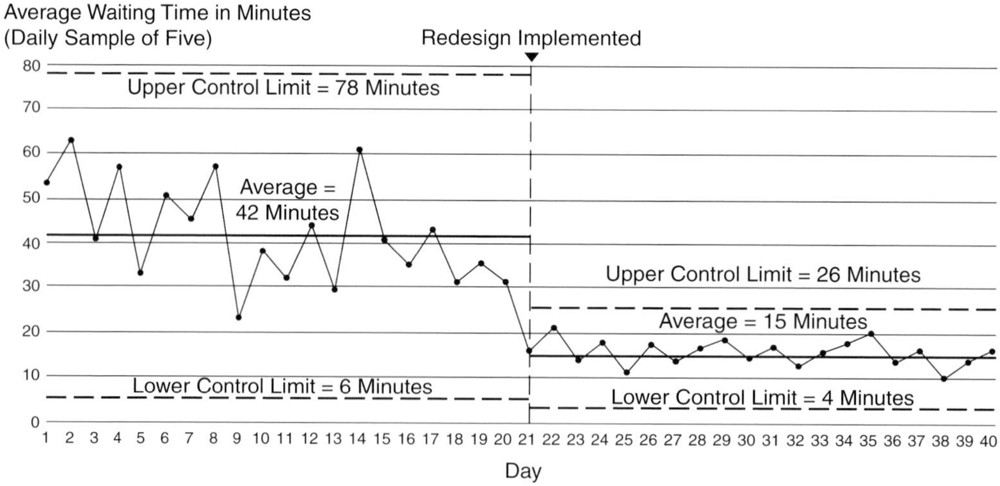

Figure 1-11 Control chart of average wait time before and after a redesign. *(Reproduced from the Quality Assurance Project.)*

activities demonstrate significantly greater performance gains than organizations that do not.

Use of continuous quality improvement tools requires significant thought regarding how to improve care structures and processes. An essential step in improving care processes, before or after initial analysis, is developing a checklist of the steps and parties involved and then creating a flowchart (Fig 1-12) of the care system. By examining the overall process for a specific outcome (eg, making sure a patient with diabetes mellitus gets an annual eye examination), the organization can identify opportunities for improving the process.

Another graphic tool is the fishbone, or cause-and-effect, diagram, which maps out the different factors that are significant inputs in each step of the care process, including

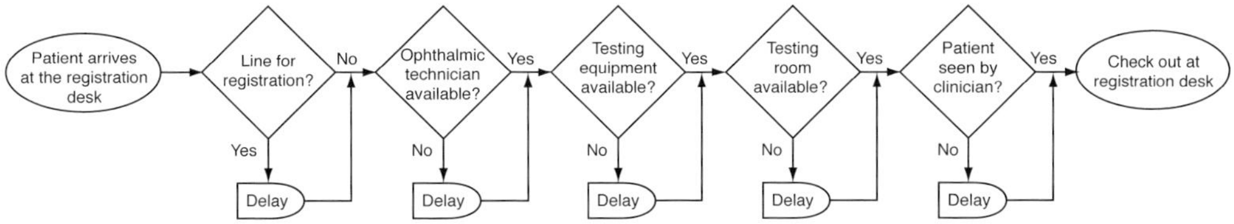

Figure 1-12 Flowchart of patient registration. *(Modified from the Quality Assurance Project.)*

personnel. Mapping each of these important factors can help clarify where problems may occur and where work may be improved. Changes in those factors can then be measured and the results monitored, providing continuous feedback to those interested in improving the quality of care.

Using Lean Techniques to Improve Clinical Practice

Health care providers are increasingly using an organizing framework called *lean* to improve patient care and experience. Toyota uses the lean methodology to produce high-volume, high-quality, low-cost automobiles in an environment with reasonable staffing. Toyota's goal is to continually increase its production volume and quality with no additional costs; this goal, implemented with lean techniques, has helped Toyota to become a dominant car company. What does automobile manufacturing have to do with health care, and specifically, what does it have to do with ophthalmology? As insurance reimbursements decrease and the volume of patients increases, ophthalmologists are tasked with delivering high-quality care to more patients at the same costs. The lean method may be a useful tool to help ophthalmology practices deliver this outcome.

Lean is a mind-set and a management toolbox to support the philosophy of delivering the right care at the right time every time. It focuses on value, in particular in determining, and then delivering, what is of value to the patient (of lesser priority, but still included, is what is of value to the physician and the institution). In other words, first ophthalmologists need to understand their patients' wants and needs, especially what the patients perceive as "value" gained from their interaction with the ophthalmology clinic. Understanding value provides key information to the goals of: increasing quality, eliminating waste, managing staffing to volume, and reducing time to complete tasks.

An example of the implementation of lean techniques in an ophthalmology practice is a glaucoma clinic in an academic center whose patients consistently reported extended wait times. Although the clinicians were excellent, with high-quality surgical results and excellent patient reviews, several patients per month reported, both formally and informally, that they waited too long to see the ophthalmic technician and doctors. The clinic's usual response to such patients included apologizing and explaining that the clinic had suffered unforeseen delays from complicated patients and/or unscheduled emergencies on the day in question. When the clinic realized that these delays were occurring too often, management decided to hire more staff members. Although the wait time improved slightly, it continued to be suboptimal; patient complaints continued, and the clinic suffered increased costs. Why did this not work? One reason that the quality of care did not improve was that the "evaluation and treatment procedures" at this clinic did not include a unifying organizing framework. In addition, management, rather than frontline workers, decided the action plans.

The following year, this clinic implemented a lean methodology to evaluate and improve their clinical practice. Their first step was to define and measure their outcome of interest. They used an electronic medical record to measure patients' wait time and discovered that it ranged from 5 to 90 minutes. Their goal was less than 10 minutes! They canceled clinic for a day and called a meeting with all management, providers, and frontline staff to solicit answers to several key lean questions regarding waste, safety, delays, and quality.

Using these answers, the clinic created "areas of focus," which had the highest-priority action plans. These action plans included structured daily huddles with staff at the beginning of clinic to discuss equipment problems, scheduling issues, missing charts, and recent quality or safety issues; at the end of the huddle, they allotted time for open discussion of any other issues. The clinic also created standardized work for each member of the team, eliminated paper printouts of schedules and patient face sheets, loaded rooms in the same order to create the same physician and patient movement, and removed any extra work that provided no value. Because lean represents "continual improvement," each day the process is reevaluated, and yearly, the staff holds a kaizen evaluation meeting with different areas of focus. If improvements do not work, the clinic evaluates these failures. Over a 5-year period, with the same amount of staff, clinic visits increased 20%; revenues increased 50%; patient delays decreased 80%; staff satisfaction soared; and patients expressed their satisfaction to the clinic on a daily basis. Overall, this example suggests that lean may be a useful method for ophthalmology clinics to "work smarter, not harder" to improve value, give the highest quality of care, and provide exceptional service with the same or decreased resources.

Simon RW, Canacari EG. A practical guide to applying lean tools and management principles to health care improvement projects. *AORN J.* 2012;95(1):85–100; quiz 101–103.

Toussaint JS, Berry LL. The promise of Lean in health care. *Mayo Clin Proc.* 2013;88(1):74–82.

Summary

Efforts to improve the quality of care—and ensure that fair and meaningful quality measures are part of this endeavor—bring key statistical concepts to the forefront. Because of the Medicare Access and CHIP Reauthorization Act (MACRA), ophthalmologist reimbursements will be more associated with quality and improvement (eg, Merit-based Incentive Payment System [MIPS]) and eligible alternative payment models (APMs). Indeed, insurance companies are already selecting providers that have documented higher quality and lower cost for participation in insurance company provider panels. Thus, clinical research and statistics are useful not only for understanding the scientific literature and providing care for patients, but also for influencing the practices and livelihoods of providers, including ophthalmologists.

Sloan FA, Brown DS, Carlisle ES, Picone GA, Lee PP. Monitoring visual status: why patients do or do not comply with practice guidelines. *Health Serv Res.* 2004;39(5):1429–1448.

CHAPTER 2

Endocrine Disorders

Highlights

- Metabolic syndrome is a serious health condition that affects about 23% of adults in the United States, putting them at higher risk of cardiovascular disease, diabetes mellitus, stroke, and diseases related to buildup of fatty plaque in artery walls.
- Diabetes mellitus is a group of metabolic diseases that increase the risk of microvascular and macrovascular complications.
- Teprotumumab, an investigational drug, may slow progression of ophthalmopathy in patients with moderate to severe thyroid eye disease.

Diabetes Mellitus

Diabetes mellitus (DM) is a group of metabolic diseases characterized by hyperglycemia resulting from defects in insulin secretion, insulin action, or both. In 2012, DM was present in 12.3% of persons over the age of 20 years in the United States and in 49% of those over the age of 65 years. A substantial percentage of affected individuals have not been diagnosed. Type 2 DM represents 90%–95% of all cases of DM, with type 1 DM and other causes representing the remaining 10%.

Persons with DM are at risk for microvascular complications, including retinopathy, nephropathy, and neuropathy, and are at increased risk for macrovascular disease. Among adult patients, type 2 DM is accompanied by hypertension (in approximately 75%) and hyperlipidemia (in more than 50%). It is considered a cardiac risk equivalent because of the high excess risk it poses for macrovascular disease, cardiovascular disease events, and mortality.

Centers for Disease Control and Prevention. National Diabetes Statistics Report, 2020. Atlanta, GA: Centers for Disease Control and Prevention, US Department of Health and Human Services; 2020. www.cdc.gov/diabetes/pdfs/data/statistics/national-diabetes-statistics-report.pdf. Accessed September 10, 2021.

Classification of Diabetes Mellitus

DM is classified into 4 clinical types.

Type 1 DM (<10% of all cases) results from a cell-mediated autoimmune destruction of β cells in the pancreas. It can present at any age; and, because of its variable clinical phenotypes, the diagnosis can be challenging in adults. The rate of destruction of β cells is rapid in infants and children and slower in adults. Therefore, ketoacidosis as an initial presentation is more common in young patients.

Latent autoimmune diabetes in adults (LADA), a subtype of type 1 DM, is characterized by mild to moderate hyperglycemia and, initially, often does not require insulin therapy. Adults with LADA have one or more β-cell–specific autoantibodies and will tend to require insulin therapy sooner than patients with classic type 2 DM. Type 1 DM should be suspected when there is a positive family history, thyroid disease, or other autoimmune disease.

Type 2 DM (>90% of cases) is characterized by insulin resistance followed by defective insulin secretion and loss of β-cell mass. The reason for this β-cell loss is unknown, but programmed cell death in response to genetic and environmental factors has been demonstrated in animal models. Type 2 disease is usually diagnosed in adults, with both incidence and prevalence increasing with age. However, it is becoming more common in children and now accounts for up to one-third of new cases of diabetes mellitus diagnosed in patients between the ages of 5 and 15 years.

This type of DM is associated with obesity, a positive family history, history of gestational diabetes or prediabetes, physical inactivity, and race/ethnicity. African American, Hispanic, and American Indian individuals have a greater risk of developing type 2 DM than White individuals. Type 2 DM may be asymptomatic and remain undiagnosed for months to years.

Gestational DM is glucose intolerance that has its onset or diagnosis during pregnancy (occurs in 5%–20% of pregnancies).

Other types of DM include those caused by genetic defects in insulin secretion or action, pancreatic surgery, disease of the exocrine pancreas (eg, cystic fibrosis), endocrinopathies (eg, Cushing syndrome), or drugs (eg, glucocorticoids, thiazide-type diuretics, and atypical antipsychotic medications).

Diagnosis of Diabetes Mellitus

DM is diagnosed by means of tests that evaluate glucose tolerance. A definitive diagnosis is made when at least 1 of the 4 following criteria is met and confirmed with repeat testing:

- HbA_{1c} ≥6.5% (<5.7% = normal), reflecting average levels of blood glucose over 3 months
- fasting plasma glucose (FPG) level ≥126 mg/dL (7.0 mmol/L)
- oral glucose tolerance test (OGTT) plasma glucose level ≥200 mg/dL (11.1 mmol/L) 2 hours after intake of a 75-g glucose load
- symptoms of diabetes mellitus (polyuria, polydipsia, fatigue, weight loss) and a random plasma glucose level ≥200 mg/dL (11.1 mmol/L)

Prediabetes

Persons with prediabetes have an increased risk for developing diabetes mellitus. The following abnormal test results suggest prediabetes:

- HbA_{1c} 5.7%–6.4%
- FPG level 100–125 mg/dL (5.6–5.9 mmol/L)

- OGTT plasma glucose level 140–199 mg/dL (7.8–11.0 mmol/L) 2 hours after intake of a 75-g glucose load

Progression from impaired fasting glucose or impaired glucose tolerance to type 2 DM occurs at a rate of about 12% per year.

Metabolic syndrome

Metabolic syndrome is a serious health condition that affects about 23% of adults in the United States, putting them at higher risk of cardiovascular disease, diabetes mellitus, stroke, and diseases related to the buildup of fatty plaques in artery walls. The underlying causes of metabolic syndrome include overweight and obesity, physical inactivity, genetic factors, and aging.

Metabolic syndrome is characterized by the presence of 3 or more of the following:

- FPG ≥100 mg/dL
- abdominal obesity (waist circumference >102 cm in men and >89 cm in women)
- triglyceride level ≥150 mg/dL or greater
- HDL cholesterol <40 mg/dL in men or <50 mg/dL in women
- systolic blood pressure ≥130 mm Hg or diastolic blood pressure ≥85 mm Hg

Individuals can decrease their risk of metabolic syndrome significantly by reducing their weight; increasing physical activity; eating a heart-healthy diet that is rich in whole grains, fruits, vegetables, and fish; and working with a health care provider or dietitian to monitor and manage blood glucose, blood cholesterol, and blood pressure.

Reduction of Risk for Diabetes Mellitus

Several clinical trials have recently shown that the risk of progression from impaired glucose tolerance to type 2 DM can be markedly reduced (by approximately 50% over several years) through lifestyle modifications such as a combination of diet and exercise therapy. The amount of weight loss and exercise required to achieve this result is surprisingly modest. For instance, in the Diabetes Prevention Program, patients who were asked to perform 150 minutes of brisk walking per week (a little over 20 minutes per day) lost only about 12 pounds of weight on average but reduced their risk of diabetes mellitus development by 50% over 6 months. Other studies have suggested that early pharmacologic intervention with oral hypoglycemic agents also decreases the risk of progression to diabetes mellitus. There are, as yet, no known ways to prevent type 1 DM, but trials of interventions to regulate immune response are under way.

The importance of glycemic control

For patients with either type 1 or type 2 DM, glycemic control is of the utmost importance. The Diabetes Control and Complications Trial showed that intensive therapy aimed at maintaining near-normal glucose levels had a large and beneficial effect on delaying the development and progression of long-term complications for patients with type 1 diabetes mellitus. For example, intensive therapy decreased the risk of the development and progression of retinopathy, nephropathy, and neuropathy by 40%–76%. The beneficial effects increased over time, but they were accompanied by a threefold increased risk of hypoglycemia. Thus, intensive therapy is recommended for most patients with type 1 DM, but these patients should be instructed to self-monitor their blood glucose levels carefully to prevent hypoglycemic episodes. See also BCSC Section 12, *Retina and Vitreous.*

Tight glycemic control has a profound effect on the development of complications. The risk of retinopathy progression rises almost exponentially as the HbA_{1c} level increases (Fig 2-1). However, patients who decrease their HbA_{1c} by 1 percentage point (eg, from 8.0% to 7.0%) reduce their risk of retinopathy by approximately 30%, and this benefit also holds for other complications of diabetes mellitus, such as nephropathy and neuropathy. When working with patients with diabetes mellitus, health care providers should emphasize the importance of tight control and encourage patients to achieve it.

For patients with type 1 DM, intensive therapy also provides protection against macrovascular complications such as cardiovascular disease. For patients with type 2 DM, however, the role of glycemic control in reducing cardiovascular risk has not been established. In this group, macrovascular disease may be affected more by other risk factors, such as smoking, obesity, and lipid abnormalities.

Action to Control Cardiovascular Risk in Diabetes Study Group; Gerstein HC, Miller ME, Byington RP, et al. Effects of intensive glucose lowering in type 2 diabetes. *N Engl J Med.* 2008;358(24):2545–2559.

Treatment

The goals of therapy are to alleviate symptoms; to achieve glycemic, blood pressure, and lipid targets; and to prevent acute and chronic complications of DM. The recommended targets for control of type 1 and type 2 DM are similar:

- fasting and preprandial capillary blood glucose 80–130 mg/dL

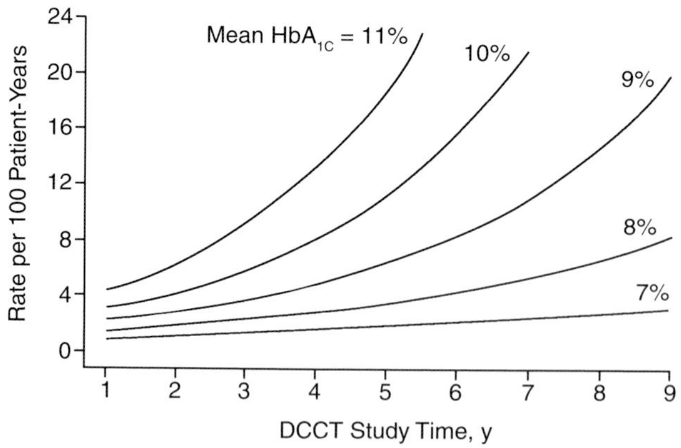

Figure 2-1 Rate of retinopathy progression relative to mean hemoglobin A_{1c}. *(Redrawn with permission from the DCCT Research Group. The relationship of glycemic exposure [HbA_{1c}] to the risk of development and progression of retinopathy in the Diabetes Control and Complications Trial.* Diabetes. *1995;44[8]:968–983.)*

- postprandial capillary blood glucose <180 mg/dL
- HbA_{1c} <6.5%

This degree of glycemic control has been associated with the lowest risk of microvascular complications in both type 1 and type 2 DM.

Type 1 diabetes mellitus

Treatment of type 1 DM requires lifelong insulin replacement and careful coordination of insulin doses with food intake and activity. Insulin can be administered by subcutaneous injection, continuous subcutaneous infusion, or inhalation. A regimen of multiple daily insulin injections that includes basal, premeal, and correction doses is preferred to obtain optimal control in patients. Capillary glucose monitoring 4 times daily, 10–30 minutes before meals and at bedtime, is required for such a regimen.

Continuous subcutaneous insulin infusion by means of an insulin pump is widely used in patients with type 1 and, increasingly, with type 2 DM. However, it does not automatically improve glycemic control without patient self-management. A typical regimen provides 50% of total daily insulin as basal insulin and the remainder as multiple preprandial boluses of insulin using a programmable insulin pump. Patients must check their blood glucose regularly because diabetic ketoacidosis can occur rapidly if the insulin infusion is disrupted.

Regular human insulin is now available in inhaled form as Technosphere insulin (Afrezza). The onset of effect occurs about 15 minutes after administration, with a peak effect in the first hour and a duration of action of 3 hours. It is contraindicated in patients with asthma or COPD because of the risk of bronchospasm. Pulmonary function tests are required prior to initiation of therapy and at regular intervals during therapy.

Pancreas transplantation For patients with type 1 DM, pancreas transplantation can be performed alone or in conjunction with kidney transplantation. With modern techniques and immunosuppression, the transplant survival rate is high, and most patients become euglycemic without the need for insulin. Although quality of life is usually improved, the patient faces risks both from the surgery and from long-term immunosuppression. Thus, pancreas transplantation alone is limited to specific situations, such as in patients with frequent metabolic complications or in whom standard insulin therapy consistently fails to control disease. However, when pancreas transplantation and kidney transplantation are combined in patients with end-stage renal disease, the benefits far outweigh the risks.

Transplantation of pancreatic islet cells has been shown to improve the quality of life for patients with type 1 DM that is difficult to control, which includes patients with DM with frequent episodes of severe and potentially fatal hypoglycemia. These cells can be injected directly into the liver without the need for formal transplantation. After injection, patients remain on lifelong immunosuppression therapy to prevent transplant rejection. A recent phase 3 clinical trial funded by the National Institute of Allergy and Infectious Diseases (NIAID) and the National Institute of Diabetes and Digestive and Kidney Diseases (NIDDK), both part of the National Institutes of Health, released results from a study of pancreatic islet cell transplantation. At 1-year follow-up after transplant, 88% of transplant recipients had no episodes of severe hypoglycemia and approximately 50% of recipients no longer needed insulin use to achieve glycemic control.

Foster ED, Bridges ND, Feurer ID, et al; Clinical Islet Transplantation Consortium. Improved health-related quality of life in a phase 3 islet transplantation trial in type 1 diabetes complicated by severe hypoglycemia. *Diabetes Care.* 2018;41(5):1001–1008.

Type 2 diabetes mellitus

The achievement of glycemic control requires individualized therapy in a comprehensive approach that incorporates lifestyle and pharmacologic interventions. Following are considerations for noninsulin therapy in patients with type 2 DM:

- Noninsulin therapy should be considered early in the course of the disease, in conjunction with diet and exercise. Metformin is the recommended first-line therapy if tolerated.
- When used as monotherapy at the maximum dose, insulin secretagogues, metformin, and thiazolidinediones (TZDs) have comparable glucose-lowering effects. The glucose-lowering effects of these medications and analogues are observed within days to weeks, except for the maximum effect of TZDs, which may not be apparent for several weeks to months.
- Combination therapy with 2 or more oral or injectable agents may be needed to achieve targets for HbA_{1C} and blood glucose in patients presenting with significant hyperglycemia and will likely become necessary as β-cell function deteriorates over time. Dual therapy may be considered when the initial HbA_{1C} is ≥7.5%, and triple therapy or insulin when the initial HbA_{1C} is >9%.
- Because all noninsulin therapies require some pancreatic β-cell function to achieve glucose-lowering effects, many patients will eventually need insulin replacement therapy.

American Diabetes Association. *Standards of Medical Care in Diabetes—2017. Diabetes Care.* 2017;40(suppl 1). http://care.diabetesjournals.org/content/diacare/suppl/2016/12/15/40.Supplement_1.DC1/DC_40_S1_final.pdf. Published January 2017. Accessed September 10, 2021.

Complications of Diabetes Mellitus

Acute complications of diabetes mellitus

The acute complications of diabetes mellitus are *nonketotic hyperglycemic hyperosmolar coma* and *diabetic ketoacidosis.* Either of these, if not recognized promptly and treated aggressively, can lead to death. These complications should be considered as part of a continuum of hyperglycemia rather than as separate entities; the main difference between the 2 is whether ketoacids accumulate. Both are often precipitated by some type of stress, such as an infection, that leads to increased production of glucagon, catecholamines, and cortisol, which in turn promotes gluconeogenesis. If not treated with adequate amounts of insulin or oral hypoglycemic agents, the elevated glucose level will lead to osmotic diuresis and volume depletion. When insulin levels are extremely low or absent (eg, in a patient with type 1 DM), catabolic processes (eg, conversion of lipids to ketones) prevail and ketoacids are produced, superimposing severe metabolic acidosis on the hyperosmotic volume-depleted state.

Long-term complications of diabetes mellitus

The long-term complications of DM are usually secondary to vascular disease. Nephropathy, neuropathy, peripheral artery disease, coronary atherosclerosis, secondary cerebral thrombosis, cardiac infarction, and retinopathy are all important causes of morbidity and mortality. The precise mechanism for the development of diabetic complications is elusive, but hyperglycemia plays a central role by triggering a number of processes that ultimately cause vascular damage. (Diabetic retinopathy is discussed in BCSC Section 12, *Retina and Vitreous.*)

The blood glucose level is not the only risk factor that can be modified to reduce the complications of DM. In particular, hypertension and lipid abnormalities seem to be inextricably intertwined with glycemic control. Thus, any attempt to minimize complications must include aggressive control of these other factors.

Nephropathy Approximately 40% of patients who have had DM for 20 or more years have nephropathy. Albuminuria greater than 300 mg/24 hours—approximately the level at which a standard urine dipstick test becomes positive—is the hallmark of diabetic nephropathy. Renal failure eventually occurs in approximately 50% of patients who developed diabetes mellitus before age 20 and in 6% of those with onset after 40 years of age. Diabetic nephropathy is the leading cause of end-stage renal disease, and the 5-year survival rate of patients with DM on maintenance dialysis is less than 20%. Almost invariably, nephropathy and retinopathy develop within a short time of each other.

The progression of diabetic nephropathy occurs in the following sequence: microalbuminuria (urine albumin levels of 30–300 mg/24 hours), macroalbuminuria (urine albumin levels >300 mg/24 hours), nephrotic syndrome, and finally end-stage renal disease. Tight control of blood glucose can delay and perhaps prevent the development of microalbuminuria. In addition, controlling hypertension (particularly with angiotensin-converting enzyme inhibitors) and adhering to low-protein diets may help slow the decline in glomerular filtration rate.

Neuropathy Diabetic neuropathy is a common problem. After 30 years of DM, about 50% of patients have signs of neuropathy, and 15%–20% have symptoms of distal symmetric polyneuropathy. Changes in nerve metabolism and function are thought to be mediated in part through increased aldose reductase activity; Schwann cell synthesis of myelin is impaired, and axonal degeneration ensues. In addition, microangiopathy of the endoneural capillaries leads to vascular abnormalities and microinfarcts of the nerves, with multifocal fiber loss.

Symptoms in the feet and lower legs are the most common manifestations. Foot pain, paresthesias, and loss of sensation occur frequently and probably result from both ischemic and metabolic nerve abnormalities. Weakness may be present as part of mononeuritis or a mononeuritis multiplex and is usually associated with pain. Cranial neuropathies may also occur (see BCSC Section 5, *Neuro-Ophthalmology*). Additional types of morbidity, stemming from autonomic dysfunction, include male and female sexual dysfunction, impaired urination, delayed gastric emptying, orthostatic hypotension, and tachycardia due to loss of vagal tone.

There is no specific treatment for diabetic neuropathy. Aldose reductase inhibitors (not yet commercially available) may improve nerve conduction slightly but do not result in major clinical improvement. Neuropathic pain may respond to tricyclic antidepressants or capsaicin cream. Anticonvulsant drugs such as carbamazepine and gabapentin may also be useful.

Large-vessel disease The risk of coronary heart disease is 2–10 times higher in patients with DM than in the general population, and the mortality rate in patients with DM who have anterior myocardial infarctions is twice that in patients who do not have DM. Because myocardial infarction may present without the classic symptom of chest pain in patients with DM, an increased index of suspicion is required to make the diagnosis. Hypertension further increases the risk of cardiovascular disease for persons with DM. Cerebral thrombosis is approximately twice as prevalent in the diabetic population as in the nondiabetic population, and peripheral artery disease is 40 times as prevalent.

Ophthalmic considerations Management of patients with diabetes mellitus can be challenging. The ophthalmologist may be the first to identify a complication related to a patient's diabetes, whether diabetic retinopathy or a transient refractive change due to glucose elevation. Moreover, an ophthalmologist may be a patient's only regular health care provider. Thus, it is important that both the patient and the ophthalmologist are aware of the patient's HbA_{1c} level, a specific and objective measure of glycemic control.

Patients may need to be educated about frequent blood glucose testing, the paramount importance of maintaining good glycemic control, and the possible consequences of poor control. In addition, patients should be reminded that other modifiable risk factors for retinopathy progression, including hypertension, lipid abnormalities, early renal failure, and anemia, are also important.

It is important for the ophthalmologist to be aware of the patient's glycemic control status, because it may affect the rate of retinopathy progression and, in turn, influence decisions on treatment and follow-up frequency. For example, studies have shown that rapid improvement in glycemic control can hasten progression of retinopathy. This finding is independent of cataract surgery, and the mechanism of action is not fully understood. Therefore, attempting to rapidly improve glycemic control in a patient prior to cataract surgery may not be beneficial, as it may speed the progression of retinopathy and affect visual outcomes.

The importance of all of the risk factors for retinopathy progression should be communicated to the patient's primary care physician so that these factors can be controlled as well as possible. The ophthalmologist should strive to keep informed on the status of these issues, because a patient with significant problems in any of these areas is likely to have less-than-optimal results with any ophthalmic surgical intervention. Educating patients who have poorly controlled DM about their prognosis before surgery may facilitate more realistic expectations. (Perioperative management in ocular surgery is reviewed in Chapter 15.)

Jingi AM, Tankeu AT, Ateba NA, Noubiap JJ. Mechanism of worsening diabetic retinopathy with rapid lowering of blood glucose: the synergistic hypothesis. *BMC Endocr Disord.* 2017;17(1):63.

Thyroid Disease

Physiology

Functionally, the thyroid gland can be thought of as having 2 parts. The *parafollicular* (or C) cells secrete calcitonin and play a role in calcium homeostasis; they do not affect thyroid physiology. Thyroid *follicles* are made up of a single layer of epithelial cells surrounding colloid, which consists mostly of thyroglobulin, the storage form of the thyroid hormones T_4 and T_3.

T_4 (thyroxine), the main secretory product of the thyroid gland, contains 4 iodine atoms. Deiodination of T_4, which occurs mainly in the liver and kidneys, gives rise to T_3 (triiodothyronine), the metabolically active form of thyroid hormone. Eighty percent of serum T_3 is derived through deiodination; the remainder is secreted by the thyroid. Only a small fraction of these hormones circulates freely in the plasma (0.02% of total T_4 and 0.30% of total T_3); the remainder is bound to the proteins thyroxine-binding globulin (TBG), transthyretin, and albumin.

Thyroid function is regulated by the interrelationship of hypothalamic, pituitary, and thyroid activity. Thyrotropin-releasing hormone (TRH), which is secreted by the hypothalamus, causes the synthesis of thyrotropin (or thyroid-stimulating hormone, TSH) and its release from the anterior pituitary. TSH, in turn, stimulates the thyroid, leading to the release of T_4 and T_3. In this negative-feedback loop, increased levels of T_4 and T_3 inhibit the release of TSH and the TSH response to TRH at the level of the pituitary.

The main role of the thyroid hormones is regulation of tissue metabolism through their effects on protein synthesis. Normal development of the central nervous system requires adequate amounts of thyroid hormone during the first 2 years of life. Congenital hypothyroidism results in irreversible cognitive disabilities (cretinism). Normal growth and bone maturation also depend on sufficient hormone levels.

Tests of Thyroid Function

Detection of thyroid disease and evaluation of the efficacy of therapy require the use of various combinations of laboratory tests. The American Thyroid Association recommends initial screening with tests of TSH and free T_4.

Measurement of serum TSH

Thyroid-stimulating hormone secretion by the pituitary is tightly controlled by negative-feedback mechanisms regulated by serum T_4 and T_3 levels. TSH levels begin to rise early in the course of hypothyroidism and fall in hyperthyroidism, even before free T_4 levels are outside the reference range. Therefore, the serum TSH level is a sensitive indicator of thyroid dysfunction.

Some extremely sensitive assays of TSH can detect levels down to 0.005 mIU/L, making it possible to differentiate low normal values from abnormally low values. The TSH test is useful for (1) screening for thyroid disease, (2) monitoring replacement therapy in hypothyroid patients (TSH levels respond 6–8 weeks after changes in hormone replacement dosage), and (3) monitoring suppressive therapy for thyroid nodules or cancer. In screening for thyroid disease, the combination of free T_4 and sensitive TSH assays has a sensitivity of 99.5% and a specificity of 98.0%. As a result, both of these tests are used together for screening in most situations. There is presently some controversy about the upper limit of normal for TSH, so endocrinologic consultation is indicated in borderline cases.

Measurement of serum T_4

Total serum T_4 comprises 2 parts: the protein-bound fraction and the free hormone. Total T_4 levels can be affected by changes in serum TBG levels, while euthyroidism is maintained and free T_4 levels remain normal. Levels of TBG and total T_4 are elevated during pregnancy and with use of oral contraceptives, while free T_4 levels remain normal. Low TBG and total T_4 levels are associated with chronic illness, protein malnutrition, hepatic failure, and use of glucocorticoids.

Measurement of serum T_3

Serum T_3 levels may not accurately reflect thyroid gland function for 2 reasons: first, T_3 is not the major secretory product of the thyroid; and, second, many factors influence T_3 levels, including nutrition, medications, and mechanisms regulating the enzymes that convert T_4 to T_3. Determination of T_3 levels is indicated in patients who may have T_3 thyrotoxicosis, an uncommon condition in which clinically hyperthyroid patients have normal T_4 and free T_4 but elevated T_3 levels.

Thyroid hormone–binding protein tests

Radioactive iodine uptake testing can be used to distinguish Graves disease from other causes of hyperthyroidism in the absence of other clinical features of Graves disease. However, it is not routinely performed.

Thyroid antibody tests

Several antibodies against thyroid antigens can be detected in the blood. The most common is thyroid peroxidase antibody, which has 99% sensitivity and specificity for Graves disease. Antibodies to thyroglobulin are also found in various thyroid diseases, including Hashimoto thyroiditis, Graves disease, and thyroid carcinoma. Patients with Graves disease usually have antibodies called thyroid-stimulating immunoglobulins (TSIs), which are directed at TSH receptors. These antibodies generally stimulate the release of thyroid hormone, but in rare cases patients have antibodies that block thyroid hormone release.

High serum levels of TSI and the absence of thyroperoxidase antibody are both risk factors for ophthalmopathy in patients with Graves disease.

Thyroid scanning

Thyroid scanning is useful in distinguishing functioning from nonfunctioning thyroid nodules and in evaluating chest and neck masses for metastatic thyroid cancer.

Thyroid ultrasonography

Ultrasonography, which can detect nodules as small as 1 mm, is used to identify the presence of cystic or solid thyroid nodules.

Biopsy

Biopsy to obtain tissue samples for evaluating thyroid nodules may be performed with fine-needle aspiration, core, or excisional techniques. Fine-needle aspiration specimens require interpretation by an experienced cytologist.

Hyperthyroidism

Hypermetabolism caused by excessive quantities of circulating thyroid hormones leads to the clinical syndrome of *hyperthyroidism (thyrotoxicosis)*. Clinical findings include exophthalmos, chest palpitations, excessive sweating, diarrhea, weight loss, and sensitivity to heat. Graves hyperthyroidism accounts for approximately 85% of cases of thyrotoxicosis. Toxic nodular goiter and thyroiditis account for most of the remaining cases.

Thyroid storm is a rare, acute hypermetabolic state that is fatal if untreated. It is often precipitated by surgery, infection, or trauma in a patient with otherwise mild hyperthyroidism. Patients typically present with fever, tachycardia, nausea, vomiting, agitation, and psychosis; and they may become comatose secondary to hypotension. Modern treatments aimed at controlling the process have dramatically reduced mortality.

Graves hyperthyroidism

Thyroid eye disease (TED) is discussed in BCSC Section 5, *Neuro-Ophthalmology,* and Section 7, *Oculofacial Plastic and Orbital Surgery.* This section focuses on the thyroid disease.

Patients with Graves hyperthyroidism (also known as *diffuse toxic goiter*) exhibit various combinations of hypermetabolism, diffuse enlargement of the thyroid gland, TED, and infiltrative dermopathy. Graves hyperthyroidism is an autoimmune disorder. Up to 90% of patients have circulating TSH receptor antibodies; furthermore, the level of TSI has been shown to correlate with the severity of clinical disease.

Graves hyperthyroidism is common, with a lifetime risk of 3.0% for women and 0.5% for men. The incidence peaks in the third to fifth decades of life, and there is a strong familial component. Risk factors including stress and smoking are associated with increased incidence of thyroid eye disease.

Common clinical symptoms include fatigue, tremor, weight loss, palpitations, and heat intolerance. Manifestations can vary by age of patient at the onset of hyperthyroidism. For instance, atrial fibrillation is rare in patients younger than 60 years but occurs in more than 10% of patients 60 years or older. A palpable goiter develops in most patients younger than

60 years old compared with less than 50% of patients older than 60 years. Approximately one-third of patients with Graves hyperthyroidism have clinically obvious TED at the time of diagnosis of the hyperthyroidism.

Treatment of Graves hyperthyroidism is aimed at returning thyroid function to normal. A significant proportion of patients (30%–50%) experience remission in association with drug treatment directed at the thyroid. Later in the course of the disease, patients may experience relapse, hypothyroidism, or both.

Thyroid secretion is suppressed using one of the thiourea derivatives, propylthiouracil or methimazole. The drugs inhibit the use of iodine by the gland. Treatment is continued until clinical and laboratory indexes show improvement. Adverse effects include rash (common), liver damage (rare), vasculitis (rare), and agranulocytosis (occurs in 0.02%–0.05% of patients).

There are several options for long-term management of Graves hyperthyroidism: the aforementioned antithyroid drugs can be continued for 12–24 months in hopes of remission; part of the gland can be surgically removed, although approximately half of such patients eventually become hypothyroid; or radioactive iodine can be used. Iodine 131 (^{131}I) is highly effective, resulting in hypothyroidism in 80% of patients within 6–12 months; some require a second treatment. Although adverse effects of ^{131}I are minimal, its use is associated with worsening of TED.

Ophthalmic considerations A new drug, teprotumumab, has been shown to slow progression of ophthalmopathy in patients with moderate to severe thyroid eye disease and is currently undergoing clinical trials. The drug, which inhibits insulin-like growth factor I receptor, represents a new therapeutic strategy for treating the underlying autoimmune pathogenesis of TED. Teprotumumab has been granted orphan drug status by the US Food and Drug Administration, and clinical trials will determine if it slows the progression of ophthalmopathy in patients with newly diagnosed TED.

Smith TJ, Hegedüs L. Graves' disease. *N Engl J Med.* 2016;375(16):1552–1565.

Smith TJ, Kahaly GJ, Ezra DG, et al. Teprotumumab for thyroid-associated ophthalmopathy. *N Engl J Med.* 2017;376(18):1748–1761.

Toxic nodular goiter

In toxic nodular goiter, thyroid hormone–producing adenomas (either single or multiple) make enough hormone to cause hyperthyroidism. These so-called *hot nodules* are almost never carcinomatous and often result in hyperthyroidism. Toxic nodules may be treated with radioactive iodine or surgery.

Hypothyroidism

Hypothyroidism is a clinical syndrome resulting from a deficiency of thyroid hormone. *Myxedema* is the nonpitting edema caused by subcutaneous accumulation of mucopolysaccharides in severe cases of hypothyroidism; the term is sometimes used to describe the entire syndrome of severe hypothyroidism.

Primary hypothyroidism accounts for more than 95% of cases and may be congenital or acquired. Most primary cases are due to Hashimoto thyroiditis (discussed in the following section), "idiopathic" myxedema (thought by many to be end-stage Hashimoto thyroiditis), and iatrogenic causes (^{131}I or surgical treatment of hyperthyroidism). *Secondary hypothyroidism,* caused by hypothalamic or pituitary dysfunction (usually after pituitary surgery), is much less common. As in hyperthyroidism, the female preponderance among adults is significant. *Subclinical hypothyroidism* is defined as a normal T_4 concentration and a slightly elevated TSH level. These patients may or may not have symptoms suggestive of hypothyroidism, and some controversy surrounds whether such patients should be treated.

Clinically, a patient with hypothyroidism presents with signs and symptoms of hypometabolism and accumulation of mucopolysaccharides in the tissues of the body. Many of the symptoms are nonspecific—they include weakness, fatigue, memory loss, dry skin, hair loss, deepening of the voice, weight gain (despite loss of appetite), cold intolerance, arthralgias, constipation, and muscle cramps—and their relationship to thyroid dysfunction may not be recognized for some time. Clinical signs include bradycardia, reduced pulse pressure, myxedema, weight gain, loss of body and scalp hair, and menstrual disorders. In severe cases, personality changes ("myxedema psychosis") and death (following "myxedema coma") may occur.

Treatment of hypothyroidism is straightforward, consisting of oral thyroid replacement medication to normalize circulating hormone levels. Levothyroxine is the most commonly used preparation. Serum T_4 and TSH levels are monitored at regular intervals to ensure that euthyroidism is maintained.

Thyroiditis

Thyroiditis may be classified as acute, subacute, or chronic. *Acute thyroiditis,* caused by bacterial infection, is extremely rare. *Subacute thyroiditis* occurs in 2 forms: granulomatous and lymphocytic. Hashimoto thyroiditis is the most common type of *chronic thyroiditis.*

Patients with *subacute granulomatous thyroiditis* present with a painful, enlarged gland associated with fever, chills, and malaise. Thyroid function tests may be helpful because they may reveal the unusual combination of an elevated T_4 level and a low radioactive iodine uptake. Patients may be hyperthyroid because of the release of hormone from areas of thyroid destruction; pathologic examination reveals granulomatous inflammation. The disease is self-limited, and treatment is symptomatic, with use of either analgesics or, in severe cases, oral corticosteroids. After resolution, transient hypothyroidism (which becomes permanent in 5%–10% of patients) may occur.

Patients with *subacute lymphocytic thyroiditis* ("painless" thyroiditis), which commonly occurs 2–4 months postpartum in mothers but may occur in isolation, present with symptoms of hyperthyroidism and a normal or slightly enlarged but nontender thyroid gland. Pathologic investigation shows lymphocytic infiltration resembling Hashimoto thyroiditis, suggesting an autoimmune cause. This disease is also self-limited, generally lasting less than 3 months, and treatment is symptomatic. Hypothyroidism may ensue.

Hashimoto thyroiditis is an autoimmune disease that causes goitrous hypothyroidism. Patients have antibodies to thyroid antigens and an increased incidence of other autoimmune diseases. Patients with Hashimoto thyroiditis may present with hypothyroidism, an enlarged thyroid, or both. Pathologic examination reveals lymphocytic infiltration. Treatment is aimed at normalizing hormone levels with thyroid replacement therapy. Patients with enlarged glands and airway obstruction who do not respond to TSH suppression may require surgery. The risk of primary thyroid lymphoma and papillary thyroid cancer is slightly increased in patients with Hashimoto thyroiditis.

Postpartum thyroiditis occurs in approximately 5% of women after delivery (often in subsequent pregnancies) and can cause hyperthyroidism or hypothyroidism (or first one problem and then the other). Postpartum thyroiditis is usually painless and self-limited and is often associated with thyroid peroxidase antibodies.

Thyroid Tumors

Virtually all tumors of the thyroid gland arise from glandular cells and are, therefore, adenomas or carcinomas. Functioning adenomas were discussed previously (see the section "Toxic nodular goiter").

On thyroid scan, 90%–95% of thyroid adenomas are cold nodules and come to attention only if they are large enough to be physically apparent. Diagnostic testing involves a combination of approaches, including ultrasonography (cysts are benign and simply aspirated), fine-needle aspiration, and surgery, depending on the clinical situation. Treatment options for benign cold nodules are suppressive therapy, in which thyroid hormone replacement is used to suppress TSH secretion and its stimulatory effect on functioning nodules, and surgery.

There are 4 types of carcinomas of the thyroid: papillary, follicular, medullary, and anaplastic (undifferentiated). *Papillary carcinoma* is the most common form of thyroid tumor. Tumors removed before extension outside the capsule of the gland appear to have no adverse effect on survival. *Follicular carcinoma* may also be associated with a normal life span if it is identified before it becomes invasive, but late metastases can occur. *Medullary carcinoma* arises from the C cells and produces calcitonin. The lesion can occur as a solitary malignant tumor or as part of multiple endocrine neoplasia type 2 (discussed at the end of the chapter). *Anaplastic carcinoma,* though rare, is the most malignant tumor of the thyroid gland and is found mainly in patients older than 60 years. For the giant cell form, the survival time is less than 6 months from time of diagnosis; for the small cell form, the 5-year survival rate is 20%–25%.

Ponto KA, Kanitz M, Olivo PD, Pitz S, Pfeiffer N, Kahaly GJ. Clinical relevance of thyroid-stimulating immunoglobulins in Graves' ophthalmopathy. *Ophthalmology.* 2011;118(11): 2279–2285.

Disorders of the Hypothalamic-Pituitary Axis

The *hypothalamus* is the coordinating center of the endocrine system. It consolidates signals from higher cortical centers, the autonomic nervous system, the environment, and systemic endocrine feedback. The hypothalamus then delivers precise instructions to the pituitary gland, which releases hormones that influence most endocrine systems in

Table 2-1 Hypothalamic Neurohormones and Neurotransmitters Involved in Anterior Pituitary Function

Thyrotropin-releasing hormone (TRH) → ↑TSH, PRL
Gonadotropin-releasing hormone (GnRH) → ↑FSH, LH
Growth hormone–releasing hormone (GHRH) → ↑GH
Corticotropin-releasing hormone (CRH) → ↑ACTH
Somatostatin → ↓GH, TSH
Dopamine → ↓PRL

ACTH = adrenocorticotrophic hormone; FSH = follicle-stimulating hormone; GH = growth hormone; LH = luteinizing hormone; PRL = prolactin; TSH = thyroid-stimulating hormone; ↑ = stimulates release of; ↓ = inhibits release of.

the body. The hypothalamic-pituitary axis directly affects the thyroid gland, the adrenal gland, and the gonads; and it influences growth, milk production, and water balance.

Table 2-1 outlines the major hypothalamic hormones and their actions on the anterior pituitary hormones. The hypothalamic hormones are released directly into a primary capillary plexus that empties into the hypophyseal portal venous circulation; they then travel down the pituitary stalk and bathe the anterior pituitary gland in a secondary capillary plexus. The hormones released by the hypothalamic neurons, therefore, reach their target cells rapidly and in high concentrations. This proximity allows a rapid, pulsatile response to signals between the hypothalamus and the anterior pituitary. The posterior pituitary is controlled by direct neuronal innervation from the hypothalamus rather than by blood-borne hormones. The main products of the posterior pituitary are vasopressin and oxytocin. *Vasopressin* (antidiuretic hormone) is primarily involved in controlling water excretion by the kidneys. *Oxytocin* stimulates uterine contractions during labor and delivery and milk ejection in lactation.

Pituitary Adenomas

Pituitary tumors account for 10%–15% of intracranial tumors. They are classified as *microadenomas* (<10 mm in the greatest diameter) or *macroadenomas* (≥10 mm in the greatest diameter). Typically benign, these tumors arise from hormone-producing cells and may be functionally active (ie, secrete large amounts of hormones) or inactive. The clinical presentation depends on what type of cell the tumor derives from and whether the tumor produces hormones. Any type of tumor may be clinically inactive and will become apparent only when it has enlarged enough to cause symptoms. Patients may present with headaches, visual symptoms such as visual field loss due to chiasmal compression, cranial neuropathies, and/or hypopituitarism from compression of normal pituitary tissue. (The ophthalmic effects of pituitary adenomas and other parasellar lesions are discussed in BCSC Section 5, *Neuro-Ophthalmology*.)

Accounting for approximately 15% of pituitary tumors, *somatotroph adenomas* produce growth hormone, which can cause gigantism in prepubertal patients and acromegaly in adults. Acromegaly often develops insidiously over several years, and patients may present with headaches and visual symptoms due to enlargement of the adenoma before the diagnosis is recognized. Characteristic findings include an enlarged jaw, coarse facial features, and enlarged and swollen hands and feet. Patients may also have cardiac disease and diabetes mellitus in addition to the typical bone and soft-tissue changes.

Lactotroph adenomas (prolactinomas) account for approximately 25% of symptomatic pituitary tumors. Hyperprolactinemia produces amenorrhea and galactorrhea in women and decreased libido and impotence in men. The symptoms tend to develop gradually in men, and patients may present with compression symptoms due to tumor enlargement before the hormonal effects are recognized.

Thyrotroph adenomas are rare, accounting for less than 1% of pituitary tumors. They may cause hyperthyroidism, hypothyroidism, or no change in thyroid function, depending on how the TSH subunits are processed in the tumor cells. These tumors tend to be large macroadenomas, and patients may present with compressive symptoms in addition to any thyroid changes.

Corticotroph adenomas account for approximately 15% of pituitary tumors. They are associated with *Cushing syndrome*, characterized by the classic features of centripetal obesity, hirsutism, and facial plethora. Fat deposits develop over the thoracocervical spine (buffalo hump) and temporal regions (moon facies). Psychiatric abnormalities occur in 50% of patients, and long-standing Cushing syndrome can cause osteoporosis. Patients bruise easily and have violet striae on the abdomen, upper thighs, and arms. Hypertension and glucose intolerance leading to diabetes mellitus can also occur. Cushing syndrome can also develop secondary to adrenal gland neoplasms and, most commonly, from iatrogenic administration of glucocorticoids.

Gonadotroph adenomas (approximately 10% of pituitary tumors) may produce serum follicle-stimulating hormone and, in rare cases, luteinizing hormone. Affected patients present with hypogonadism related to gonadal downregulation. Gonadotropin-producing pituitary tumors may also be clinically inactive, and patients may present with compression symptoms.

Accounting for approximately 15% of pituitary tumors, *plurihormonal adenomas,* as the name implies, produce more than 1 type of hormone. Common combinations include elevated growth hormone with prolactin and growth hormone with TSH.

Null-cell adenomas (approximately 20% of pituitary tumors) do not have any pathologic markers to suggest a certain cell type and do not produce excess hormone. Most tumors that present with signs of enlargement and compression are gonadotroph or null-cell adenomas.

Tumors of the pituitary gland are best diagnosed by means of contrast magnetic resonance imaging focused on the pituitary region. Endocrinologic testing is warranted when hypersecretion syndromes are suspected or when the patient has evidence of hypopituitarism. The treatment approach is complex and depends on a number of factors, including the size of the tumor and the nature of the hormonal activity. Treatment is discussed further in BCSC Section 5, *Neuro-Ophthalmology.*

Pituitary Apoplexy

Pituitary apoplexy results from hemorrhage or infarction in a pituitary adenoma; it can occur spontaneously or after head trauma. In its most dramatic presentation, apoplexy causes the sudden onset of excruciating headache, visual field loss, diplopia due to pressure on the oculomotor nerves, and hypopituitarism. Any type of pituitary hormone deficiency can occur, but cortisol deficiency is the most serious because it can cause life-threatening hypotension. Imaging of the pituitary may show intra-adenomal hemorrhage and deviation of the pituitary stalk. Most patients recover but experience long-term pituitary insufficiency. Signs of reduced vision and altered mental status are indications for transsphenoidal surgical decompression. Ophthalmologists need to be aware of this entity because of the high incidence of visual symptoms on presentation.

Multiple Endocrine Neoplasia Syndromes

Multiple endocrine neoplasia (MEN) syndromes are rare hereditary disorders of benign and malignant endocrine neoplasms. There are 2 syndromes, MEN 1 and MEN 2. Both are typically autosomal dominant, but sporadic cases exist. MEN 2 is further divided into types 2A, 2B (Figs 2-2, 2-3), and medullary thyroid cancer (MTC) alone.

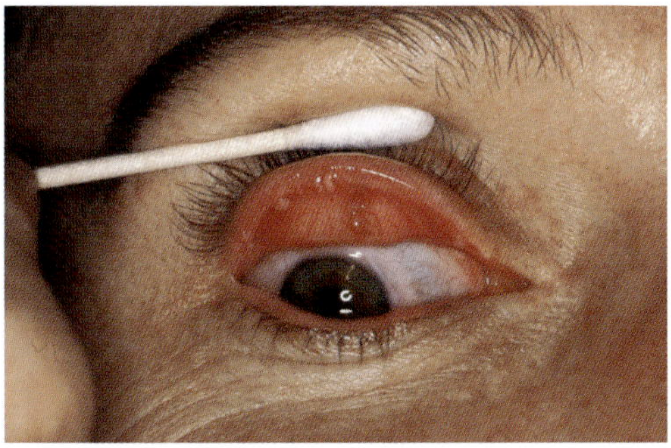

Figure 2-2 Eyelid nodules in multiple endocrine neoplasia (MEN) 2B. *(Courtesy of Jason M. Jacobs, MD, and Michael J. Hawes, MD.)*

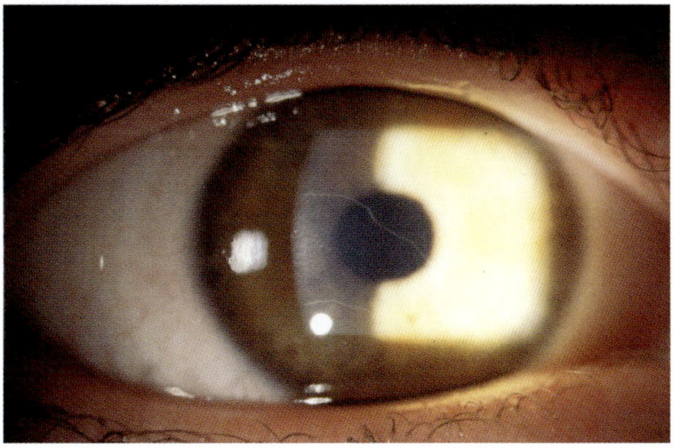

Figure 2-3 Enlarged corneal nerves in MEN 2B. *(Courtesy of Jason M. Jacobs, MD, and Michael J. Hawes, MD.)*

The most common features of MEN 1 are parathyroid, enteropancreatic, and pituitary tumors. Hyperparathyroidism is the most common endocrine abnormality. Enteropancreatic tumors include *gastrinomas*, which cause increased gastric acid output (Zollinger-Ellison syndrome), and *insulinomas*, which cause fasting hypoglycemia. Pituitary adenomas can also be present; they are usually prolactinomas, but other types can occur. Carcinoid and adrenal tumors can develop as well.

MEN 2A and 2B are characterized by the presence of MTC, which occurs in 90%–100% of patients and is the main cause of morbidity. The lifetime incidence of pheochromocytoma is approximately 50%. Hyperparathyroidism is seen in approximately 20%–30% of patients with MEN 2A but is rarely seen in patients with MEN 2B.

MEN 2B is characterized by ganglioneuromas, which occur in 95% of patients. They can be present on the lips, eyelids, and tongue, giving these patients a characteristic phenotype that may be apparent at birth. Patients with MEN 2B may also have marfanoid features including pectus excavatum and scoliosis, but without lens subluxation and aortic disease. The eyelid margins may be nodular as a result of multiple small tumors (see Fig 2-2); subconjunctival neuromas have also been reported. Perhaps the most striking ophthalmic finding is the presence of prominent corneal nerves in a clear stroma (see Fig 2-3), a phenomenon reported in 100% of cases. Because MTC may not appear until the patient's second or third decade, ophthalmic manifestations may be the initial sign of MEN 2B, making ophthalmologists potentially instrumental in the diagnosis of this disease.

The management of MEN depends on the nature of the tumors and usually involves medical treatment to control hormonal effects and/or surgical excision when possible. The genes that cause all types of MEN have been located, and genetic testing can identify patients at risk. Identification of affected family members is particularly important in MEN 2 because prophylactic thyroidectomy can decrease the risk of death from MTC. Screening for pheochromocytoma is also warranted in order to identify problems that could lead to the development of complications such as hypertension.

Walls, GV. Multiple endocrine neoplasia (MEN) syndromes. *Semin Pediatr Surg.* 2014;23(2): 96–101.

CHAPTER 3

Hypertension

Highlights

- The American College of Cardiology (ACC) and the American Heart Association (AHA) guidelines published in November 2017 state that in adults, a normal blood pressure (BP) is less than 120/80 mm Hg. Treatment with lifestyle modifications and medications is now recommended in some individuals with a BP greater than or equal to 130/80 mm Hg.
- The *prehypertension* category has been eliminated in the 2017 ACC/AHA guidelines. The BP goals set by many subspecialty associations are more aggressive than those of JNC 7, especially for patients with diabetes mellitus, proteinuria, congestive heart failure, or renal insufficiency.
- The risk of cardiovascular disease, which begins at a BP of 115/75 mm Hg, doubles with each 20/10 mm Hg increase in BP.
- Masked hypertension (BP that is normal in the office but elevated when measured at home) carries a worse prognosis than "white coat" hypertension with regard to development of arteriosclerosis.
- Thiazide-type diuretics are no longer the first-line therapy for hypertension, except in patients with cardiovascular issues. Depending on the history and comorbidities of the patient with hypertension, treatment with a renin-angiotensin system (RAS) blockade, β-blockers, or calcium channel blockers (CCBs) may be initiated.
- Combination therapy, or 2 or more medications, at onset of hypertension is indicated for patients whose BP is 20/10 mm Hg or more above goal.
- Hypertension is increasingly common in children and adolescents as well as in women aged 45 years and older and has substantial long-term health implications.

Introduction

Hypertension (HTN) affects an estimated 103 million persons aged 20 years or older in the United States and approximately 1.39 billion individuals worldwide. Individuals with hypertension are at greater risk for stroke, myocardial infarction (MI), heart failure, peripheral vascular disease, kidney disease, and retinal vascular complications. The prevalence of hypertension increases with age; it is typically familial and is also related to lifestyle behaviors. HTN is more common in non-Hispanic Black persons than in Hispanic persons, and it is higher in both of those groups than in White persons. BP control rates are lowest in Mexican American and American Indian individuals. The prevalence and severity of hypertension are increased in Black persons, in whom β-blockers, angiotensin-converting enzyme (ACE) inhibitors, and angiotensin II receptor blockers (ARBs) are less effective than diuretics and CCBs in lowering BP. High blood pressure prevalence is also increasing in the Hispanic population. The incidence of devastating complications is higher in lower socioeconomic groups because of greater prevalence, delayed detection, and poor control rates of multifactorial etiology. Antihypertensive therapy is effective in reducing cardiovascular morbidity and mortality, but only 59% of individuals with hypertension are treated, and only 69% of those individuals achieve a blood pressure of 140/90 mm Hg or lower, according to National Health and Nutrition Examination Surveys (NHANES) in the United States and similar cohorts in Canada and Europe. Under the new definition of hypertension (systolic pressure greater than or equal to 130 mm Hg and/or a diastolic greater than or equal to 80 mm Hg), only 47% of individuals undergoing hypertensive therapy will achieve controlled blood pressure. Unfortunately, for many minority patients, socioeconomic and lifestyle factors continue to be barriers to treatment.

Classification of Blood Pressure and Diagnosis of Hypertension

In 2003, the Joint National Committee on Prevention, Detection, Evaluation, and Treatment of High Blood Pressure (JNC 7) published a classification of BP for adults aged 18 years or older. The November 2017 ACC/AHA guidelines update this classification. Normal blood pressure is still defined as blood pressure that is less than 120/80 mm Hg. The prehypertension category has been eliminated entirely. Elevated blood pressure is now classified as systolic blood pressure between 120–129 mm Hg and diastolic blood pressure less than 80 mm Hg. Stage 1 hypertension is defined as systolic BP between 130–139 mm Hg or diastolic BP between 80–89 mm Hg. Stage 2 HTN refers to systolic BP of at least 140 mm Hg or diastolic BP of at least 90 mm Hg (Table 3-1). These classifications are

Table 3-1 2017 Blood Pressure Classification

BP Category	Systolic BP		Diastolic BP
Normal	<120 mm Hg	and	<80 mm Hg
Elevated	120–129 mm Hg	and	<80 mm Hg
Hypertension			
Stage 1	130–139 mm Hg	or	80–89 mm Hg
Stage 2	≥140 mm Hg	or	≥90 mm Hg

Individuals with systolic BP and diastolic BP in 2 categories should be designated to the higher BP category.
BP indicates blood pressure (based on an average of at least 2 careful readings obtained on at least 2 separate occasions).

Modified from Whelton PK, Carey RM, Aronow WS, et al. 2017 ACC/AHA/AAPA/ABC/ACPM/AGS/APhA/ASH/ASPC/NMA/PCNA Guideline for the prevention, detection, evaluation and management of high blood pressure in adults: a report of the American College of Cardiology/American Heart Association Task Force on Clinical Practice Guidelines. *Hypertension.* 2018; 71(6):22.

based on the average of 2 or more properly measured seated BP readings during each of 2 or more office visits or other outpatient assessments such as ambulatory blood pressure monitoring or home blood pressure monitoring with an approved device.

In 10%–15% of patients, BP increases only while in a physician's office; these patients are said to have "white coat" hypertension. Home BP monitoring or 24-hour ambulatory BP measurement (ABPM) is warranted in these individuals and in patients with labile hypertension, resistant hypertension, hypotensive episodes, or postural hypotension, as well as in patients with masked hypertension (normal blood pressure in the office setting but abnormal readings at home). ABPM, which is more widely used in Europe, provides data on circadian variations of BP. ABPM readings are usually lower than measurements taken in a physician's office, and they correlate better with target-organ injury than do office measurements. BP in most individuals decreases by 10%–20% during sleep (dipping pattern); those without such a decrease (nondipping pattern) are at greater risk for cardiovascular and neurovascular events. Masked hypertension may occur in 10%–30% of patients and carries a worse prognosis than white coat hypertension with regard to the development of atherosclerosis. Thus, it is important to recognize that a normal office BP does not exclude hypertension. Individuals with a mean self-measured daytime BP above 135/85 mm Hg or a nighttime BP of 120/70 mm Hg at home are generally considered to be hypertensive.

Chobanian AV, Bakris GL, Black HR, et al; National Heart, Lung, and Blood Institute Joint National Committee on Prevention, Detection, Evaluation, and Treatment of High Blood Pressure; National High Blood Pressure Education Program Coordinating Committee. The Seventh Report of the Joint National Committee on Prevention, Detection, Evaluation, and Treatment of High Blood Pressure: the JNC 7 report. *JAMA*. 2003;289(19):2560–2572.

Whelton PK, Carey RM, Aronow WS, et al. 2017 ACC/AHA/AAPA/ABC/ACPM/AGS/APhA/ASH/ASPC/NMA/PCNA Guideline for the prevention, detection, evaluation and management of high blood pressure in adults: a report of the American College of Cardiology/American Heart Association Task Force on Clinical Practice Guidelines. *Hypertension*. 2018; 71(6):e13–e115.

Etiology and Pathogenesis of Hypertension

Approximately 90% of cases of hypertension are *primary (essential),* in which the etiology is unknown, and 10% are secondary to identifiable causes. Primary hypertension most likely results from a dysregulation of various renal, hormonal, and cellular processes in conjunction with environmental factors such as diet and exercise. These processes include abnormal sodium transport, increased sympathetic nervous system activity, abnormal vasodilation, excess transforming growth factors β (TGF-βs), and abnormalities in the renin-angiotensin-aldosterone system (Fig 3-1).

Causes of *secondary hypertension* vary. Following are some of these causes, along with signs associated with secondary hypertension:

- *polycystic kidney disease:* flank mass
- *renovascular disease:* unilateral abdominal bruit in a young patient with marked hypertension; new-onset hypertension with severe end-organ disease

- *pheochromocytoma:* markedly labile BP with tachycardia and headache
- *hyperaldosteronism:* persistent hypokalemia in the absence of diuretic therapy or marked drop with low-dose diuretics
- *coarctation of the aorta:* delayed or absent femoral pulses in a young patient
- *Cushing syndrome:* truncal obesity and abdominal striae

Secondary causes of hypertension should be suspected in persons who have accelerating hypertension or hypertension unresponsive to medication or in those who have a sudden change in previously well-controlled BP. Patients with secondary hypertension are more likely to have *resistant hypertension*, which is defined as a failure to achieve goal BP even when the patient adheres to the optimal doses of 3 antihypertensive drugs, including a diuretic. The prevalence of resistant hypertension is currently not known, but indirect population study evidence suggests it is more common than previously suspected. This prevalence may be secondary to an aging population, and the increased prevalence of obesity, diabetes mellitus, obstructive sleep apnea syndrome, and chronic kidney disease.

Most cases of diagnosed resistant hypertension are due to inadequate dosing of medication and patient nonadherence to treatment. The most common factors contributing to resistant hypertension are excess sodium intake, volume overload, and failure to treat the

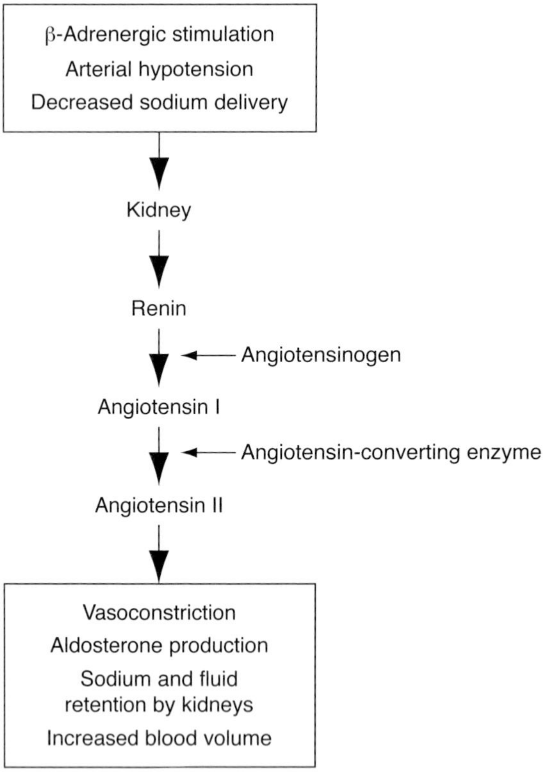

Figure 3-1 Renin-angiotensin-aldosterone system.

Table 3-2 Causes of Secondary Hypertension and Resistant Hypertension

Chronic kidney disease
Obstructive uropathy
Renovascular disease
Genetic mutations
Primary hyperaldosteronism and other mineralocorticoid excess states
Pheochromocytoma
Cushing syndrome and corticosteroid excess
Coarctation of the aorta
Thyroid or parathyroid disease
Sleep apnea
Drugs (oral contraceptives, sympathomimetics, antidepressants, NSAIDs, erythropoietin-stimulating agents, calcineurin inhibitors [cyclosporine, tacrolimus], over-the-counter medicines, ephedra, ma huang, bitter orange)
Alcohol

NSAIDS = nonsteroidal anti-inflammatory drugs.

Data from Chobanian AV, Bakris GL, Black HR, et al; National High Blood Pressure Education Program Coordinating Committee. The Seventh Report of the Joint National Committee on Prevention, Detection, Evaluation, and Treatment of High Blood Pressure: the JNC 7 report. *JAMA.* 2003;289(19):2563.

condition, whether with dietary modification or the proper diuretic and dosage. Other causes of secondary hypertension and resistant hypertension are listed in Table 3-2.

Evaluation of Patients With Hypertension

The 2017 ACC/AHA guidelines expanded the recommended procedures for evaluation of patients with hypertension; the recommended evaluation includes an assessment of lifestyle and the identification of other cardiovascular risk factors (Table 3-3), a search for causes of secondary hypertension, and determination of the presence or absence of target-organ damage and cardiovascular disease.

The physical examination of the patient should include measurement of BP in both arms (from at least 2 readings taken on 2 or 3 different occasions); measurement of orthostatic BP; ophthalmoscopic examination; calculation of body mass index; measurement of waist circumference, which is considered the most important anthropometric factor associated with hypertensive risk; auscultation for carotid, abdominal, and femoral bruits; examination of the thyroid gland; examination of the heart and lungs; examination of the abdomen for masses and aortic pulsation; examination of the lower extremities for edema and pulses; and neurologic assessment.

Laboratory tests to screen for secondary causes and exclude comorbidity (recommended before starting treatment) include an electrocardiogram, urinalysis, complete blood count, and serum chemistry studies, including uric acid tests and a fasting lipid profile. Patients with suspected cardiac morbidities should have a 2-dimensional echocardiogram. More extensive testing for identifiable causes of hypertension is usually not

Table 3-3 Cardiovascular Risk Factors

Major risk factors	
Hypertension[a]	
Cigarette smoking	
Obesity (BMI ≥30)[a]	
Physical inactivity	
Dyslipidemia[a]	
Diabetes mellitus[a]	
Microalbuminuria or estimated GFR <60 mL/min in early-morning urine specimen	
Age (>55 years for men, >65 years for women)	
Family history of premature cardiovascular disease (men <55 years of age or women <65 years of age)	
Target-organ damage	
Heart	
	Left ventricular hypertrophy
	Angina or prior myocardial infarction
	Prior coronary revascularization
	Heart failure
Brain	
	Stroke or transient ischemic attack
Chronic kidney disease	
Peripheral arterial disease	
Retinopathy	

BMI = body mass index, calculated as weight in kilograms divided by the square of height in meters; GFR = glomerular filtration rate.
[a] Components of metabolic syndrome.

Adapted with permission from Chobanian AV, Bakris GL, Black HR, et al; National High Blood Pressure Education Program Coordinating Committee. The Seventh Report of the Joint National Committee on Prevention, Detection, Evaluation, and Treatment of High Blood Pressure: the JNC 7 report. *JAMA.* 2003; 289(19):2563.

indicated unless BP control is not achieved or if other clinical findings warrant further evaluation.

Berrington de Gonzalez A, Hartge P, Cerhan JR, et al. Body-mass index and mortality among 1.46 million White adults. *N Engl J Med.* 2010;363(23):2211–2219.

Treatment of Hypertension

The primary objective of antihypertensive therapy is to reduce cardiovascular and renal morbidity and mortality. Controlling systolic BP is the major concern because, in patients older than 50 years, systolic BP greater than 140 mm Hg is a more important cardiovascular risk factor than diastolic BP. In addition, diastolic BP is usually controlled when the systolic goal is reached. Maintaining BP at less than 130/80 mm Hg decreases cardiovascular complications. In hypertensive patients with diabetes mellitus or renal disease, the BP goal is less than 120/80 mm Hg. These patients have a higher incidence of proteinuria, which is associated with hyperlipidemia, cardiovascular events, and overall higher morbidity. Effective BP control can be attained in most patients with hypertension, but the majority of these patients require 2 or more medications to achieve this control. It is important for patients to understand that lifelong treatment is usually necessary and that symptoms are not a reliable indicator of the severity of hypertension.

When selecting the appropriate therapy for a patient, the physician should consider multiple factors: stage of hypertension, target-organ disease, cardiovascular risk factors, cost, adherence, adverse effects, and comorbid conditions. In general, the higher the BP, the greater the damage to target organs; and the greater the risk factors for cardiovascular disease, the sooner treatment should be initiated. For example, patients with severe hypertension and encephalopathy require urgent treatment, whereas those with mild hypertension may wish to attempt lifestyle modifications before drug therapy is initiated along with consideration of comorbid conditions such as diabetes mellitus and obesity.

Lifestyle Modifications

Obesity, sedentary lifestyle, excessive sodium intake, moderate daily alcohol consumption, and inadequate intake of vitamins and minerals, including potassium, calcium, magnesium, and folate, can contribute to the development of hypertension. Smoking is also a major contributor to cardiovascular disease in patients with hypertension. Lifestyle modifications, including reducing weight, adopting the DASH (Dietary Approaches to Stop Hypertension) eating plan, reducing dietary sodium intake, increasing physical activity, and moderating alcohol and caffeine consumption can decrease BP, enhance the effectiveness of antihypertensive drugs, and lower the risk of cardiovascular disease; Table 3-4 presents further details. The PREMIER trial investigated the benefit of adding behavioral modifications such as increased physical activity to the DASH diet. At 18 months, the prevalence of hypertension remained lowest in this group compared with those on the DASH program alone and with those who had only received advice once on dietary and behavioral intervention. Such healthful lifestyle habits are essential for the prevention and control of hypertension.

Pharmacologic Treatment

Several classes of drugs effectively lower BP and reduce the complications resulting from hypertension. The most commonly prescribed antihypertensive drugs include diuretics, β-blockers, ACE inhibitors, ARBs, and CCBs. Table 3-5 lists these and other types of oral antihypertensive drugs. Figure 3-2 provides an algorithm for the treatment of hypertension.

The 2017 ACC/AHA guidelines focus on the pharmacologic treatment of hypertension. The JNC 7 guidelines recommended thiazide-type diuretics as the initial drug therapy unless compelling reasons dictated otherwise. In the 2017 ACC/AHA guidelines, thiazides are not necessarily the first-line therapy; CCBs, ACE inhibitors, ARBs, and β-blockers are alternatives. The initial drug choice for non-Black patients may be selected from 4 drug classes, based on clinical setting and comorbidities: thiazide-type diuretics, CCBs, ACE inhibitors, and ARBs. For Black patients, the initial drug choice may be selected from 2 drug classes: thiazide-type diuretics and CCBs.

Table 3-4 2017 Recommended Nonpharmacologic Interventions for Prevention and Treatment of Hypertension[a]

	Nonpharmacologic Intervention	Dose	Approximate Impact on Systolic BP: Hypertension	Approximate Impact on Systolic BP: Normal Blood Pressure
Weight loss	Weight/body fat	Expect a reduction of about 1 mm Hg for every 1-kg reduction in body weight in overweight patients.	–5 mm Hg	–2 to –3 mm Hg
Healthy diet	DASH eating plan	A diet rich in fruits, vegetables, whole grains, and low-fat dairy products, with reduced content of saturated and total fat.	–11 mm Hg	–3 mm Hg
Reduced intake of dietary sodium	Dietary sodium	Optimal goal is <1500 mg/day, but aim for at least a 1000-mg reduction in most adults.	–5 to –6 mm Hg	–2 to –3 mm Hg
Enhanced intake of dietary potassium	Dietary potassium	Aim for 3500–5000 mg/day, preferably by consumption of a diet rich in potassium.	–4 to –5 mm Hg	–2 mm Hg
Increased physical activity	Aerobic	90–150 min/week 65%–75% heart rate reserve	–5 to –8 mm Hg	–2 to –4 mm Hg
	Dynamic resistance	90–150 min/week 50%–80% 1 rep maximum	–4 mm Hg	–2 mm Hg
	Isometric resistance	3 sessions/week for 8–10 weeks	–5 mm Hg	–4 mm Hg
Moderation in alcohol intake	Alcohol consumption	In individuals who drink alcohol, reduce alcohol[b] to: Men: ≤2 drinks daily Women: ≤1 drink daily	–4 mm Hg	–3 mm Hg

[a] Type, dose, and expected impact on BP in adults with a normal BP and with hypertension.
[b] In the United States, 1 "standard" drink contains roughly 14 g of pure alcohol, which is typically found in 12 oz of regular beer (usually about 5% alcohol), 5 oz of wine (usually about 12% alcohol), and 1.5 oz of distilled spirits (usually about 40% alcohol).
DASH = Dietary Approaches to Stop Hypertension; BP = blood pressure.

Table 3-5 Oral Antihypertensive Drugs

Class	Drugs
Thiazide-type diuretics	Chlorothiazide, chlorthalidone, hydrochlorothiazide, indapamide, metolazone, polythiazide
Loop diuretics	Bumetanide, furosemide, torsemide
Potassium-sparing diuretics	Amiloride, triamterene
Aldosterone-receptor blockers	Eplerenone, spironolactone
β-Blockers	Atenolol, betaxolol, bisoprolol, metoprolol, metoprolol extended release, nadolol, nebivolol, propranolol, propranolol long-acting, timolol
β-Blockers with intrinsic sympathomimetic activity	Acebutolol, penbutolol, pindolol
ACE inhibitors	Benazepril, captopril, enalapril, fosinopril, lisinopril, moexipril, perindopril, quinapril, ramipril, trandolapril
Angiotensin II antagonists	Azilsartan, candesartan, eprosartan, irbesartan, losartan, olmesartan, telmisartan, valsartan
Calcium channel blockers: nondihydropyridines	Diltiazem, verapamil
Calcium channel blockers: dihydropyridines	Amlodipine, felodipine, isradipine, nicardipine, nifedipine, nisoldipine
α_1-Blockers	Doxazosin, prazosin, terazosin
Combined α- and β-blockers	Carvedilol, labetalol
Central α_2-agonists and other centrally acting drugs	Clonidine, clonidine patch, guanfacine, methyldopa, reserpine
Direct vasodilators	Hydralazine, minoxidil
Direct renin inhibitor	Aliskiren[a]

ACE = angiotensin-converting enzyme.

[a] Aliskiren is an oral renin inhibitor that effectively lowers BP when used either alone or with other antihypertensive agents. It is the first new class of antihypertensive drug approved by the FDA in more than a decade, and its role in the management of patients with hypertension is yet to be established.

Data from Chobanian AV, Bakris GL, Black HR, et al; National High Blood Pressure Education Program Coordinating Committee. The Seventh Report of the Joint National Committee on Prevention, Detection, Evaluation, and Treatment of High Blood Pressure: the JNC 7 report. *JAMA.* 2003;289(19):2565–2566.

Antihypertensive Drugs

Diuretics Diuretics are categorized by their site of action in the kidney and are divided into thiazide, loop, and potassium-sparing types.

Thiazide-type diuretics send more of a sodium load to the kidney's distal tubules, initially decreasing plasma volume and cardiac output through natriuresis. As the renin-angiotensin-aldosterone system compensates for the diminished plasma volume, cardiac output returns to normal and peripheral vascular resistance is lowered. Chlorthalidone, 12.5–25 mg, can be used in patients with a glomerular filtration rate (GFR) of less than 30 mL/min and has a strong safety and cardio-protective profile.

Loop diuretics act on the ascending loop of Henle and block sodium resorption, increasing free water loss, resulting in an initial decrease in plasma volume. As with thiazide-type

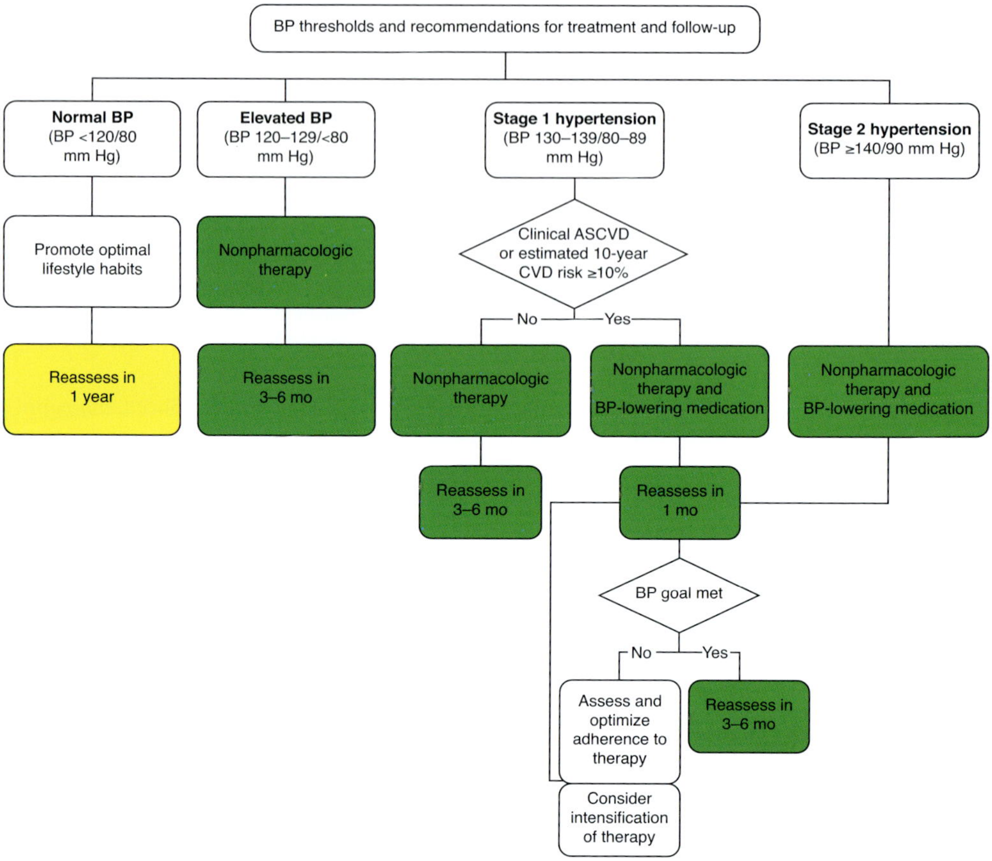

Figure 3-2 Blood pressure (BP) thresholds and recommendations for treatment and follow-up. *(Modified with permission from Whelton PK, Carey RM, Aronow WS, et al. 2017 ACC/AHA/AAPA/ABC/ACPM/AGS/APhA/ASH/ASPC/NMA/PCNA Guideline for the prevention, detection, evaluation and management of high blood pressure in adults: a report of the American College of Cardiology/American Heart Association Task Force on Clinical Practice Guidelines.* Hypertension. *2018; 71[6]:e74.)*

diuretics, BP is eventually lowered because of decreased peripheral vascular resistance. Loop diuretics are used primarily in treating patients with moderate renal insufficiency.

Potassium-sparing diuretics may block the actions of aldosterone to prevent potassium loss from the distal tubule, or they may act directly on the distal tubule to inhibit aldosterone-induced sodium resorption in exchange for potassium. They are often used as adjuncts to the thiazide-type or loop diuretics to counteract potassium depletion, but in patients with suspected hyperaldosterone states they may be used alone.

Side effects of diuretics vary according to class. Thiazide-type diuretics can cause weakness, muscle cramps, impotence, hypokalemia, hyperglycemia, hyperlipidemia, hyperuricemia, hypercalcemia, hypomagnesemia, hyponatremia, azotemia, and pancreatitis. Thiazide-type diuretics may also unmask type 2 diabetes and aggravate lipid disorders. On a positive note, they may also slow the demineralization that occurs with osteoporosis. Loop diuretics can cause ototoxicity, as well as electrolyte abnormalities such as hypokalemia, hypocalcemia, and hypomagnesemia. Potassium-sparing diuretics can cause hyperkalemia, renal calculi, renal tubular damage, and gynecomastia. Diuretics are particularly effective in individuals with salt-sensitive hypertension such as older persons and in Black persons.

Angiotensin-converting enzyme inhibitors Angiotensin-converting enzyme (ACE) catalyzes the conversion of angiotensin I to angiotensin II. Angiotensin II, a potent vasoconstrictor, is the primary vasoactive hormone of the renin-angiotensin-aldosterone system, and it plays a major role in the pathophysiology of hypertension. ACE inhibitors block the conversion of angiotensin I to angiotensin II, resulting in vasodilation with decreased peripheral vascular resistance and natriuresis. They also decrease aldosterone production and increase levels of vasodilating bradykinins. Some ACE inhibitors stimulate production of vasodilatory prostaglandins. The efficacy of ACE inhibitors is enhanced when they are used in combination with diuretics, reducing hypokalemia, hypercholesterolemia, hyperglycemia, and hyperuricemia caused by diuretic therapy. ACE inhibitors are beneficial in patients with left ventricular dysfunction and with proteinuria, especially in patients with diabetes. ACE inhibitors may also help improve insulin sensitivity.

Adverse effects of ACE inhibitors include a dry cough (5%–20% of patients), angioneurotic edema, hypotension, hyperkalemia, abnormal taste, leukopenia, and proteinuria; in addition, patients may have a reduced GFR (30% of patients). Preexisting renal artery stenosis should be considered in this clinical situation. In patients with volume-reduced states, ACE inhibitors should be suspended and reassessed later. ACE inhibitors should be avoided in patients with a history of angioedema or known renal artery stenosis (RAS). They are contraindicated during pregnancy and in patients trying to become pregnant because of the adverse effects on fetal renal function and risk of fetal death.

Angiotensin II receptor blockers Angiotensin II receptor blockers (ARBs) inhibit the vasoconstrictive and aldosterone-secreting effects of angiotensin II by selectively blocking the angiotensin II receptors that are found in such tissues as vascular smooth muscle and the adrenal gland, resulting in decreased peripheral vascular resistance. ARBs are effective in managing hypertension in a variety of situations, including in patients with heart failure who are unable to tolerate ACE inhibitors. ARBs also have been associated with a reduced incidence of new-onset diabetes mellitus and, like ACE inhibitors, improve insulin sensitivity.

The adverse effects of ARBs are similar to those occurring with ACE inhibitors, though they occur less commonly with ARBs. The dry cough caused by ACE inhibitors generally does not occur with use of ARBs, and angioedema is rare. Like ACE inhibitors, ARBs are contraindicated in pregnancy unless there is profound proteinuria, and then use is very closely monitored. ACE inhibitors should not be combined with ARBs.

Calcium channel blockers Calcium channel blockers (CCBs) block the entry of calcium into vascular smooth muscle cells, resulting in reduced myocardial contractility and decreased systemic vascular resistance. CCBs are divided into 2 types: dihydropyridine and nondihydropyridine. Dihydropyridine (DHP) CCBs tend to be more potent vasodilators, whereas the nondihydropyridine CCBs have more marked negative inotropic effects.

Adverse effects of CCBs vary according to the agent but include constipation, headache, fatigue, dizziness, nausea, palpitations, flushing, edema, gingival hyperplasia, arrhythmias, and cardiac ischemia. Because of their negative inotropic effects, nondihydropyridine CCBs should generally be avoided in patients with cardiac conduction abnormalities such as atrial fibrillation or heart failure associated with left ventricular dysfunction and in patients with acute MI. Dihydropyridine CCBs may be helpful in patients with Raynaud syndrome and in some arrhythmias.

β-Blockers There are 2 types of β-adrenergic receptor sites: β_1 is present in vascular and cardiac tissue, and β_2 is found in the bronchial system. Circulating or locally released catecholamines stimulate β sites, resulting in vasoconstriction, bronchodilation, tachycardia, and increased myocardial contractility. β-Blockers inhibit these effects. They also decrease plasma renin, reset baroreceptors to facilitate lower BP, induce the release of vasodilatory prostaglandins, and decrease plasma volume, and they may have a central nervous system–mediated antihypertensive effect.

β-Blockers are divided into those that are nonselective (β_1 and β_2), those that are cardioselective (primarily β_1), and those that have intrinsic sympathomimetic activity (ISA). The cardioselective agents may be prescribed with caution in patients with pulmonary disease, diabetes mellitus, or peripheral arterial disease, but at higher doses they lose their β_1 selectivity and can cause adverse effects in these patients. Those agents with ISA minimize the bradycardia caused by other β-blockers. β-Blockers with α-blocking properties, such as carvedilol or labetalol, have additional vasodilatory effects caused by selective α_1-receptor blockade. In patients with heart failure due to systolic dysfunction, the use of certain β-blockers—particularly carvedilol, metoprolol succinate, and bisoprolol—reduces hospitalizations for heart failure and improves survival rates. Nebivolol has nitric oxide–potentiating vasodilatory effects. β-Blockers are beneficial in the treatment of atrial fibrillation and tachyarrhythmias, migraine, thyrotoxicosis, and essential tremor.

Adverse effects of β-blockers include bronchospasm, bradycardia, masking of insulin-induced hypoglycemia, insomnia, fatigue, depression, impotence, impaired peripheral circulation, impaired exercise tolerance, nasal congestion, and hypertriglyceridemia (except for β-blockers with ISA). Angina pectoris and increased BP can be precipitated by abrupt cessation of β-blocker therapy. β-Blockers should generally be avoided in patients with asthma, reactive airway disease, or second-degree or third-degree heart block.

Ophthalmic considerations β-Blockers are used in the treatment of glaucoma and are effective in lowering intraocular pressure; they have a long duration of action. Systemic adverse effects resulting from the use of these topical agents may occur; these can be minimized by nasolacrimal occlusion for 3 minutes after drop instillation.

α_1-Blockers α_1-Adrenergic antagonists block postsynaptic α-receptors, resulting in arterial and venous vasodilation. Selective α_1-blockers have replaced older nonselective agents in the treatment of hypertension. Although these agents are not as effective as diuretics, CCBs, and ACE inhibitors, they may be prescribed as adjunct therapy in selected cases, not as a primary agent.

Adverse effects include the "first-dose effect," in which BP is decreased more with the initial dose than with subsequent doses; orthostatic hypotension; headache; dizziness; and drowsiness.

Combined α-adrenergic and β-adrenergic antagonists Combined α-adrenergic and β-adrenergic antagonists block the action of catecholamines at both α-adrenergic and β-adrenergic receptor sites. Adverse effects are similar to those of other α-adrenergic and β-adrenergic antagonists.

Centrally acting adrenergic drugs Centrally acting adrenergic drugs are potent antihypertensive agents that stimulate presynaptic α_2-adrenergic receptors in the central nervous system (CNS), causing reductions in the tone and contractility of smooth muscle, cardiac output, and peripheral vascular resistance.

Adverse effects include fluid retention, dry mouth, drowsiness, dizziness, orthostatic hypotension, rash, impotence, and hepatitis; positive results on the direct antiglobulin (Coombs) test and the antinuclear antibody (ANA) test; and heart failure in patients with decreased left ventricular dysfunction. There may also be severe rebound hypertension if the drug is abruptly discontinued.

Methyldopa continues to be widely used in pregnancy because of its proven safety. Older centrally acting sympatholytic agents (eg, reserpine) have significant adverse effects and are seldom used.

Direct vasodilators Direct-acting vasodilators such as minoxidil and hydralazine decrease peripheral vascular resistance by direct arterial vasodilation. They are generally reserved for special situations, such as pregnancy or intractable hypertension. They should be avoided or used with caution in patients with ischemic heart disease.

Adverse effects include headache, tachycardia, edema, nausea, vomiting, a lupuslike syndrome, and hypertrichosis. Because of the sympathetic hyperactivity and the sodium and fluid retention caused by direct vasodilators, they are often used in conjunction with diuretics or β-blockers.

Combination therapy Combination therapy usually includes small doses of a diuretic, which potentiates the effects of other drugs such as ACE inhibitors, ARBs, and β-blockers. This therapy may improve patient adherence and reduce BP to target levels more quickly than other classes of drugs. Another advantage of combination therapy is that low-dose therapy with 2 antihypertensive drugs is associated with fewer adverse effects than is higher-dose therapy with a single agent.

Direct renin inhibitors Aliskiren is the first orally active renin inhibitor launched to treat hypertension. It has a high specificity for renin and has a long half-life (approximately 24 hours), which makes it ideal for once-daily treatment of hypertension. Direct renin inhibitors (DRIs) are more likely to be effective in younger White patients, who, in general, have a more active renin system, and in any patients receiving diuretics or CCBs, in whom the renin system has been activated. The main adverse effect of DRIs is possible diarrhea at higher doses.

Parenteral antihypertensive drugs Parenteral antihypertensive therapy is indicated for immediate reduction of BP in hypertensive emergencies.

Sodium nitroprusside, a direct arterial and venous vasodilator, is the drug of choice for most hypertensive emergencies. Nitroglycerin may be preferable in patients with severe coronary insufficiency or advanced kidney or liver disease. Labetalol is also effective and is the drug of choice in hypertensive emergencies that occur in pregnancy. Esmolol is a cardioselective β-adrenergic antagonist that can be used in hypertensive emergencies when β-blocker intolerance is a concern; it is also useful in treating aortic dissection. Phentolamine is effective in managing hypertension with acute drug intoxication or withdrawal. Nicardipine is a CCB that can be administered intravenously for postoperative hypertension. Intravenous enalapril is an ACE inhibitor that can be effective in the treatment of postoperative hypertension, although unpredictable results have been reported with its use. Diazoxide and hydralazine are used infrequently now, but hydralazine does have a long-established safety profile and may be useful in pregnancy-related hypertensive emergencies.

Future Treatments and Targets for Hypertension

Data from the Conduit Artery Function Endpoint (CAFE) study showed that different classes of antihypertensive drugs have different effects on brachial versus central aortic systolic and pulse pressures and that central pressures may be a better predictor of cardiovascular outcomes in response to treatment. The Strong Heart Study also showed that central aortic pressures may be a better predictor of target end-organ damage and outcomes than are conventional brachial pressures.

Thus, it is worth mentioning several other drugs, such as soluble guanylate cyclase activators, that would lower central aortic pressures. These increase cyclic guanosine monophosphate levels in target tissues, resulting in vasodilation and an antiproliferative effect. One study found that such an activator lowered BP and inhibited cardiac hypertrophy in rats with angiotensin II–induced hypertension. This drug may also potentially reduce large-artery stiffness, lowering central aortic systolic pressures beyond the benefits observed on brachial BP.

Other experimental agents, known as *advanced glycation cross-link breakers,* target vascular wall thickness and its effects on BP. We know that increased large-artery stiffness occurs with aging and disease and is associated with increased brachial systolic pressure. This increased pressure is due to the accumulation of advanced glycation end products (AGEs) within the vascular wall. AGEs also impair endothelial function, leading to arterial stiffness. Therefore, targeting these molecules to reduce their levels or indeed their presence in vascular walls may have an effect on decreasing vessel stiffness and lowering BP.

Other intriguing studies have involved attempts to develop a vaccine for hypertension and the use of acupuncture in treatment of hypertension. Nonpharmacologic device-based therapies are being investigated to treat resistant hypertension, including renal denervation, baroreflex activation therapy, carotid body ablation, central iliac arteriovenous anastomosis, deep brain stimulation, median nerve stimulation, and vagal nerve stimulation. Catheter-based radiofrequency ablation of the renal sympathetic nerves can lower BP in patients with resistant hypertension. The initial results look promising, but it is not yet known whether the antihypertensive effect of radiofrequency ablation is due in part to improved patient adherence to the medication regimen. These techniques have been found to be of limited efficacy. Long-term data regarding these modalities are still lacking.

Ng FL, Saxena M, Mahfoud F, Pathak A, Lobo MD. Device-based therapy for hypertension. *Curr Hypertens Rep.* 2016;18(8):61.

Williams B, Lacy PS, Thom SM, et al; CAFE Investigators; Anglo-Scandinavian Cardiac Outcomes Trial Investigators; CAFE Steering Committee and Writing Committee. Differential impact of blood pressure-lowering drugs on central aortic pressure and clinical outcomes: principal results of the Conduit Artery Function Evaluation (CAFE) study. *Circulation.* 2006;113(9):1213–1225.

Special Considerations

Ischemic Heart Disease

For patients with hypertension and stable angina pectoris, a β-blocker is generally the initial drug of choice; alternatively, CCBs can be used. ACE inhibitors and β-blockers are recommended as first-line drugs in hypertensive patients with acute coronary syndromes (unstable angina or MI). In post-MI patients, β-blockers, ACE inhibitors, and potassium-sparing diuretics (aldosterone antagonists) are beneficial.

Heart Failure

In asymptomatic patients with hypertension and ventricular dysfunction, ACE inhibitors and β-blockers are recommended. In patients with symptomatic ventricular dysfunction or end-stage heart failure, ACE inhibitors, ARBs, aldosterone antagonists, loop diuretics, and β-blockers—especially carvedilol, bisoprolol, or nebivolol—are useful.

Diabetes Mellitus and Hypertension

As mentioned earlier, hypertensive patients with diabetes mellitus usually require 2 or more antihypertensive drugs to achieve a BP goal of less than 130/80 mm Hg. Chlorthalidone (the preferred thiazide diuretic), β-blockers, ACE inhibitors, ARBs, and CCBs reduce cardiovascular complications in these patients. ACE inhibitors or ARBs are beneficial for those with diabetic nephropathy.

Chronic Renal Disease

Aggressive treatment, often with 3 or more drugs, may be necessary to achieve a BP goal of less than 130/80 mm Hg and to prevent deterioration of renal function and cardiovascular complications in hypertensive patients with chronic renal disease. ACE inhibitors and ARBs favorably alter the progression of diabetic and nondiabetic nephropathy. However, as the GFR nears 20 mL/min, less aggressive treatment may be appropriate, particularly in patients with renin-angiotensin-aldosterone system suppression.

Cerebrovascular Disease

The combination of an ACE inhibitor and the appropriate diuretic lowers the risk of recurrent stroke. The optimal BP level during an acute stroke remains undetermined, but consensus favors intermediate control in the range of 160/100 mm Hg until patient stabilization is achieved.

Obesity and Metabolic Syndrome

Obesity (body mass index ≥30) is a risk factor for the development of hypertension and has become a major concern in the United States, where an estimated 160 million adults are overweight or obese. Closely related to obesity is *metabolic syndrome.* This syndrome is characterized by the presence of 3 or more of these conditions: central (abdominal) obesity, elevated triglyceride level, reduced high-density lipoprotein cholesterol level, hypertension, and elevated fasting blood glucose levels. Patients with these conditions should adopt healthful lifestyle habits and, if necessary, use drug therapy, excepting thiazide-type diuretics, which may aggravate this syndrome. See Chapter 2 for additional discussion of metabolic syndrome.

Obstructive Sleep Apnea Syndrome

Hypertension and obstructive sleep apnea syndrome (OSAS) often coexist. OSAS is a sleep-related breathing disorder with cardinal signs, including obstructive apneas; hypopneas; and sleep disturbances with snoring, restlessness, or resuscitative snorts. This disrupted sleep leads to daytime fatigue, poor concentration, and sleeplessness and has been associated with the development of heart disease and metabolic syndrome. There is an increased prevalence and incidence of hypertension in these patients and an observed dose-response effect between the severity of OSAS and the likelihood of hypertension. Treatment of OSAS can lower BP by clinically significant levels.

Left Ventricular Hypertrophy

Left ventricular hypertrophy is a risk factor for cardiovascular disease, but regression is possible with treatment of hypertension. All antihypertensive drug classes, except the direct vasodilators, are effective in treating left ventricular hypertrophy.

Peripheral Arterial Disease

The risk factors for peripheral arterial disease parallel those for ischemic heart disease in patients with hypertension. All classes of antihypertensive agents are useful in treating hypertensive patients with peripheral arterial disease.

Ophthalmic considerations Most individuals experience a physiological drop in systemic BP (dipping pattern) during sleep; BP normalizes when these individuals awaken. This decrease in BP may be exacerbated when antihypertensive medications are taken at night. Systemic nocturnal hypotension may be a risk factor for low-tension glaucoma. There is also some evidence that nocturnal arterial hypotension may play a role in the development of nonarteritic anterior ischemic optic neuropathy (NAION), which has been associated with obstructive sleep apnea syndrome (OSAS). OSAS may increase the risk of NAION and low-tension glaucoma via several potential mechanisms, including impaired autoregulation of optic nerve head blood flow, optic nerve vascular dysregulation, and direct optic nerve damage due to prolonged hypoxia. OSAS also plays a role in the development of various retinal findings, including microaneurysms, hypertensive retinopathy, and intraocular production of postischemic molecules that are associated with neovascularization, apoptosis, and macular edema.

Orthostatic Hypotension

Orthostatic hypotension is defined as a postural drop in systolic blood pressure of more than 10 mm Hg associated with dizziness or fainting. It occurs more frequently in older patients with systolic hypertension; in patients with diabetes mellitus; and in those taking diuretics, vasodilators, or certain psychotropic drugs. In these individuals, BP should be monitored while they are in the upright position, and hypovolemia should be avoided. Also, medication dosages should be carefully titrated and various shorter-acting drugs considered for these patients.

Hypertension in Older Patients

Hypertension is present in most individuals older than 65 years. Treatment recommendations for patients in this age group are generally the same as for others with hypertension. In older patients with isolated systolic hypertension, the preferred treatment is a diuretic with or without a β-blocker, or a dihydropyridine CCB alone. Diastolic BP less than 75 mm Hg increases these patients' risk of stroke and should be avoided.

Antihypertensive drug therapy in older patients can cause adverse effects that increase the risk of falls, such as dizziness and hypotension. Appropriate precautions should be taken to reduce this risk and enhance patient safety.

Dementia occurs more commonly in individuals with hypertension. In some patients, antihypertensive therapy may slow the progression of cognitive impairment.

Women and Pregnancy

Because the use of oral contraceptives increases the risk of hypertension, women taking oral contraceptives should have regular BP checks. Hypertension in women who are pregnant may be classified as follows:

- *preeclampsia or eclampsia:* preeclampsia—hypertension, proteinuria, generalized edema, and possibly coagulation and liver function abnormalities after 20 weeks' gestation; eclampsia—those same abnormalities plus generalized seizures
- *chronic hypertension:* BP greater than 140/90 mm Hg before 20 weeks' gestation

- *chronic hypertension with superimposed preeclampsia or eclampsia*
- *transient hypertension:* hypertension without proteinuria or CNS manifestations during pregnancy; the return of normal BP within 10 days of delivery

Hypertension in women who are pregnant can potentially increase maternal and fetal morbidity and mortality. The possible adverse effects of antihypertensive drug therapy on fetal development must be considered, however, when pharmacologic treatment is planned. Methyldopa, β-blockers, and vasodilators are the recommended drugs for treatment of hypertension in pregnancy. ACE inhibitors and ARBs are contraindicated in pregnancy because of teratogenic effects; they should also be avoided in women who are likely to become pregnant.

Children and Adolescents

Considerable advances have been made in the detection, evaluation, and management of hypertension in children and adolescents. Current evidence indicates that primary hypertension in young individuals occurs more commonly than previously recognized and has substantial long-term health implications. There is little doubt that obesity in young people is a predictor for developing hypertension as well as associated metabolic risk factors. Hypertension in individuals aged 3–18 years is defined as average systolic BP and/or diastolic BP that is in the 95th percentile or higher for sex, age, and height, taken on 3 or more occasions. BP between the 90th percentile and the 95th percentile in childhood is designated as *elevated* and is an indication for lifestyle modifications. It is recommended that children older than 3 years have their BP measured when they are examined in a medical setting.

Children and adolescents who are hypertensive are frequently overweight, and some may have sleep disorders. Secondary hypertension occurs more commonly in children than in adults.

Indications for initiating antihypertensive drug therapy in children include uncontrolled hypertension despite nonpharmacologic measures, symptomatic hypertension, secondary hypertension, hypertensive target-organ damage, and hypertension in patients with diabetes mellitus. Acceptable drug choices for treating hypertension in children include diuretics, β-blockers, ACE inhibitors, ARBs, and CCBs.

Flynn JT, Kaelber DC, Baker-Smith CM, et al; Subcommittee on Screening and Management of High Blood Pressure in Children. Clinical practice guideline for screening and management of high blood pressure in children and adolescents. *Pediatrics.* 2017;140(3):ii.

National High Blood Pressure Education Program Working Group on High Blood Pressure in Children and Adolescents. The fourth report on the diagnosis, evaluation, and treatment of high blood pressure in children and adolescents. *Pediatrics.* 2004;114(2 Suppl 4th report):555–576.

Withdrawal Syndromes

Hypertension can be associated with withdrawal from alcohol or drugs such as cocaine, amphetamines, and opioid analgesics. Withdrawal syndromes can occur with acute drug intoxication or as the result of abrupt discontinuation of a drug after long-term use. Phentolamine, sodium nitroprusside, and nitroglycerin are all effective in the immediate management of hypertension in these situations. β-Blockers should not be used, because unopposed α-adrenergic stimulation may exacerbate the hypertension.

Monoamine oxidase inhibitors taken with certain drugs or with tyramine-containing foods can increase catecholamine levels, thereby causing accelerated hypertension. Phentolamine, sodium nitroprusside, and labetalol are effective for treating this type of hypertension.

Abrupt discontinuation of antihypertensive therapy can cause severe rebound hypertension. This occurs most commonly in patients taking centrally acting adrenergic agents (particularly clonidine) or β-blockers, but it can occur with other drug classes as well, including diuretics. When an acute withdrawal syndrome occurs, and parenteral antihypertensive treatment is necessary, sodium nitroprusside is the drug of choice.

Hypertensive Crisis

Patients with severe BP elevation and acute target-organ damage (eg, encephalopathy, MI, unstable angina, pulmonary edema, stroke, head trauma, eclampsia, or aortic dissection) should be admitted to the hospital for emergency parenteral antihypertensive therapy. Patients with marked BP elevation but without target-organ damage may not require hospital admission, but they should be treated urgently with combination oral antihypertensive drugs. Identifiable causes of hypertension should be sought, and these patients should be carefully monitored for target-organ damage.

Ophthalmic considerations Retinal vascular complications (hypertensive retinopathy, retinal vein occlusions, retinal arterial occlusions), glaucoma, ischemic optic neuropathy, microvascular cranial nerve palsies, and stroke-related disorders of the afferent and efferent pathways of the visual system are commonly associated with hypertension. Moreover, ophthalmic surgery patients with poorly controlled hypertension may be more susceptible to intraoperative and postoperative complications.

There is strong evidence that certain signs of hypertensive retinopathy, independent of other risk factors, are associated with increased cardiovascular risk. Based on these reported associations, a simplified classification of hypertensive retinopathy was proposed in 2004 (Table 3-6).

In addition to the kidney, the renin angiotensin system (RAS) exists in ocular tissues and are overexpressed in the retina of individuals with diabetes. In the retina, angiotensin II activates receptors that stimulate pathways involved in diabetic retinopathy, such as inflammation, oxidative stress, cell proliferation, pericyte migration, remodeling of extracellular matrix, angiogenesis, and fibrosis. RAS blockade is thought to attenuate or inhibit these pathogenic effects.

The 2017 ACC/AHA guidelines emphasize the importance of patient assessment and education, echoing earlier reviews from the JNC 7 and

Table 3-6 Classification of Hypertensive Retinopathy With Systemic Associations

Grade of Retinopathy	Retinal Signs	Systemic Associations
None	No detectable signs	None
Mild	Generalized and/or focal arteriolar narrowing, arteriovenous nicking, opacity ("copper wiring") due to thickening of arteriolar wall, or a combination of these signs	Modest association with risk of stroke, coronary artery disease, and death
Moderate	Hemorrhage (blot, dot, or flame-shaped), microaneurysm, cotton-wool spot, hard exudates, or a combination of these signs	Strong association with stroke, cognitive decline, and death from cardiovascular causes
Malignant	Signs of moderate retinopathy plus swelling of the optic nerve head	Strong association with death

Modified with permission from Wong TY, Mitchell P. Hypertensive retinopathy. *N Engl J Med.* 2004;351(22):2314. ©2004 Massachusetts Medical Society.

several other societies (European Society of Hypertension, European Society of Cardiology, American Society of Hypertension, International Society of Hypertension). These organizations generally agree that control of hypertension is possible only if patients are motivated to take their prescribed medications and to maintain healthful lifestyle habits. Motivation improves when individuals develop empathy with and trust in their physicians. As members of the health care team, ophthalmologists have an important role in the identification, monitoring, and shared management of patients with hypertension.

Wong TY, Mitchell P. Hypertensive retinopathy. *N Engl J Med.* 2004;351(22):2310–2317.

CHAPTER 4

Hyperlipidemia and Cardiovascular Risk

Highlights

- Therapeutic lifestyle changes remain an essential modality in the management of hyperlipidemia.
- More aggressive management of serum cholesterol and modifiable risk factors has been emphasized by the US National Cholesterol Education Program (NCEP) and the European Society of Cardiology (ESC).
- A number of tools (eg, HeartScore, the American Heart Association's pooled cohort equations, QRISK, MESA) are available to assess the cardiovascular risk for an individual patient.
- Numerous clinical trials have shown that effective reduction of low-density-lipoprotein cholesterol (LDL-C) levels substantially reduces the risk of coronary heart disease and stroke.
- Patients at very-high risk of a cardiovascular event benefit from an LDL-C reduction of at least 50% or below 70 mg/dL.
- Statin therapy is recommended for most dyslipoproteinemic adult patients with cardiometabolic risk.
- Use of statins in acute coronary syndromes reduces the risk of recurrent coronary events.

Introduction

Coronary heart disease (CHD) is the leading cause of death in the United States and in most of the developed world, accounting for more deaths than all forms of cancer combined. Numerous major studies have confirmed earlier reports that lowering elevated LDL-C levels reduces the risk of CHD. The NCEP provided 3 sets of guidelines for treating elevated blood cholesterol levels in adults: Adult Treatment Panel (ATP) I, II, and III. ATP I proposed a strategy for primary prevention of CHD in persons with high levels of LDL-C (≥160 mg/dL) or with borderline high levels of LDL-C (130–159 mg/dL) and multiple (at least 2) risk factors (discussed in the section Risk Assessment). ATP II added intensive management of LDL-C in persons with established CHD. The ATP III guidelines recommended total cholesterol levels of less than 200 mg/dL, LDL cholesterol levels of less than 100 mg/dL, HDL cholesterol levels that are greater than or equal to 60 mg/dL (for HDL, more is better), and triglyceride levels of less than 150 mg/dL.

In 2013, a series of reports published in the United States questioned the value of having specific targets for LDL-C levels. These reports instead recommended the individual assessment of each patient's cardiovascular risk, followed by aggressive treatment with statin drugs in those most likely to benefit. These recommendations are discussed later in this chapter.

Lipoproteins, Cholesterol, and Cardiovascular Disease

Cholesterol and triglycerides are transported in the body by *lipoproteins.* The various classes of lipoprotein differ in the relative concentrations of their components: cholesterol, triglycerides, phospholipids, and proteins *(apolipoproteins).* Chylomicrons carry triglycerides following dietary lipid absorption, whereas *very-low-density lipoproteins (VLDLs),* which are produced by the liver, carry most circulating triglycerides. LDL, or "bad cholesterol," is a product of the metabolism of VLDL and intermediate-density lipoprotein and is the primary carrier of cholesterol. High-density lipoprotein (HDL), or "good cholesterol," is the smallest and densest lipoprotein particle. The result of the inflammatory interaction among these lipoproteins, macrophages, and the cellular components of the arterial wall is called *atherosclerosis.* Although patients' cholesterol levels are what is typically measured, it is the lipoproteins that interact with the arterial wall, producing plaques. The narrowing of the arterial lumen that results from plaque growth or the rupture of a plaque with subsequent thrombosis leads to cardiovascular disease (CVD), including myocardial infarction (MI), stroke, and peripheral arterial disease.

Risk Assessment

The cholesterol level of approximately half the US population puts these individuals at significant risk. A fasting lipoprotein profile (measuring total cholesterol, LDL-C, HDL-C, and triglyceride levels) helps determine an individual's risk status. The US Preventive Services Task Force recommends screening for lipid disorders in men 20–35 years of age and women aged 45 years and older when other risk factors exist, and all men aged 35 years and older regardless of other risk factors. Experimental studies directly support the central role of LDL in atherogenesis, and lowering LDL-C levels is associated with a reduction in CVD risk. Conversely, HDL-C appears protective against atherosclerosis because of its anti-inflammatory properties and its ability to transport cholesterol from vessel walls to the liver for disposal. In general, current guidelines recommend a high-HDL and low-LDL concentration to decrease CVD risk.

Other CHD risk factors, such as hypertension, smoking, diabetes mellitus, short sleep duration, obesity, and limited physical activity should be assessed and managed appropriately in all adults (Table 4-1). The INTERHEART study, which involved 15,000 patients with acute MI versus 15,000 controls in 52 countries, found that current smoking,

Table 4-1 Risk Factor Modification Treatment Goals

Risk Factor	Goal	Intervention
Blood pressure	<130/80 mm Hg Lower goal if patient has chronic kidney disease or diabetes mellitus	Weight control, increased physical activity, alcohol moderation, sodium reduction, medications
Smoking	Smoking cessation Avoid environmental tobacco smoke	Smoking cessation programs, nicotine replacement, bupropion, varenicline
Lipid management	Decreased LDL-C with goal based on overall cardio-vascular risk	Diet low in saturated fat, increased omega-3 fatty acids, weight control, increased physical activity, statins
Diabetes mellitus	HbA_{1c} <7% or tailored to individual patient	Diet, weight control, oral hypoglycemic agents, insulin
Physical activity	150 mins/week moderate exercise or 75 mins/week vigorous exercise	Walking, biking, swimming, gardening, household work, weight training
Weight management	BMI 18.5–24.9 kg/m^2 Waist circumference: ≤102 cm men ≤88 cm women	Physical activity, caloric intake, behavioral programs

BMI = body mass index; HbA_{1c} = hemoglobin A_{1c}; HDL-C = high-density-lipoprotein cholesterol; LDL-C = low-density-lipoprotein cholesterol.

Modified with permission from Smith S, Allen J. AHA/ACC secondary prevention for patients with coronary and other atherosclerotic vascular disease: 2005 update. *Circulation.* 2006;113:2363–2372 (92).

hypertension, diabetes mellitus, abdominal obesity, psychosocial factors, and a raised apolipoprotein B/apolipoprotein A-I ratio increased the risk of acute MI, while moderate or strenuous exercise, daily consumption of fruits and vegetables, and daily consumption of small amounts of alcohol were protective.

A number of risk assessment tools are available to estimate the 10-year risk of a cardiovascular event, including the pooled cohort equations on the American Heart Association (AHA) website (United States); QRISK (United Kingdom); HeartScore (Europe); and MESA (Multi-Ethnic Study of Atherosclerosis; United States). Physicians are encouraged to use the risk tool best suited to the individual patient, because relative cardiac risk varies among national, ethnic, and racial groups. Use of these tools guides the clinician in identifying patients requiring aggressive treatment and those most likely to benefit from such treatment.

2018 prevention guidelines tools: CV risk calculator. AHA website. https://static.heart.org/riskcalc/app/index.html#!/baseline-risk. Accessed September 10, 2021.

Goff DC Jr, Lloyd-Jones DM, Bennet G, et al; American College of Cardiology/American Heart Association Task Force on Practice Guidelines. 2013 ACC/AHA guideline on the assessment of cardiovascular risk: a report of the American College of Cardiology/American Heart Association Task Force on Practice Guidelines. *Circulation.* 2014; 129(25 Suppl 2):S49–73.

Graham I, Atar D, Borch-Johnsen K, et al; European Society of Cardiology (ESC) Committee for Practice Guidelines (CPG). European guidelines on cardiovascular disease prevention in clinical practice: executive summary: Fourth joint task force of the European Society of Cardiology and other societies on cardiovascular disease prevention in clinical practice (constituted by representatives of nine societies and by invited experts). *Eur Heart J.* 2007; 28(19):2375–2414.

HeartScore. European Association of Preventive Cardiology website. www.heartscore.org. Accessed September 10, 2021.

MESA risk calculator. https://mesa-nhlbi.org/MESACHDRisk/MesaRiskScore/RiskScore.aspx. Accessed September 10, 2021.

QRISK3-2018 risk calculator. ClinRisk website. http://qrisk.org/three. Accessed September 10, 2021.

Management

In its simplest terms, the management of hyperlipidemia consists of matching the intensity of LDL-lowering therapy with the absolute risk: the higher the risk, the lower the target LDL level. This approach is based primarily on data from clinical trials and epidemiological studies, which, as mentioned previously, have suggested that a direct relationship exists between the level of LDL-C and the risk of CHD. The ATP III guidelines suggested measuring fasting lipoprotein levels in patients with hyperlipidemia and/or hyperlipoproteinemia. The clinician should also assess the patient for the presence of other risk factors (see Table 4-1) and the presence of clinical atherosclerotic disease, including clinical CHD, cerebrovascular or peripheral arterial disease, or abdominal aortic aneurysm. A risk calculator can help the clinician determine a patient's 10-year risk for CHD based on these factors on a scale from lower risk to high risk. LDL treatment goals are determined based on the patient's risk level. When treatment with a statin drug is indicated, the 2013 guidelines from the American College of Cardiology and the American Heart Association (ACC/AHA) recommend that patients be given the maximum tolerated intensity of the statin. Similarly, in 2016, the European Society of Cardiology recommended that each patient undergo a risk assessment (systematic coronary risk evaluation, or SCORE) and lowering of LDL cholesterol levels to 100 mg/dL in high-risk patients and 70 mg/dL in very-high-risk patients. These groups no longer advocate treatment to a preset generalized goal but instead recognize that any reduction in LDL-C is beneficial, and that some patients should be treated more aggressively because of their higher cardiovascular risk.

Therapeutic lifestyle changes, including dietary modifications, weight management, and increased physical activity, should be initiated. A diet high in fruits, vegetables, fiber, omega-3 fatty acids, and foods with a low glycemic index, and substituting monounsaturated fats for polyunsaturated or trans fats, have repeatedly been shown to lower cardiovascular risk. If LDL goals are not achieved by lifestyle changes alone, drug therapy should be introduced and, if necessary, advanced. Current US and European guidelines strongly support the use of statin drugs as the primary intervention. Tables 4-2 and 4-3 present information about specific drugs, their lipid-lowering effects, and possible adverse effects.

Table 4-2 Drugs Affecting Lipoprotein Metabolism

Drug Class	Agents	Lipid/Lipoprotein Effects	Adverse Effects
HMG-CoA reductase inhibitors	Statins (see Table 4-3)	LDL ↓ 20%–60% HDL ↑ 5%–10% TG ↓ 10%–30%	Myopathy, increased levels of liver enzymes
Bile acid sequestrants	Cholestyramine Colestipol Colesevelam	LDL ↓ 15%–30% HDL ↑ 3%–5% TG no change or increase	GI distress, constipation, decreased absorption of other drugs
Nicotinic acid	Immediate-, extended-, or sustained-release nicotinic acid	LDL ↓ 10%–25% HDL ↑ 15%–35% TG ↓ 20%–30%	Flushing, hyperglycemia, hyperuricemia (gout), upper GI tract distress, hepatotoxicity
Fibric acids	Gemfibrozil Fenofibrate Clofibrate Bezafibrate Ciprofibrate	LDL ↓ 5%–20% (may be increased in patients with high TG) HDL ↑ 10%–20% TG ↓ 30%–50%	Dyspepsia, gallstones, myopathy; unexplained non-CHD deaths in WHO study
Cholesterol absorption inhibitor	Ezetimibe	LDL ↓ 14%–17% HDL ↑ 1% TG ↓7–8%	Myopathy, increased liver enzymes, possible increased cancer risk

CHD = coronary heart disease; GI = gastrointestinal; HDL = high-density lipoprotein; HMG-CoA = 3-hydroxy-3-methylglutaryl coenzyme A; LDL = low-density lipoprotein; TG = triglycerides; WHO = World Health Organization; ↓ = decrease; ↑ = increase.

Table 4-3 Intensity of Statin Therapy With Daily Dosing

High-intensity statin therapy (reduces LDL-C by ≥50%)	
Atorvastatin 40–80 mg	Rosuvastatin 20–40 mg
Moderate-intensity statin therapy (reduces LDL-C by 30%–50%)	
Atorvastatin 10–20 mg	Pitavastatin 2–4 mg
Fluvastatin 40 mg twice daily	Pravastatin 40–80 mg
Fluvastatin XL 80 mg	Rosuvastatin 5–10 mg
Lovastatin 40 mg	Simvastatin 20–40 mg

Modified with permission from Stone NJ, Robinson JG, Lichtenstein AH, et al. 2013 ACC/AHA guideline on the treatment of blood cholesterol to reduce atherosclerotic cardiovascular disease risk in adults: a report of the American College of Cardiology/American Heart Association Task Force on Practice Guidelines. *J Am Coll Cardiol.* 2014;63(25 Pt B):2889–2934.

Once the goal LDL levels have been achieved, other lipid and nonlipid risk factors can be modified. Elevated triglyceride levels may respond to increased physical activity or weight management, but if the triglyceride levels are greater than or equal to 200 mg/dL after the LDL goal is reached, a secondary treatment goal would be a non–HDL-C (total – HDL) level of 30 mg/dL higher than the LDL goal.

Eckel RH, Jakicic JM, Ard JD, et al; American College of Cardiology/American Heart Association Task Force on Practice Guidelines. 2013 AHA/ACC guideline on lifestyle management to reduce cardiovascular risk: a report of the American College of Cardiology/American Heart Association Task Force on Practice Guidelines. *Circulation.* 2014; 129(25 Suppl 2):S76–99.

Catapano AL, Graham I, De Backer G, et al. 2016 ESC/EAS guidelines for the management of dyslipidaemias. *Eur Heart J.* 2016; 37(39):2999–3058.

The Role of Statins

For virtually all patients whose LDL-C goals cannot be achieved by therapeutic lifestyle changes alone, 3-hydroxy-3-methylglutaryl coenzyme A (HMG-CoA) reductase inhibitors, more popularly known as *statins,* are the first choice for medical therapy. Multiple trials involving the use of statin drugs have reinforced the value of LDL-lowering therapy in reducing the risk of cardiometabolic disease. Moreover, the statins are the only class of oral drugs whose use has been shown to improve overall mortality in primary and secondary prevention. The Heart Protection Study, Myocardial Ischemia Reduction with Acute Cholesterol Lowering (MIRACL) study, and the PROVE IT study, among others, each demonstrated a decreased risk of major cardiovascular events in patients whose LDL-C levels had been lowered with statins. Findings from the Justification for the Use of Statins in Primary Prevention: An Intervention Trial Evaluating Rosuvastatin (JUPITER) suggest that statins—which are known to lower C-reactive protein levels in addition to having positive effects on hyperlipidemia—may decrease the risk of stroke, coronary artery disease, and death in apparently healthy persons without hyperlipidemia but with a C-reactive protein level greater than 2.0 mg/L. The beneficial effects of statins arise from the reduction of LDL-C levels, stabilization of atherosclerotic plaques, and decreased atherogenic inflammation.

The 2013 ACC/AHA guidelines identified 4 patient groups likely to benefit from statin use:

- individuals with clinical atherosclerotic cardiovascular disease (ASCVD)
- individuals with LDL-C levels of ≥190 mg/dL
- individuals aged 40–75 years with diabetes (but without ASCVD) and LDL-C levels of 70–189 mg/dL
- individuals aged 40–75 years without diabetes or ASCVD with LDL-C levels of 70–189 mg/dL and an estimated 10-year ASCVD risk of >7.5%.

In these patients, the ACC/AHA recommendation is moderate to maximal intensity statin therapy (see Table 4-3), while those intolerant of high-intensity therapy or those at lower estimated cardiovascular risk may be treated with moderate intensity therapy. Current ESC and other international guidelines are similar, and they also recommend assessment of the risk for each patient with LDL-C goals tailored to the patient's level of cardiovascular risk. Large studies have not established exact LDL-C goals, but many study authors recommend an LDL-C of less than 100 mg/dL for high-risk patients and less than 70 mg/dL in very-high-risk individuals.

Other drugs used to lower LDL-C levels (see Table 4-2) include nicotinic acid, bile acid sequestrants, fibric acids, and cholesterol absorption inhibitors. Although many of these drugs have been shown to lower LDL-C levels, there is a general lack of large randomized controlled trials demonstrating their effects on ASCVD or mortality. These drugs are often used worldwide; however, the most recent ACC/AHA and ESC guidelines do not support the use of these drugs in place of statins when statin therapy is effective and well tolerated. The role of these drugs when added to high-intensity statin treatment is still to be elucidated. A new class of injectable drugs consisting of monoclonal antibodies to proprotein convertase subtilisin kexin 9 (PCSK9-abs) shows promise in lowering LDL levels and reducing the risk of CV events, even when added to maximal statin therapy. Although the PCSK9-abs agents have been shown to reduce LDL-C levels by 60%–70%, their expense and delivery method (injection) have limited their outpatient use thus far.

Although statin drugs are largely safe and effective, patients taking them must be monitored for serious adverse effects, especially in the first few months of treatment. Adverse effects of statin use are rare but can include elevated hepatic transaminases, diarrhea, liver failure, polyneuropathy, and myopathy. Simvastatin should not be started at or increased to a dose of 80 mg per day because of the high risk of muscle injury. The risk of myopathy is also increased when simvastatin is used in conjunction with other medications, including amiodarone, some fibrates (gemfibrozil), and some calcium channel blockers. Cerivastatin was voluntarily withdrawn from the market after more than 52 reports of rhabdomyolysis and death related to its use. Pregnant women should not take statin drugs due to possible teratogenic effects.

Chou R, Dana T, Blazina I, Daeges M, Jeanne TL. Statins for prevention of cardiovascular disease in adults: evidence report and systematic review for the US Preventive Services Task Force. *JAMA.* 2016; 316(19):2008–2024.

ESC Clinical Practice Guidelines. European Society of Cardiology website. www.escardio.org/Guidelines/Clinical-Practice-Guidelines. Accessed September 10, 2021.

Stone NJ, Robinson JG, Lichtenstein AH, et al; American College of Cardiology/American Heart Association Task Force on Practice Guidelines. 2013 ACC/AHA guideline on the treatment of blood cholesterol to reduce atherosclerotic cardiovascular risk in adults: a report of the American College of Cardiology/American Heart Association Task Force on Practice Guidelines. *Circulation.* 2014; 129(25 Suppl 2):S1–S45.

Metabolic Syndrome

Metabolic syndrome comprises a constellation of lipid and nonlipid risk factors of metabolic origin. In 2006, the International Diabetes Federation developed a consensus definition for metabolic syndrome that includes central (abdominal) obesity (as measured by waist circumference), elevated triglyceride levels, high blood pressure, reduced HDL cholesterol, and elevated fasting blood glucose.

Metabolic syndrome is closely linked to insulin resistance. Excess body fat (particularly abdominal fat) and physical inactivity promote impaired responses to insulin; these impaired responses may also result from genetic predisposition. The risk factors for metabolic syndrome are highly concordant; in aggregate, they increase the risk of CHD at any given LDL level. Management of metabolic syndrome includes those measures previously discussed for elevated LDL and triglyceride levels, as well as treatment of hypertension and the use of aspirin to reduce the prothrombotic state in CHD patients. For further discussion of metabolic syndrome, please see Chapter 2.

Alberti KG, Eckel RH, Grundy SM, et al. Harmonizing the metabolic syndrome: a joint interim statement of the International Diabetes Federation Task Force on Epidemiology and Prevention; National Heart, Lung, and Blood Institute; American Heart Association; World Heart Federation; International Atherosclerosis Society; and International Association for the Study of Obesity. *Circulation.* 2009; 120(16):1640–1645.

The IDF consensus worldwide definition of the metabolic syndrome. International Diabetes Federation website. www.idf.org/e-library/consensus-statements/60-idfconsensus-worldwide-definitionof-the-metabolic-syndrome.html. Published 2006. Accessed September 10, 2021.

Ophthalmic considerations Hyperlipidemia is a significant risk factor for ischemic heart disease, cerebrovascular disease, and peripheral arterial disease. The ophthalmologist may be the first physician to detect or recognize manifestations of atherosclerosis, particularly transient monocular visual loss, retinal vascular emboli or occlusions, ischemic optic neuropathy, or cortical visual field deficits from a previous cerebral infarction. Detection of atherosclerosis may initiate a diagnostic evaluation that reveals significant carotid artery stenosis or coronary artery disease.

Corneal arcus, a nonreversible lipid deposit at the corneal limbus, is associated with age and hyperlipidemia. In the Blue Mountains Eye Study, the presence of arcus in persons aged 49 years and older was associated with higher total cholesterol and triglyceride levels.

The Action to Control Cardiovascular Risk in Diabetes (ACCORD) trial was designed to assess the effect of tight glycemic, dyslipidemic, and blood pressure control on cardiovascular events in patients with type 2 diabetes. A subset of these patients (ACCORD EYE) was examined to assess the effects of this control on the progression of diabetic retinopathy (DR). Previous studies had shown mixed results of the effect of tight glycemic control on DR. In the ACCORD EYE study, the tight control of glycemia resulted in a 33% reduction in the relative risk of progression of DR, although it did not decrease the risk of moderate vision loss. Treating patients with simvastatin plus fenofibrate for dyslipidemia control yielded a 40% reduction in the risk of DR progression. Tight blood pressure control did not appear to affect DR progression in ACCORD. Previous studies (eg, the Fenofibrate Intervention and Event Lowering in Diabetes [FIELD] study) have also suggested a possible protective effect of the use of fenofibrate on DR.

Statin use may also be associated with a reduction in intraocular pressure and potentially a protective effect against glaucoma. Additional clinical research is needed. Patients with ocular hypertension or glaucoma being treated with topical timolol have a small but statistically significant elevation of serum LDL and reduction in HDL, but do not appear to have increased mortality.

The relationship of statin use to age-related macular degeneration (AMD) is unresolved. Several population-based studies (Atherosclerosis Risk in Communities [ARIC], the Melbourne Collaborative Cohort Study, Blue Mountains Eye Study) have suggested that the use of statins is associated with a decreased risk of advanced AMD, whereas other studies (Beaver Dam, Age-Related Eye Disease Study 2 [AREDS2]) suggest there is no change in AMD risk with statin use. More data are required to assess the nature of this relationship.

The effect of statins on the development of cataracts is unclear. Although the Blue Mountains study suggested a protective effect, the AREDS2 study points to an increased risk of cataract development in patients taking a statin, particularly in women over age 75.

Al-Holou SN, Tucker WR, Agron E, et al; Age-Related Eye Disease Study 2 Research Group. The association of statin use with age-related macular degeneration progression: The Age-Related Eye Disease Study 2 Report Number 9. *Ophthalmol.* 2015; 122(12):2490–2496.

Al-Holou SN, Tucker WR, Agron E et al; Age-Related Eye Disease Study 2 Research Group. The association of statin use with cataract progression and cataract surgery: The AREDS2 Report Number 8. *Ophthalmol.* 2016; 123(4):916–917.

American Academy of Ophthalmology website; www.aao.org.

American Heart Association website; www.heart.org.

CardioSource. American College of Cardiology website; www.acc.org.

Chew EY, Ambrosius WT, Davis MD, et al; ACCORD Study group, ACCORD Eye Study group. Effects of medical therapies on retinopathy progression in type 2 diabetes. *N Engl J Med.* 2010; 363(3):233–244.

European Society of Cardiology website; www.escardio.org.

Talwar N, Musch DC, Stein JD. Association of daily dosage and type of statin agent with risk of open-angle glaucoma. *JAMA Ophthalmol.* 2017; 135(3):263–267.

Tan JS, Mitchell P, Rochtchina E, Wang JJ. Statin use and the long-term risk of incident cataract: The Blue Mountains Eye Study. *Am J Ophthalmol.* 2007;143(4):687–689.

CHAPTER 5

Acquired Heart Disease

Highlights

- Atherosclerotic *coronary heart disease (CHD)* remains by far the leading killer in the United States and around the world.
- Primary prevention of CHD at a public health level requires lifestyle changes, including reduced intake of saturated fat and cholesterol, increased physical activity, and weight control.
- Smoking remains the number-one preventable risk factor worldwide for *vascular disease*, which includes CHD, cerebrovascular disease, and peripheral vascular disease.
- Randomized trials suggest that, regardless of cholesterol level, any patient at significant risk for vascular events should be prescribed a statin.
- Primary *percutaneous coronary intervention (PCI)* performed by experienced operators is superior to thrombolysis for the treatment of acute myocardial infarction (MI).
- *Stenting* with either a bare-metal stent or a drug-eluting stent is useful for managing patients with acute MI and for preventing MI in selected patients. It requires a postprocedural period of dual antiplatelet therapy (DAT).
- Prophylactic *implantable cardioverter-defibrillators (ICDs)* are indicated for patients who have survived a cardiac arrest or an episode of hemodynamically unstable ventricular tachycardia. ICDs are also indicated for severe left ventricular dysfunction after MI.

Ischemic Heart Disease

Atherosclerotic CHD is by far the number-one killer not only in the United States but also in the world. In the United States, it is estimated that 1 person dies of CHD every minute. The number of women who die of CHD is 10 times that of women who die of breast cancer.

Pathophysiology

Abnormal cholesterol intake and metabolism leading to atherosclerosis are central factors in the development of ischemic heart disease (IHD). The "fatty streak," an early sign of atherosclerosis, is an accumulation of lipids and lipid-laden macrophages, called *foam cells*, under the endothelium of the coronary arteries. These cells organize into a plaque, and as the plaque becomes calcified, the lumen of the vessel narrows. The plaque can also become unstable and rupture, leading to turbulence and activation of the coagulation cascade and, ultimately, to intravascular thrombosis. The result is partial or complete vessel occlusion, which causes the symptoms of unstable angina or MI.

Ischemia is defined as local, temporary oxygen deprivation associated with inadequate removal of metabolites due to reduced tissue perfusion. IHD is typically caused by decreased perfusion of the myocardium secondary to stenotic or obstructed coronary arteries. The balance between arterial supply of and myocardial demand for oxygen determines whether ischemia occurs. Significant coronary stenosis, thrombosis, occlusion, reduced arterial pressure, hypoxemia, or severe anemia can impede the supply of oxygen to the myocardium. On the demand side, an increase in heart rate, ventricular contractility, or wall tension (which is determined by systolic arterial pressure, ventricular volume, and ventricular wall thickness) may increase utilization of oxygen. When the demand for oxygen exceeds the supply, ischemia occurs. If the ischemia is prolonged, infarction and myocardial necrosis result. The necrotic process begins in the subendocardium, usually after approximately 20 minutes of coronary obstruction, and progresses to transmural and complete infarction in 4–6 hours.

Risk Factors for Coronary Heart Disease

The majority of patients with CHD have identifiable risk factors. Epidemiologic studies have implicated a positive family history, male sex, lipid abnormalities, diabetes mellitus, hypertension, physical inactivity, short sleep duration, obesity, and smoking as risk factors. Many of these factors are modifiable; see Chapter 4 for a more detailed discussion on how to reduce risk. Markers of inflammation, particularly high-sensitivity C-reactive protein (CRP), may also represent strong risk factors for CHD.

CHD is the leading cause of death in women, accounting for one-third of all deaths, and kills more women than men each year. The average lifetime risk of CHD in women is very high, nearly 1 in 2. Compared with a man of the same age, a 50-year-old woman with a single additional risk factor has a substantially higher lifetime risk for CHD. Fortunately, most CHD risk in women is modifiable with the recommendations previously discussed; optimizing modifiable risk is of crucial importance in women.

In addition, postmenopausal women are disproportionately affected by a stress-induced cardiomyopathy called *takotsubo cardiomyopathy*, or broken-heart syndrome. This disorder may mimic an acute MI, but testing reveals no occlusive vascular disease. The etiology is unclear.

Clinical Syndromes

Clinical presentations of CHD include angina pectoris (ie, stable angina and variant, or Prinzmetal, angina), the acute coronary syndromes (ie, unstable angina, acute MI), congestive heart failure (CHF), sudden cardiac death, and asymptomatic CHD.

Angina pectoris

The cardinal symptom in patients with CHD is *angina pectoris*. It is usually manifested as precordial chest pain or tightness that is often triggered by physical exertion, emotional distress, or eating. Angina pectoris is usually due to atherosclerotic heart disease. Coronary vasospasm may occur at the site of a lesion or even in otherwise normal coronary arteries. Angina typically lasts 5–10 minutes and is usually relieved by rest, nitroglycerin, or both. Patients may present with pain radiating into other areas, including the jaw, arm, neck, shoulder, back, chest wall, or abdomen.

Often, angina is misinterpreted as indigestion or musculoskeletal pain. The level of physical activity that results in angina pectoris is clinically significant and is useful in determining the severity of CHD, as well as its treatment and prognosis. Because myocardial ischemia may be painless in diabetic patients and in women, the diagnosis is often delayed in these patients until the disease is more advanced. The pain associated with myocardial infarction is similar to that of angina but is usually more severe and more prolonged.

Stable angina pectoris Angina is considered stable if it responds to rest or nitroglycerin and if the patterns of frequency, ease of onset, duration, and response to medication have not changed substantially over 3 months.

Variant (Prinzmetal) angina Variant angina occurs at rest and is not related to physical exertion. The ST segment is elevated on electrocardiography during the anginal episodes, which are caused by coronary artery spasm. Underlying atherosclerosis is present in 60%–80% of cases, and thrombosis and occlusion may result during the episodes of coronary artery spasm.

Acute coronary syndrome

Acute coronary syndrome (ACS) comprises the spectrum of unstable cardiac ischemia, from unstable angina to acute MI. Plaque rupture is considered the common underlying event. Unstable angina and acute MI should be considered closely related events, clinically differentiated by the presence or absence of markers of myocardial injury. In 2007, a task force representing groups from the United States and Europe established a definition of MI; it includes the detection of cardiac biomarkers (eg, troponin), ischemia symptoms, electrocardiogram (ECG) changes indicating new ischemia, pathologic Q waves on ECG, and evidence of loss of viable myocardium or wall-motion abnormalities on imaging.

If an occlusive coronary thrombus persists, MI can result. The location and extent of the infarction depend on the anatomical distribution of the occluded vessel, the presence of additional stenotic lesions, and the adequacy of collateral circulation. If the patient has chest pain at rest, unstable angina is the diagnosis. If the ischemia is severe enough to cause myocardial necrosis, infarction results. *Acute MI* is further differentiated into *non–ST-segment elevation MI (NSTEMI)* and *ST-segment elevation MI (STEMI)*. Typical findings used to differentiate between these include the following:

- *Unstable angina (chest pain at rest).* The ECG shows ST-segment depression and/or T-wave inversion. No cardiac biomarkers are detected, indicating the absence of myocardial necrosis.
- *NSTEMI (subendocardial, nontransmural).* The ECG shows ST-segment depression and/or T-wave inversion. Cardiac biomarkers are present. The MI may be considered

incomplete; thus, patients may be more susceptible to reinfarction or extension. Aggressive workup and treatment are required to prevent progression to STEMI.

- *STEMI.* The ECG shows early ST-segment elevation (Figs 5-1, 5-2) and later Q waves. This condition involves full-thickness or nearly full-thickness necrosis of the ventricular wall. If the necrosis has not yet involved the full thickness of the ventricular wall, early reperfusion therapy is required to avoid progression to full-thickness necrosis.

Myocardial infarction may occur suddenly, without warning, in a previously asymptomatic patient or in a patient with stable or variant angina; MI may also follow a period of unstable angina. Patients commonly experience chest pain, nausea, vomiting, diaphoresis, weakness, anxiety, dyspnea, lightheadedness, and palpitations. However, nearly 25% of myocardial infarcts are painless. Symptoms may begin during or after exertion or at rest.

The clinical findings in MI vary and depend on the location and severity of the ischemia or injury. Approximately half of all infarctions involve the inferior myocardial wall, and most of the remaining half involve the anterior regions. Examination may reveal pallor, coolness of the extremities, low-grade fever, signs of pulmonary congestion and increased central venous pressure (if left ventricular dysfunction is present), an S_3 or S_4 gallop, an apical systolic murmur (caused by papillary muscle dysfunction), hypertension, or hypotension. The ECG may demonstrate a variety of ST-segment and T-wave changes and arrhythmias.

Approximately 60% of patients who die of cardiac disease die suddenly, before reaching the hospital. However, the prognosis for patients hospitalized with MI has become

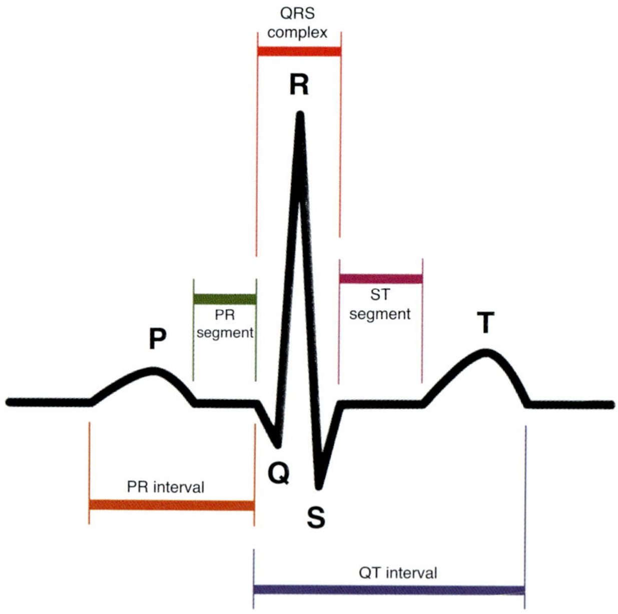

Figure 5-1 Nomenclature of the deflections, intervals, and segments of the normal electrocardiogram (ECG). *(Courtesy of Petr Heřman.)*

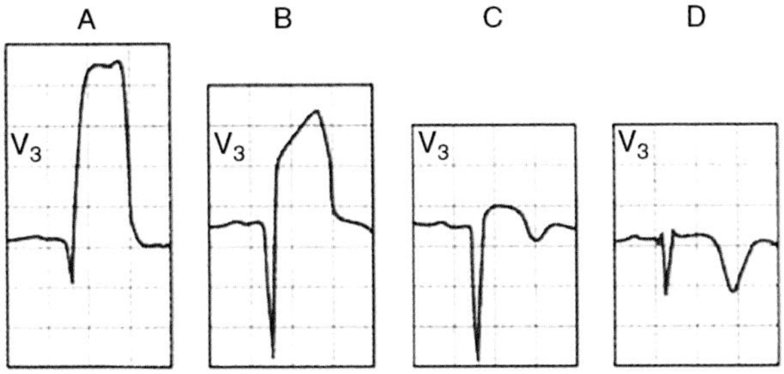

Figure 5-2 ST segment and T-wave abnormalities. The changes in an ECG during myocardial infarction (ie, ST elevation, QRS reduction, and inverted T waves) occur in specific leads that determine its site. In the meantime, reciprocal changes can be observed in the opposite site. *(Reproduced with permission from Fuster V, Walsh RA, Harrington RA, eds.* Hurst's The Heart. *13th ed. New York: McGraw-Hill; 2011.)*

remarkably good. Some studies in which thrombolytic therapy or PCI was used reported a mortality rate in the range of 5%–8%. Mortality is affected by a wide variety of factors, such as the degree of heart failure, extent of myocardial damage, severity of the underlying atherosclerotic process, heart size, and previous ischemia.

Immediate coronary angiography and primary PCI (including stenting) of the infarct-involved artery have been shown to be superior to thrombolysis when done promptly by experienced operators in high-volume centers. If the time from first medical contact to intervention ("door to balloon" time) is kept under 90 minutes, the outcome is improved and is superior to that of thrombolysis. This intervention, in conjunction with antiplatelet and anticoagulant therapy, is widely used in patients with acute MI.

The complications of MI depend on its severity and may include CHF (see the section Congestive Heart Failure), rupture of the ventricular wall, pericarditis, and arrhythmias. Regional and global ventricular contractile dysfunction may result in CHF or pulmonary edema. Mild to moderate heart failure occurs in nearly 50% of patients following MI. Some patients experience post-MI pericarditis, characterized by a pericardial friction rub 2–3 days after infarction. Injury along the conduction pathways of the atria or ventricles may lead to bradycardia, heart block, supraventricular tachycardias, or ventricular arrhythmias. Arrhythmias often exacerbate ischemic injury by reducing the perfusion pressure in the coronary arteries. Most acute deaths from MI are caused by arrhythmia.

Thygesen K, Alpert JS, Jaffe AS, et al; Executive Group on behalf of the Joint European Society of Cardiology (ESC)/American College of Cardiology (ACC)/American Heart Association (AHA)/World Heart Federation (WHF) Task Force for the Universal Definition of Myocardial Infarction. Fourth universal definition of myocardial infarction (2018). *J Am Coll Cardiol.* 2018;72(18):2231–2264.

Sudden cardiac death

Sudden cardiac death (SCD) is defined as unexpected, nontraumatic death that occurs within 1 hour after onset of symptoms in clinically stable individuals. A disproportionate number of SCDs take place in the early morning hours. SCD is usually caused by a severe arrhythmia, such as ventricular tachycardia, ventricular fibrillation, profound bradycardia, or asystole. SCD may result from MI, occur during an episode of angina, or strike without warning in a patient with frequent arrhythmias secondary to underlying IHD or ventricular dysfunction. Other causes of SCD are Wolff-Parkinson-White syndrome, long QT syndrome, torsades de pointes, atrioventricular block, aortic stenosis, myocarditis, cardiomyopathy, ruptured or dissecting aortic aneurysm, and pulmonary embolism. An implantable cardioverter-defibrillator (ICD) is recommended for patients who have survived a cardiac arrest or an episode of hemodynamically unstable ventricular tachycardia and for patients with severe left ventricular dysfunction after MI.

Asymptomatic ischemic heart disease

Asymptomatic patients with CHD are at particular risk for unexpected MI, life-threatening arrhythmias, and SCD. Advanced CHD may develop in these patients, and they may experience multiple infarcts before the correct diagnosis is made and appropriate treatment is initiated. Older adults, women, and individuals with diabetes mellitus are more likely to have painless ischemia. Approximately 25% of MIs are asymptomatic, but they may be detected on a subsequent ECG. A patient who has unexplained dyspnea, weakness, arrhythmias, or poor exercise tolerance requires cardiac testing to evaluate for the presence of undiagnosed CHD.

Noninvasive Cardiac Diagnostic Procedures

Noninvasive diagnostic testing for patients with CHD includes electrocardiography, serum biomarker measurements, echocardiography, various types of stress testing, and imaging studies. Assessment of cardiac risk using various measures (see Chapter 4 in this volume) will identify those patients most likely to benefit from testing.

Electrocardiography

The ECG may appear normal between episodes of ischemia in patients with angina. During angina, the ST segments often become elevated or depressed by up to 5 mm. T waves may be inverted, they may become tall and peaked, or inverted T waves may normalize. These ECG findings, when associated with characteristic anginal pain, are virtually diagnostic of IHD. However, absence of ECG changes does not definitively exclude myocardial ischemia.

During myocardial infarction, QT-interval prolongation and peaked T waves may appear. The ST segments may be depressed or elevated (see Fig 5-2). ST-segment elevation may persist for several days to weeks before returning to normal. T-wave inversion appears in the leads corresponding to the site of the infarct. Q waves or a reduction in the QRS amplitude appears with the onset of myocardial necrosis. Q waves are typically absent in a subendocardial (nontransmural) infarction. Tachycardia and ventricular arrhythmias are most common within the first few hours after the onset of infarction. Bradyarrhythmias, such as heart block, are more common with inferior infarction; ventricular tachycardia and fibrillation are more common with anteroseptal infarction.

Serum biomarker testing

Cardiac enzymes are released into the bloodstream when myocardial necrosis occurs and, therefore, are valuable in differentiating MI from unstable angina and noncardiac causes of chest pain. With the advent of assays for cardiac-specific troponins, serum biomarker testing has also proved useful in identifying patients with ACS who are at greatest risk for adverse outcomes.

Cardiac-specific troponins are accepted as the most sensitive and specific biochemical cardiac markers in ACS. Cardiac isoforms of troponins (troponins T and I) are important regulatory elements in myocardial cells and, unlike creatine kinase MB (CK-MB), are not normally present in the serum of healthy individuals. Moreover, unlike CK-MB levels, troponin levels are not elevated in patients with skeletal muscle injury. Troponins T and I have been shown to be more cardiac-specific and cardiac-sensitive than CK-MB, allowing for more accurate diagnosis of cardiac injury. Troponin levels remain elevated from 3 hours to 14 days after MI. Mildly elevated troponin levels may be found in patients with NSTEMI who otherwise would be considered to have unstable angina. Troponin levels are elevated after MI, but they may also be elevated in patients with myocarditis, stress cardiomyopathy, and chronic kidney disease.

In addition to being diagnostically valuable, troponin levels provide prognostic information. Patients with an ACS who present with elevated troponin levels have an increased risk of CHF, cardiogenic shock, death, recurrent nonfatal infarction, and need for revascularization with PCI or coronary artery bypass grafting (CABG, discussed later in this chapter). Finally, a quantitative relationship has been demonstrated between the peak amount of troponin measured and the risk of death in patients who present with ACS. Patients who are at greatest risk for adverse outcomes can be identified in the emergency department, allowing for more appropriate medical decisions and therapeutic triage.

Serum myoglobin is the first marker to rise following myocardial damage, and levels can be elevated between 1 and 20 hours after infarction. Although myoglobin might appear to be ideal for early detection of MI, its performance is not consistent and its specificity for cardiac events is poor. The cardiac-specific troponins remain the optimal biomarker test in the setting of ACS.

Echocardiography

Echocardiography employs 1- and 2-dimensional ultrasound and color flow Doppler techniques to image the ventricles and atria, the heart valves, left ventricular contraction and wall-motion abnormalities, left ventricular ejection fraction, and the pericardium. Patients with IHD, particularly following infarction, commonly have regional wall-motion abnormalities that correspond to the areas of myocardial injury. Other, less frequent complications of infarction, such as mitral regurgitation from papillary muscle injury, ventricular septal defect, ventricular aneurysm, ventricular thrombus, and pericardial effusion, can also be detected with echocardiography. Color flow Doppler imaging provides information on the flow of blood across abnormal valves, pressure differences within the chambers, intracardiac shunts, and cardiac output. However, cardiac biomarkers are far more sensitive and specific than echocardiography in detecting cardiac injury.

Stress echocardiography (exercise echocardiography) is useful for imaging cardiac-valve and wall-motion abnormalities and ventricular dysfunction induced by ischemia during exercise or after pharmacologic challenge. Predischarge exercise stress echocardiography provides useful prognostic information following acute MI.

Exercise stress testing

Patients with angina may have normal findings on clinical examination, electrocardiography, and echocardiography between episodes of ischemia. Standardized exercise tests have been developed to induce myocardial ischemia under controlled conditions. The ECG, heart rate, blood pressure, and general physical status of the patient are monitored during the procedure. The endpoint in angina patients is a symptom or sign of cardiac ischemia, such as chest pain, dyspnea, ST-segment depression, arrhythmia, or hypotension. A modified exercise stress test can also be performed in patients with a recent MI to help determine functional status and prognosis. Stress testing is useful both in establishing the diagnosis of ischemic heart disease and in assessing its severity.

Radionuclide scintigraphy and scans

Radionuclide techniques can be used to increase the sensitivity of exercise testing. Left ventricular dysfunction can result from necrotic tissue, myocardial hibernation after injury, or myocardial stunning. Approximately 20%–40% of patients with left ventricular dysfunction on echo or stress testing still have viable myocardial tissue, which may improve with reperfusion. Several agents are available for injection during testing, including thallium-201, technetium-99m (Tc99m) sestamibi, and technetium-99m tetrofosmin.

Thallium accumulates in healthy myocardium and reveals a perfusion defect in areas of myocardial ischemia. Thallium scans have a high sensitivity and specificity for CHD. Reversible thallium or Tc99m sestamibi defects are those that are present during exercise but resolve during rest. This correlates with myocardial ischemia. In contrast, a fixed thallium or Tc99m defect is present during both exercise and rest and represents a region of prior infarction or nonviable tissue. For patients unable to exercise vigorously enough to reach the required heart rates during the exercise stress test, a thallium scan or echocardiogram in conjunction with a pharmacologic stress test may provide information similar to that of an exercise examination. Tomographic imaging of myocardial perfusion is possible with thallium-201 or Tc99m via a technique called *single-photon emission computed tomography (SPECT),* which provides better imaging of infarcts, enhanced detection of multivessel disease, and fewer artifacts.

Other imaging technologies that may add clinically useful information include the following:

- *Positron emission tomography,* which differentiates metabolically active myocardium from scar tissue.
- *Coronary CT angiography,* which is useful in evaluating occlusive vascular disease and ruling out atherosclerotic disease.
- *Electron beam CT;* this quantifies coronary artery calcification, which correlates with atherosclerosis and is highly sensitive but not specific. It may be an alternative to angiography in some patients.
- *Cardiac MRI,* which provides excellent imaging, and perfusion testing with gadolinium. MRI may be contraindicated in some patients with ICDs or pacemakers, but it can be safely used in the presence of coronary stents. Cardiac CT and MRI are also useful in assessing congenital or acquired coronary abnormalities.

Invasive Cardiac Diagnostic Procedures

Coronary arteriography and *ventriculography* provide valuable information about the presence and severity of CHD and about ventricular function. These techniques can indicate the specific areas of coronary artery stenosis or occlusion, the number of involved vessels, the ventricular systolic and diastolic volumes, the ejection fraction, and regional wall-motion abnormalities. *Multiple gated acquisition (MUGA)* scans can also be performed for these purposes. This information helps the cardiologist and cardiac surgeon plan appropriate treatment for the patient. *Intravascular ultrasound imaging* is an evolving invasive modality for studying the intraluminal coronary anatomy and may be particularly useful in evaluating the effects of stents or angioplasty.

Coronary artery stenosis is hemodynamically significant when the arterial lumen diameter is narrowed by more than 50%, or the cross-sectional area is reduced by more than 75%. Common indications for coronary arteriography are ACS, post-MI angina, stable angina unresponsive to medical therapy or revascularization, a markedly positive exercise stress test result, and a recent MI in a patient younger than 40 years. The technique may also be useful in evaluating valvular heart disease, ventricular septal defect, papillary muscle dysfunction, cardiomyopathy of unknown cause, or unexplained ventricular arrhythmias.

Management of Ischemic Heart Disease

The goals of disease management for the patient with CHD are to reduce the frequency of or eliminate angina, prevent myocardial damage, and prolong life. The first line of attack should include eliminating or reducing risk factors for atherosclerosis. Smoking cessation, dietary modification, weight loss, exercise, and improved control of diabetes mellitus and hypertension are critical steps. Fraker and colleagues have reported regression of atherosclerotic lesions following intensive lipid-lowering therapy; and, unless contraindicated, statins are recommended for all CHD patients. Antiplatelet therapy with low-dose daily aspirin has also been advocated for all patients with CHD because it significantly reduces the risk of MI.

Aspirin appears to offer equal benefit to women and men in reducing primary MI risk, and it is also useful in secondary prevention. Aspirin may also help protect against stroke; however, in low-risk patients, the risk of bleeding complications may outweigh the benefits. Aspirin use should be guided by an assessment of the patient's risk of stroke or MI. Hormone therapy, antioxidant vitamin supplementation, and folic acid therapy do not appear to provide any benefit in preventing CVD.

Antithrombotic agents

Prevention of stroke, heart attack, and numerous other thromboembolic diseases requires selective inhibition of the hemostasis process. Numerous products have been developed to inhibit platelet aggregation or block specific steps in the coagulation cascade (Fig 5-3), including several oral agents, which are frequently used in the outpatient setting (Table 5-1). Those drugs requiring intravenous or subcutaneous injection are predominantly used in an inpatient setting (Table 5-2).

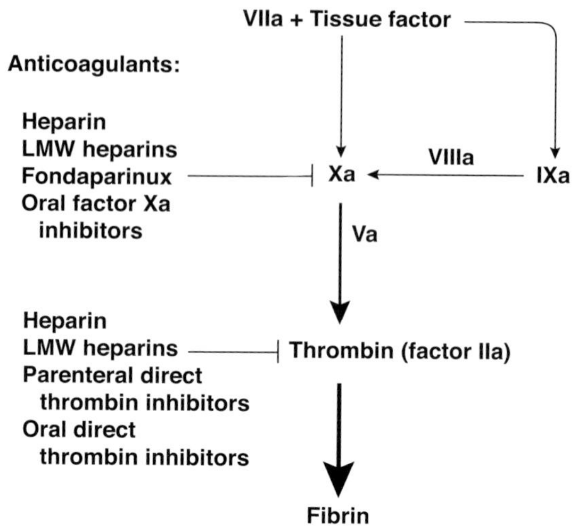

Figure 5-3 Coagulation cascade. The various anticoagulant drugs interrupt the cascade at different points in the process. *(Reproduced with permission from Leung LLK. Direct oral anticoagulants and parenteral direct thrombin inhibitors: dosing and adverse effects. In:* UpToDate, *Mannucci PM, Tirnauer JS [eds]. Available at www.uptodate.com. Accessed August 15, 2018.)*

Table 5-1 Direct Oral Antithrombotic Agents

Class	Drug (trade name)	Mechanism of Action
Antiplatelet agents	Aspirin	Blocks cyclo-oxygenase and inhibits platelet aggregation
Antiplatelet agents (P2Y12 receptor blockers)	Cangrelor (Kengreal) Clopidogrel (Plavix) Prasugrel (Effient) Ticagrelor (Brilinta) Ticlopidine (not available in US)	Prevent activation of glycoprotein IIb/IIIa and inhibit platelet aggregation
Vitamin K antagonists	Coumarins (not available in US) including acenocoumarol, phenprocoumon, fluindione Warfarin (Coumadin)	Reduce the synthesis of numerous clotting factors that require vitamin K
Direct thrombin inhibitors	Dabigatran (Pradaxa)	Prevent thrombin from cleaving fibrinogen to fibrin; can be reversed with idarucixumab (Praxbind)
Factor Xa inhibitors (Note: all drugs in this class end in "-xaban")	Apixaban (Eliquis) Betrixaban (Bevyxxa) Edoxaban (Lixiana, Savaysa) Rivaroxaban (Xarelto)	Prevent factor Xa from cleaving prothrombin to thrombin; rivavoxaban and apixaban can be reversed with andexanet alfa (Andexxa)

Table 5-2 Intravenous and Subcutaneous Antithrombotic Agents

Class	Drug (Trade Name)	Mechanism of Action
Heparin and low-molecular-weight heparins	Dalteparin (Fragmin) Enoxaparin (Lovenox) Fondaparinux (Arixtra) Heparin Nadroparin (Fraxiparine) Tinzaparin (Innohep)	Inactivate thrombin and factor Xa by enhancing activity of serum antithrombin; fondaparinux is a synthetic pentasaccharide with a similar mechanism of action
Direct thrombin inhibitors	Argatroban (Acova) Bivalirudin (Angiomax) Desirudin (Iprivasc)	Prevent thrombin from cleaving fibrinogen to fibrin
Glycoprotein IIb/IIIa inhibitors	Abciximab (ReoPro) Eptifibatide (Integrelin) Tirofiban (Aggrastat)	Prevent platelet aggregation by blocking fibrinogen binding to platelets

Treatment of stable angina pectoris

Medical management of angina pectoris is designed to deliver as much oxygen as possible to the potentially ischemic myocardium, to decrease the oxygen demand to a level at which symptoms are eliminated or reduced to a comfortable level, or both.

Therapeutic agents include the following:

- *β-Adrenergic blockers.* Also called *β-blockers,* these drugs represent the first line of treatment. They reduce heart rate and contractility (decreasing oxygen demand) and are demonstrated to prolong life in CHD patients. They should be avoided in patients with Prinzmetal angina.
- *Slow calcium channel blockers.* These agents, including diltiazem, verapamil, and amlodipine, are useful for long-term angina treatment. They should be used with caution in patients with left ventricular dysfunction.
- *Nitrates and nitroglycerin.* These agents increase oxygen delivery through coronary vasodilation. Systemic effects (eg, venous dilation, reduction in blood pressure) decrease oxygen demand. They should be used with caution in patients taking erectile dysfunction drugs.
- *Aspirin with or without clopidogrel, prasugrel, or ticagrelor.* These drugs can be used for anticoagulation. The regimen of aspirin plus 1 of these other drugs is called *dual antiplatelet therapy (DAT).*
- *Statins. Statins* are recommended for use in virtually all ACS patients, regardless of serum lipid levels, if not contraindicated.

Improving the oxygen-carrying capacity of the blood by treating anemia or coexisting pulmonary disease provides some additional benefit. Patients in whom medical therapy is unsuccessful may be candidates for revascularization procedures.

Revascularization Procedures for revascularization include *percutaneous coronary intervention (PCI)* with or without stenting or *coronary artery bypass grafting (CABG).* These approaches may improve coronary blood flow, control angina, and increase exercise tolerance. In high-risk patients, the risk of infarction is reduced, and long-term survival is enhanced. Revascularization is indicated in otherwise healthy patients with advanced left main coronary artery disease, left ventricular dysfunction with 3-vessel disease, or angina that is not adequately controlled with medical treatment. Either PCI or CABG is effective for relieving angina; however, CABG is superior to PCI in terms of survival for some patients who have significant areas of at-risk myocardium or substantial left ventricular dysfunction. Recently, some authors have questioned whether PCI is superior to maximal medical therapy in the treatment of stable angina.

PCI was developed as an alternative to surgical revascularization. One PCI technique, *angioplasty,* involves passing a balloon catheter into a stenosed vessel and inflating the balloon at the site of the narrowing to widen the lumen. Although 85%–90% of vessels can be opened with PCI, the rate of restenosis is approximately 25%–40% at 6 months. The insertion of a wire-mesh *stent* at the time of PCI improves patency and reduces the risk of restenosis by nearly 50%. Drug-eluting stents are superior to bare-metal stents in preventing restenosis but are also more likely to lead to late stent thrombosis. Stent thrombosis may result in MI or death, so patients receiving stents should be given aggressive anticoagulation at the time of placement. European and US guidelines for anticoagulant use during stent placement are similar. DAT (aspirin plus clopidogrel, prasugrel, or ticagrelor) should continue for at least 1 month after stenting for a bare-metal stent and 6–12 months for a drug-eluting stent. DAT should not be stopped during this period, and elective surgery should be postponed unless the patient is able to continue on DAT. Patients intolerant of aspirin may use clopidogrel alone.

When angioplasty is inappropriate or ineffective and medical therapy has failed to control symptoms in patients with severe multivessel disease, CABG may be considered. CABG may be indicated in patients with high-risk disease, including those with significant left main, proximal left anterior descending, or 3-vessel disease, especially if accompanied by left ventricular dysfunction. During CABG, a shunt is installed from the aorta to the diseased coronary artery to bypass the area of obstruction and increase blood flow. CABG has been shown to increase left ventricular function, improve quality of life, relieve angina, and, often, reduce the risk of infarction and cardiac death. Some patients now receive "off-pump bypass surgery," in which the grafts are sewn onto the beating heart. This technique decreases the risk of adverse effects of cardiopulmonary bypass, which include memory, cognitive, and other neurologic deficits.

PCI and CABG have similar mortality rates; but patients undergoing PCI are more likely to require a second procedure, and CABG has better long-term survival outcomes than PCI in most studies.

Although revascularization may produce good outcomes, the underlying disease process requires ongoing management. The Bypass Angioplasty Revascularization Investigation demonstrated that even after PCI or CABG, arterial disease will continue to progress unless cardiac risk factors are reduced. Optimal medical management is also required.

Al-Lamee R, Thompson D, Dehbi H-M, et al. Percutaneous coronary intervention in stable angina (ORBITA): a double-blind, randomised controlled trial. *Lancet.* 2018;391(10115):31–40.

Fihn SD, Blankenship JC, Alexander KP, et al. 2014 ACC/AHA/AATS/PCNA/SCAI/STS focused update of the guideline for the diagnosis and management of patients with stable ischemic heart disease. *J Am Coll Cardiol.* 2014;64(18):1929–1949.

Task Force members; Montalescot G, Sechtem U, Achenback S, et al. 2013 ESC guidelines on the management of stable coronary artery disease. *Eur Heart J.* 2013;34(38):2949–3003.

Thygesen K, Alpert JS, White HD; Joint ESC/ACCF/AHA/WHF Task Force for the Redefinition of Myocardial Infarction. Universal definition of myocardial infarction. *Circulation.* 2007;116(22):2634–2653.

Treatment of acute coronary syndromes

Patients with an ACS are admitted to a hospital or a chest pain observation unit for monitoring and treatment. They are initially treated aggressively with anti-ischemic pharmacotherapy. Once these initial measures are instituted, further management and triage of patients with an ACS are based on the presence or absence of ST-segment elevation. Patients with ST-segment elevation undergo reperfusion therapy with thrombolysis, CABG, or catheter-based interventions; patients with non–ST-segment elevation may be managed with medical treatment alone or a more aggressive interventional approach. The use of a risk calculator (eg, TIMI, GRACE, PURSUIT) may help identify high-risk patients and determine subsequent management; the TIMI and GRACE risk calculators are available at www.timi.org/calculators and www.mdcalc.com/grace-acs-risk-mortality-calculator, respectively.

Management of non–ST-segment elevation ACS During the initial evaluation, before biomarker results are available, unstable angina and NSTEMI may be indistinguishable and, if so, are treated the same way. In general, myocardial oxygen demands are managed with medications and supplemental oxygen. β-Blocker therapy, which reduces myocardial oxygen demands and improves survival, should be considered for all patients with evolving MI in the absence of contraindications. Medical therapy for NSTEMI includes

- β-blockers in nearly all patients (avoid in cases of cocaine-associated MI or if patient is already hemodynamically compromised)
- nitrates and/or nitroglycerin
- DAT
- anticoagulant therapy (heparins, factor Xa, and direct thrombin inhibitors)
- statins, regardless of serum lipid levels, if not contraindicated
- possible use of angiotensin-converting enzyme (ACE) inhibitors (eg, captopril, enalapril, lisinopril, ramipril)

CHF and pulmonary edema should be treated if present. If β-blockers cannot be used, the clinician may consider verapamil or diltiazem. ACE inhibitors decrease the risk of death if given within 24 hours of MI, but they should be avoided in patients with hypotension or renal insufficiency.

Anticoagulant therapy is beneficial in ACS. It involves a variety of agents, including unfractionated heparin; low-molecular-weight heparins; direct thrombin inhibitors; and factor Xa inhibitors (see Table 5-1). Choice of the optimal regimen depends on what other medications are being used and whether the treatment strategy is conservative or interventional. Glycoprotein IIb/IIIa inhibitors are of limited use in patients with NSTEMI, although they may be tried if other agents have failed to provide sufficient anticoagulation.

Once unstable angina and NSTEMI have been managed as described, patients may be treated with either a conservative noninvasive approach or an early invasive (angiographic) strategy, depending on their level of risk for adverse outcomes. Controlled trials have shown the superiority of an invasive approach in managing ACS patients, particularly those who have refractory angina, hemodynamic instability, or elevated risk as measured by bedside risk stratification tools (eg, TIMI, GRACE). The decision to proceed from diagnostic angiography to revascularization (PCI or CABG) is influenced not only by the coronary anatomy but also by several other factors, including anticipated life expectancy, ventricular function, comorbidity, functional capacity, severity of symptoms, and quantity of viable myocardium at risk. Fibrinolysis should *not* be performed on patients with unstable angina or NSTEMI.

Management of ST-segment elevation ACS Current therapy for evolving Q-wave MI involves rapid and effective reperfusion because necrosis is a time-dependent process. Optimal myocardial salvage requires nearly complete reperfusion as soon as possible: reperfusion within 1 hour of symptom onset yields maximal benefit. The benefit of reperfusion therapy 12 hours after symptom onset has not been established.

Methods of reperfusion include thrombolysis and catheter-based PCIs (balloon angioplasty with or without stent placement). Numerous clinical trials have shown the superiority of early PCI over thrombolysis, particularly if performed in the first 90 minutes following medical contact. Hospitals without PCI capability should transfer the patient to a facility that can perform PCI if the procedure can be done within 120 minutes after first medical contact. Otherwise, thrombolytic therapy should be started within 30 minutes of first medical contact. PCI following full-dose thrombolytics carries significant risks but may be done in high-risk patients or if thrombolytic therapy has failed ("rescue PCI"). Totally occluded arteries generally do not benefit from PCI.

CABG may be considered if PCI or fibrinolysis fails, but the potential benefits must be weighed against an increased mortality risk in the first 3–7 days after STEMI.

Initial medical management before and after reperfusion therapy should include aspirin, clopidogrel, morphine (for pain), nitrates, statins, and β-blockers if there are no contraindications. Except for aspirin, nonsteroidal agents should not be used acutely or during hospitalization, because they increase the risk of CHF and death. Other adjuncts to therapy may include low-molecular-weight heparins and glycoprotein IIb/IIIa inhibitors, particularly if PCI is anticipated.

Thrombolysis Patients with a STEMI who are treated with thrombolytics in the first 3 hours show a 50% reduction in mortality; those treated at 12 hours show a 10% reduction. Thrombolytic agents lyse coronary thrombi and restore coronary blood flow in most patients. *Tissue plasminogen activators (tPAs)* are the most commonly used thrombolytics; they are more effective than streptokinase in opening arteries and reducing mortality. When any tPA is used, aspirin and intravenous unfractionated heparin should be administered concurrently.

Major bleeding complications occur in up to 5% of patients undergoing thrombolytic therapy. Contraindications to thrombolysis include known sites of potential bleeding, a history of cerebrovascular accident, recent surgery, and prolonged cardiopulmonary resuscitation efforts. Thrombolysis should *not* be used in the treatment of NSTEMI due to decreased benefits and, possibly, increased hemorrhagic risks.

Ibanez B, James S, Agewall S, et al; ESC Scientific Document Group. 2017 ESC guidelines for the management of acute myocardial infarction in patients presenting with ST-segment elevation: the Task Force for the management of acute myocardial infarction in patients presenting with ST-segment elevation of the European Society of Cardiology (ESC). *Eur Heart J.* 2018;39(2):119–177.

O'Gara PT, Kushner FG, Ascheim DD, et al. 2013 ACCF/AHA guideline for the management of ST-elevation myocardial infarction. *Circulation.* 2013;127(4):e362–e425.

Congestive Heart Failure

The epidemiologic magnitude of CHF is staggering. Approximately 5 million patients in the United States have CHF, and there are 500,000 new cases per year. It is estimated that CHF will develop in 20% of the population older than 40 years. Many patients who consult an ophthalmologist belong to the older age group that is particularly prone to this condition. Heart failure occurs when the heart cannot meet the metabolic demands of the tissues. The cardiac pump itself may be failing, or it may be nearly normal but unable to keep up with demand. The direct result of heart failure is circulatory failure.

Classification

Heart failure is classified into 4 stages, including stages for patients at risk for heart failure and those without current signs or symptoms (Fig 5-4). Symptomatic heart failure is subdivided according to *ejection fraction (EF),* which is the calculated proportion of blood ejected by the ventricle during a single or average contraction. The EF is more than 50% in an average person without HF. A left ventricular EF less than or equal to 40% is classified as *heart failure with a reduced ejection fraction (HFrEF),* and a patient in heart failure with an EF greater than 50% is classified as *heart failure with a preserved ejection fraction (HFpEF).* HFrEF is sometimes called left-sided, or systolic heart, failure, and HFpEF as right-sided, or diastolic, heart failure. Approximately two-thirds of all CHF is HFrEF, but HFpEF is more common in women.

Symptoms

Although heart failure may be asymptomatic in its earliest stages, a variety of symptoms may develop, depending on the severity of ventricular dysfunction. Symptoms may result from inadequate tissue perfusion caused by pump failure or from the failing heart's inability to empty adequately, leading to edema and fluid accumulation in the lungs, extremities, and other sites. The most frequent symptoms of left ventricular failure are dyspnea with exertion or at rest, orthopnea, paroxysmal nocturnal dyspnea, diaphoresis, generalized weakness, fatigue, anxiety, and lightheadedness. With more severe CHF, the patient may also experience a productive cough; copious pink, frothy sputum; and confusion. Angina may also occur if the CHF results from ischemia. Right-sided heart failure may

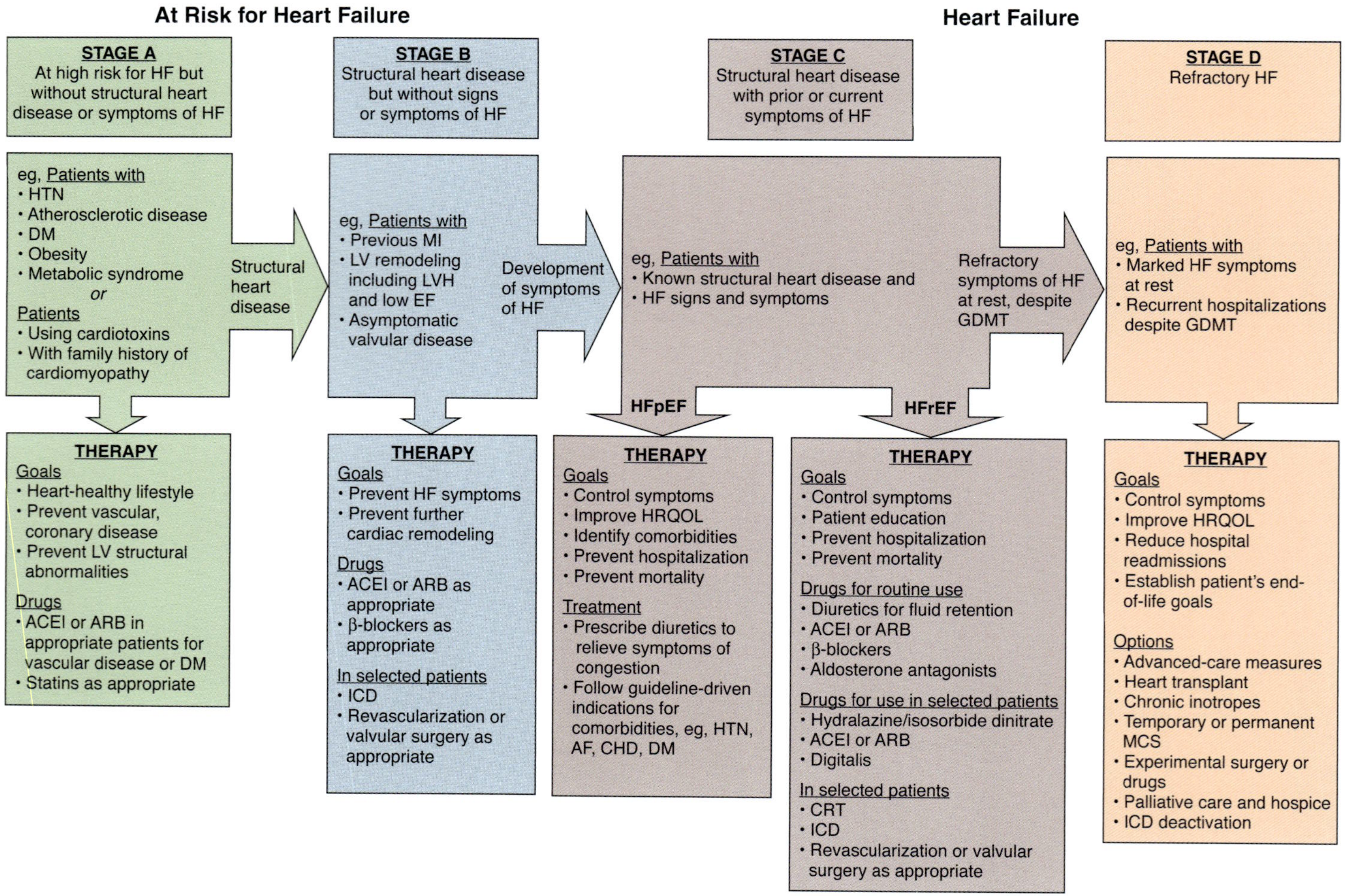

Figure 5-4 Stages in the development of heart failure. ACEI = ACE inhibitors; AF = atrial fibrillation; ARB = angiotensin II receptor blocker; CHD = coronary heart disease; CRT = cardiac resynchronization therapy; DM = diabetes mellitus; EF = ejection fraction; GDMT = guideline-directed medical therapy; HF = heart failure; HFpEF = heart failure with preserved ejection fraction; HFrEF = heart failure with reduced ejection fraction; HRQOL = health-related quality of life; HTN = hypertension; ICD = implantable cardioverter-defibrillator; LV = left ventricular; LVH = left ventricular hypertrophy; MCS = mechanical circulatory support; MI = myocardial infarction. *(Modified with permission from Yancy CW, Jessup M, Bozkurt B, et al. 2013 ACCF/AHA guideline for the management of heart failure: executive summary: a report of the American College of Cardiology Foundation/American Heart Association Task Force on Practice Guidelines.* Circulation. *2013;128[16]:1810–1852.)*

occur separately from or secondary to chronic left-sided heart failure. Peripheral edema typically develops in patients with right-sided heart failure.

Clinical Signs

Examination findings in acute left ventricular failure may include respiratory distress, use of the respiratory accessory muscles, pinkish sputum or frank hemoptysis, coarse rales on pulmonary auscultation, expiratory wheezes, a rapid heart rate, an S gallop, diaphoresis, and deterioration in mental status. Blood pressure is often markedly elevated but may be reduced during MI. Long-standing cases of CHF show signs of right ventricular failure, especially elevated central venous pressure, pedal edema, hepatomegaly, and cyanosis. In some patients, pleural effusion or ascites may be detected.

Diagnostic Evaluation

The history and clinical examination are the most important components in the diagnosis of CHF. Diagnostic studies that are helpful in evaluating CHF and its underlying causes include echocardiography, chest radiography, electrocardiography, blood gas analysis, complete blood counts, serum electrolyte tests, blood urea nitrogen and creatinine tests, liver function tests, and urinalysis.

Echocardiography is critically important in identifying the many cardiac causes and comorbidities of CHF (eg, IHD, valvular heart disease, cardiomyopathies, cardiac arrhythmias) and measuring the left ventricular EF. Although the EF can also be measured by radionuclide ventriculography or contrast ventriculography, echocardiography is the most useful and least invasive method for determining and sequentially following EF and the systolic state of the ventricles. Measuring the EF allows the clinician to differentiate between HFrEF and HFpEF, a distinction that is of paramount significance in managing the CHF patient.

Measurement of serum brain natriuretic peptide (BNP) or its metabolite (NT-proBNP), a peptide associated with reduced left ventricular EF and increased left ventricular filling pressure, may be helpful in confirming the diagnosis of CHF, assessing its severity and prognosis, and guiding the treatment. BNP may also be useful as a screening tool to identify early CHF or prevent its development. If the primary mechanism of heart failure is unclear, additional tests may prove useful in selected patients. Such tests may include exercise stress testing, cardiac nuclear imaging studies, right-sided and/or left-sided heart catheterization, Holter monitoring, pulmonary function tests, HIV testing, and thyroid function tests. Coronary angiography can be helpful in identifying patients with ongoing cardiac ischemia and CHF, for which revascularization may lead to symptomatic improvement.

The ECG may reveal acute ischemic changes, acute or previous ventricular hypertrophy, chamber enlargement, and atrial fibrillation or other arrhythmias. Typical chest radiograph findings are prominent pulmonary vessels, interstitial or alveolar pulmonary edema, cardiomegaly, and pleural effusions. Patients with severe pump failure may have abnormal serum electrolyte levels owing to poor renal perfusion. Abnormalities in the blood or urine may help detect severe anemia or renal failure as precipitating factors in CHF. Abnormal liver enzyme levels are common if venous congestion is present as a result of right ventricular failure.

Etiology

As noted previously, IHD is the most common cause of CHF. Cumulative injury to the ventricular myocardium from ischemia and infarction can lead to impaired ventricular systolic and diastolic function and, ultimately, pump failure. Additional causes of systolic dysfunction include

- valvular heart disease (aortic stenosis and aortic or mitral regurgitation)
- cardiomyopathies (idiopathic, metabolic, infectious, toxic, or connective tissue disease)
- myocarditis (secondary to viral or inflammatory diseases)
- infiltrative diseases (amyloidosis, sarcoidosis, and metastatic disease)
- left ventricular hypertrophy

Right- and left-sided heart failure often occur simultaneously in the common causes of CHF—namely, IHD, valvular disease, and the congestive cardiomyopathies. The causes of HFpEF include severe anemia, hyperthyroidism, arteriovenous fistulas, beriberi, and Paget disease.

In HFpEF, the demand for oxygen is so great that the heart eventually fails because it cannot maintain the excessive cardiac output indefinitely. In some patients, heart failure may be more complex; for example, CHF may develop in a patient with IHD who has become severely anemic. Pure right ventricular failure may result from chronic obstructive pulmonary disease, pulmonary hypertension, tricuspid or pulmonary valve disease, right ventricular infarction, or constrictive pericarditis.

Medical and Nonsurgical Management

Appropriate treatment at each stage of CHF is summarized in Figure 5-4. In both HFrEF and HFpEF, treatment of underlying causes and exacerbating conditions (cardiac ischemia, hypertension, diabetes, thyroid dysfunction, sleep apnea) is of critical importance in managing symptoms and preventing deterioration. Patients with systolic failure or HFrEF will also benefit from treatment specifically for their CHF, while diastolic or HFpEF patients rely almost solely on the treatment of their individual disease processes.

Management of HFrEF (systolic dysfunction)

In most clinical situations, reducing afterload is the most effective way to manage heart failure with a reduced EF. Lowering vascular resistance and arterial blood pressure decreases the burden on the left ventricle and enhances contraction and ejection. Regardless of the baseline values, reducing blood pressure (while maintaining adequate tissue perfusion) is the mainstay of treatment of HFrEF. Therapeutic options include the following:

- *ACE inhibitors.* The most effective agents for reducing afterload are captopril, enalapril, lisinopril, and ramipril. They decrease clinical signs of CHF as well as rates of morbidity and mortality.
- *β-Blockers.* These drugs include carvedilol, bisoprolol, and metoprolol. They decrease mortality and hospitalization rates and, if not contraindicated, should be used in almost all CHF patients.

- *Angiotensin II receptor blockers.* Candesartan and valsartan may be used when hypotension from ACE inhibitors would not be tolerated.
- *Amlodipine.* Other calcium channel blockers should be avoided in CHF.
- *Other afterload-reducing agents.* These include hydralazine, clonidine, and, for patients intolerant of ACE inhibitors due to renal disease, α-adrenergic blockers (eg, prazosin, doxazosin).
- *Treatment of anemia.* Intravenous iron replacement may be used to treat anemia, but erythropoietin should be avoided.
- *Lifestyle modification.* Helpful lifestyle changes include smoking cessation, salt restriction, weight loss, exercise, and cardiac rehabilitation.

For patients with HFrEF, the contractility of the left ventricle can be enhanced with inotropic agents. *Digoxin* is reserved mainly for patients who remain symptomatic despite the use of diuretics and ACE inhibitors and for patients with CHF and atrial fibrillation requiring rate control. The other oral inotropic agents have not proved safe or effective in patients with chronic CHF; however, intravenous inotropic agents play a key role in treating hospitalized patients with worsening heart failure. Digoxin should not be used in patients with HFpEF (diastolic failure).

Management of HFpEF (diastolic dysfunction)

Heart failure with preserved EF can be improved by reducing preload, which in turn lowers filling pressures in the ventricle. Preload can be reduced by decreasing circulating blood volume, by increasing the capacitance of the venous bed, and by improving systolic function to empty the ventricle more effectively. Therapy for patients with HFpEF should focus on managing the contributing disease processes. For example:

- Hypertension may be managed with diuretics (spironolactone) and β-blockers.
- Atrial fibrillation is present in two-thirds of HFpEF patients. Consider treatment to control rate and rhythm.
- Cardiac ischemia is present in two-thirds of these patients. Consider use of PCI or CABG.
- Hyperlipidemia may be treated with statins in patients with HFpEF (they are not beneficial in HFrEF).
- Obesity may be managed with weight loss, exercise training, and cardiac rehabilitation.

Other approaches to CHF

Whenever possible, the underlying causes and/or contributing factors for CHF should be identified and addressed. Precipitating factors can include excessive salt or fluid intake, poor medication adherence, excessive activity, obesity, pulmonary infection or embolism, MI, renal disease, anemia, thyrotoxicosis, and arrhythmias.

Intermittent arrhythmias may seriously compromise ventricular function. Tachyarrhythmias may aggravate ischemia; bradyarrhythmias may decrease cardiac output and blood pressure further. As previously discussed, β-blockers should be considered for all patients with CHF for their effects on overall mortality, although they appear to be more effective in HFrEF than in HFpEF. Amiodarone was not found to be beneficial in the Sudden Cardiac Death in Heart Failure Trial (SCD-HeFT), and most other antiarrhythmic agents are contraindicated in CHF because they may decrease cardiac function and be paradoxically proarrhythmic. ICDs can be useful adjuncts to medical therapy in patients with CHF, cardiomyopathy, and an EF of 35% or less; and they improved mortality in both the MADIT II and SCD-HeFT trials. Biventricular pacing also improves mortality rates and decreases rehospitalization rates in patients with CHF and a wide QRS complex by improving contraction efficiency. Patients with heart block or other severe bradyarrhythmias may also require cardiac pacing.

Patients with a dilated cardiomyopathy and atrial fibrillation should receive anticoagulation therapy unless contraindications exist. Many physicians also prescribe anticoagulation for patients with a dilated cardiomyopathy, low EF, and normal sinus rhythm, if there are no contraindications. Options include warfarin, DAT, and newer agents such as dabigatran, apixaban, and rivaroxaban. Risk factors, cost, tolerability, and potential drug interactions should all be considered during agent selection.

Other measures that can help in managing CHF are restricting dietary sodium, avoiding fluid overload by carefully monitoring oral and intravenous fluid intake, controlling pain and anxiety, treating concomitant metabolic and pulmonary diseases, and providing supplemental oxygen to hypoxemic patients. Finally, all patients with CHF should receive an influenza vaccination and the pneumococcal vaccine.

Invasive or Surgical Management

Patients with CHD, the leading cause of CHF, may benefit from coronary revascularization by either CABG or PCI. Depending on the underlying causes, other surgical procedures that may be helpful in CHF include percutaneous balloon valvuloplasty, mitral or aortic valve replacement, and pericardiectomy. Left ventricular reconstruction to reduce the volume of a dilated left ventricle has been performed but has not had favorable outcomes in the STICH and other trials. Cardiac transplantation can be an effective surgical treatment for patients with refractory or end-stage CHF, but the availability of organs and facilities is limited. Many transplant centers have achieved a 1-year survival rate that exceeds 85% for a first graft. Implantable ventricular assist devices may help to maintain patients awaiting cardiac transplantation.

Finally, because many patients with advanced CHF are older and have multiple comorbidities, palliative care directed only at symptomatic improvement should also be considered.

Ponikowski P, Voors AA, Anker SD, et al. 2016 ESC guidelines for the diagnosis and treatment of acute and chronic heart failure. *Eur Heart J.* 2016;37(27):2129–2200.

Yancy CW, Jessup M, Bozkurt B, et al. 2013 ACCF/AHA guideline for the management of heart failure. *J Am Coll Cardiol.* 2013;62(16):e147–e239.

Yancy CW, Jessup M, Bozkurt B, et al. 2017 ACC/AHA/HFSA focused update of the 2013 ACCF/AHA guideline for the management of heart failure. *J Am Coll Cardiol.* 2017;70(6):776–803.

Disorders of Cardiac Rhythm

Abnormalities of cardiac rhythm can vary widely, from asymptomatic premature atrial complexes and mild sinus bradycardia to life-threatening ventricular tachycardia and fibrillation. Disorders of cardiac rhythm can be categorized into several groups, including bradyarrhythmias and conduction disturbances, ectopic or premature contractions, and tachyarrhythmias.

Although many rhythm and conduction disturbances are caused by underlying IHD, they are also attributable to valvular heart disease, myocarditis, cardiomyopathy, congenital aberrant conduction pathways, pulmonary disease, toxic or metabolic disorders, neurogenic causes, and cardiac trauma.

The electrical impulse that initiates each heartbeat normally begins in the *sinoatrial (SA) node* and is conducted down through the atria and ventricles, resulting in a coordinated series of contractions of these chambers. The SA node is the primary pacemaker of the heart. It controls the heart rate and is influenced by neural, biochemical, and pharmacologic factors. If the SA node function is depressed or absent, secondary pacemakers in the *atrioventricular (AV) junction,* the *bundle of His,* or the *ventricular muscle* can generate stimuli and maintain the heartbeat. Normally, stimulus formation in these secondary pacemaker sites is slower than in the SA node. However, abnormal stimuli can also be generated at any of these sites at a rapid pace, resulting in tachycardia.

Bradyarrhythmias and Conduction Disturbances

A *bradyarrhythmia* is any rhythm resulting in a ventricular rate of less than 60 beats per minute (bpm). *Conduction block,* or *heart block,* is a condition in which electrical signals are slowed or interrupted between the atria and ventricles. Bradyarrhythmias and conduction blocks are generally asymptomatic, although they may cause lightheadedness or syncope in rare cases. If the condition is linked to medication use, simply discontinuing the inciting medication may lead to resolution of the bradycardia. Treatment is generally unnecessary except in patients with syncope or hemodynamic instability. In those cases, placement of a cardiac pacemaker is usually the definitive treatment.

Premature Contractions

The principal types of premature contractions are *premature atrial complexes (PACs), premature junctional complexes (PJCs),* and *premature ventricular complexes (PVCs).* These complexes result from ectopic premature depolarization arising from the atria (PACs), the AV node or proximal His-Purkinje system (PJCs), or the ventricles (PVCs). Often, patients have no symptoms, or they may have a sensation of "skipped beats." In many cases, no treatment is needed, but β-blockers or calcium channel blockers can be helpful in symptomatic patients. The correction of underlying abnormalities (eg, drug toxicity, electrolyte imbalance, hyperthyroidism) is often curative.

Premature ventricular complexes typically require no therapy. However, frequent or complex PVCs in the presence of cardiac disease are markers of an increased risk of

Table 5-3 Vaughan Williams Classification of Antiarrhythmic Drugs

Class	Drugs	Mechanism of Action	Indications for Use
Class Ia	Disopyramide, procainamide, quinidine	Sodium channel blockers slow conduction velocity, prolong APD	SVT and VT, prevent VF, symptomatic PVCs
Class Ib	Lidocaine, mexiletine, phenytoin	Shorten APD, no effect on conduction velocity	VT, symptomatic PVCs, prevent VF
Class Ic	Flecainide, propafenone	Slow conduction velocity, may mildly prolong APD	Refractory SVT, VT, or VF
Class II	Carvedilol, esmolol, metoprolol, propranolol	β-Blockers block β-adrenergic receptors	SVT, prevent VF, prevent recurrent AF
Class III	Amiodarone, dofetilide, dronedarone, ibutilide, sotalol	Prolong APD, no effect on conduction	Amiodarone: VT, VF, SVT, AF Dofetilide, dronedarone, or ibutilide: AF, atrial flutter Sotalol: VT, AF
Class IV	Diltiazem, verapamil	Nondihydropyridine slow calcium channel blockers	SVT

AF = atrial fibrillation; APD = action potential duration; PVC = premature ventricular contraction; SVT = supraventricular tachycardia; VF = ventricular fibrillation; VT = ventricular tachycardia.

Data from Makielski JC. Myocardial action potential and action of antiarrhythmic drugs. In: *UpToDate*, Levy S (ed), Waltham, MA. Available at www.uptodate.com. Accessed August 9, 2017.

SCD. Symptomatic patients requiring treatment are best managed with class II drugs (β-blockers) because class I drugs (sodium channel blockers) and class III drugs (potassium channel blockers) appear to worsen the arrhythmia in 5%–20% of patients. Although it is clinically useful, the Vaughan Williams classification of antiarrhythmic drugs (Table 5-3) represents an oversimplification, because many of these medications may have multiple mechanisms of action.

Tachyarrhythmias

Tachyarrhythmia is defined as a heart rate in excess of 100 bpm in an individual at rest. Tachycardias are classified as *supraventricular* or *ventricular*, depending on the mechanism and site of origin. *Narrow complex tachycardias* are almost exclusively supraventricular in origin; *wide complex tachycardias* may be either supraventricular or ventricular in origin. Correct identification of the origin and mechanisms of the tachycardia is critical to selecting appropriate treatment. The exact site of the pacing focus may be difficult to determine when the heart rate is very rapid.

Supraventricular tachycardias

The category of supraventricular tachycardias includes *paroxysmal atrial tachycardia, AV junctional tachycardia, atrial flutter,* and *atrial fibrillation.* Supraventricular tachycardias may be paroxysmal or chronic, as with chronic atrial fibrillation. Causes include emotional stress; caffeine, alcohol, or drug use; thyrotoxicosis; lung disease; and cardiac disease. A patient with a supraventricular tachycardia often experiences palpitations and, in some cases, syncope. β-Blockers are often useful in the management of these disorders, and catheter-guided radiofrequency ablation may be curative in patients with refractory supraventricular tachycardia. The prognosis for supraventricular tachycardia is usually better than that associated with ventricular tachycardia.

Atrial fibrillation Atrial fibrillation is caused by multiple simultaneous wavelets occurring in both the right and the left atria, leading to a chaotic electrical rhythm with ineffective atrial contraction (Fig 5-5). Cardiac output may be markedly reduced when the ventricular rate is very rapid, possibly resulting in CHF. Atrial thrombi may accumulate from stagnation of blood in the atrial appendages. These thrombi may embolize to the lungs, brain, or other organs. Anticoagulation therapy is indicated for patients with chronic atrial fibrillation and chronic atrial flutter associated with valvular disease, cardiomyopathy, or cardiomegaly and before conversion to sinus rhythm is attempted. Several risk stratification tools (eg, CHADS2) have been devised to weigh the risk of embolism against the risk of bleeding in these patients. Newer classes of oral anticoagulants, including direct thrombin inhibitors (dabigatran) and factor Xa inhibitors (rivaroxaban, apixaban, edoxaban), are superior to warfarin in prevention of stroke, with comparable bleeding risks.

Conversion of atrial fibrillation can be attempted with flecainide, dofetilide, propafenone, ibutilide, or direct-current (DC) cardioversion. In many patients with chronic atrial fibrillation, maintenance therapy is directed toward controlling the ventricular rate, which can usually be accomplished with verapamil, β-blockers, or amiodarone.

Other curative approaches have been developed for both atrial fibrillation and atrial flutter. These treatments include radiofrequency catheter ablation and the surgical maze procedure. The *maze procedure* interrupts all possible reentry circuits to the atrium with multiple incisions. A single uninterrupted pathway is left intact to allow normal conduction from the SA node to the AV node. This and other ablative procedures can be performed at the time of CABG or valvular surgery to restore sinus rhythm.

January CT, Wann LS, Alpert JS, et al. 2014 AHA/ACC/HRS guideline for the management of patients with atrial fibrillation. *Circulation.* 2014;130(23):e199–e267. Erratum in: *Circulation.* 2014;130(23):e272–e274.

Kirchhof P, Benussi S, Kotecha D, et al; ESC Scientific Documentation Group. 2016 ESC guidelines for the management of atrial fibrillation developed in collaboration with EACTS. *Eur Heart J.* 2016;37(38):2893–2962.

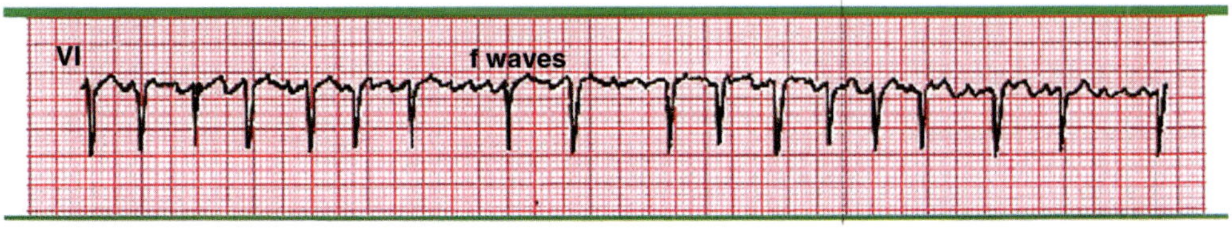

Figure 5-5 Single-lead ECG showing atrial fibrillation. Note the characteristic irregularly irregular rate and rhythm. *(Reproduced with permission from Olshansky B. The electrocardiogram in atrial fibrillation. In:* UpToDate, *Goldberger AL, Saperia GM [eds]. Available at www.uptodate.com. Accessed August 15, 2018.)*

Ventricular tachyarrhythmias

Ventricular tachycardia The ventricular tachyarrhythmias include *ventricular tachycardia (VT), torsades de pointes* (a variant of VT), *ventricular flutter,* and *ventricular fibrillation.* These arrhythmias may present with palpitations, heart failure, or syncope or may progress rapidly to sudden cardiac death. VT occurs infrequently in young patients with no organic heart disease. Brief episodes of VT cause palpitations; prolonged attacks in patients with organic cardiac disease can lead to heart failure or cardiac shock. If the rate is not very high, and there is no significant underlying heart disease, VT may be well tolerated. However, it may degenerate into ventricular fibrillation, resulting in hemodynamic collapse and death.

Treatment with immediate synchronized DC cardioversion is indicated for sustained VT associated with hemodynamic compromise, severe CHF, or ongoing ischemia or infarction. Pharmacologic cardioversion with β-blockers, calcium channel blockers (verapamil, diltiazem), or amiodarone may be attempted in patients with clinically stable VT. Amiodarone is generally the agent of choice for recurrent VT if its adverse effects are tolerated.

Electrophysiologic testing is often performed in patients with suspected or documented ventricular arrhythmias. In this procedure, direct transcatheter electrical stimulation is applied to various sites in the ventricle to induce arrhythmias. Given their efficacy and the low risk associated with implantation, ICDs, in conjunction with antiarrhythmic drugs, have become the treatment of choice for patients with life-threatening ventricular arrhythmias. Radiofrequency catheter ablation can also be performed in patients resistant to medical therapy.

Ventricular fibrillation Ventricular fibrillation (VF) is the most ominous of all the cardiac arrhythmias because it is fatal when untreated or when refractory to treatment. It is a major cause of SCD outside the hospital. The ventricular contractions are rapid and uncoordinated, resulting in ineffective ventricular pumping that soon leads to syncope, convulsions, and death if the VF is not interrupted. The prognosis is generally poor because each episode can be fatal.

Cardiopulmonary resuscitation efforts must be initiated emergently. Immediate unsynchronized DC cardioversion is the primary therapy. After successful cardioversion, continuous intravenous infusion of effective antiarrhythmic therapy should be maintained until any reversible causes have been corrected. The choice of long-term antiarrhythmic therapy depends on the conditions responsible for the initial VF episode. Primary VF occurring within the first few hours of an acute MI is not associated with an elevated risk of recurrence and does not require long-term antiarrhythmic therapy. However, VF without an identifiable and reversible cause requires implantation of an automatic defibrillator. If a patient refuses an ICD, prophylactic antiarrhythmic drug therapy (eg, amiodarone, sotalol) may be used, but multiple studies have demonstrated that an ICD is more effective in preventing SCD.

Implantable cardioverter-defibrillators

ICDs monitor heart rhythm and, when a potentially lethal tachyarrhythmia is identified, deliver therapy. Their evolution has been impressive. Initially, a thoracotomy was necessary to implant an epicardial patch or patches. Most patients now receive a transvenous system, which significantly reduces the morbidity and mortality associated with the implantation of these devices. Current-generation ICDs are generally implanted in the prepectoral region (similar to pacemaker implantation). Although first-generation ICDs delivered only high-energy defibrillating shocks, current-generation devices provide tiered therapy, including pacing algorithms for tachycardia, low-energy cardioversion for stable VT, high-energy cardioversion for VT or VF, single-chamber or dual-chamber pacing support for bradycardia, and stored diagnostic information for rhythm discrimination.

ICDs treat arrhythmias when they occur but do not prevent them. Most patients require concomitant antiarrhythmic therapy (β-blockers, amiodarone) to reduce the frequency of device discharges or to facilitate antitachycardia pacing by slowing the ventricular rate. If the device fails to terminate an arrhythmia, cardiopulmonary resuscitation and external defibrillation should proceed normally. Three randomized prospective studies have demonstrated that automatic ICDs are the preferred first-line therapy for patients who have survived a cardiac arrest or an episode of hemodynamically unstable VT, with a 20%–30% relative reduction in the risk of death. The MUSTT and MADIT trials have also proved the benefit of ICDs for primary prevention of sudden death in patients with CHD, reduced EFs, nonsustained VT, or inducible ventricular arrhythmias during electrophysiologic testing. Following an MI, ICDs appear to be the best available therapy for preventing SCD. An ICD should be considered for patients on optimal medical therapy who have left ventricular dysfunction from an MI that occurred at least 40 days previously and an expected survival with good functional status of at least 1 year. Ongoing trials may expand the role of ICDs in the primary prevention of sudden death.

Camm AJ, Lip GY, De Caterina R, et al; ESC Committee for Practice Guidelines. 2012 focused update of the ESC guidelines for the management of atrial fibrillation. *Eur Heart J.* 2012;33(21):2719–2747.

Russo AM, Stainback RF, Bailey SR, et al. ACCF/HRS/AHA/ASE/HFSA/SCAI/SCCT/SCMR 2013 appropriate use criteria for implantable cardioverter-defibrillators and cardiac resynchronization therapy. *J Am Coll Cardiol.* 2013;61(12):1318–1368.

Ophthalmic considerations Many of the adult patients seen and treated by ophthalmologists are in the age group at risk for IHD and its many complications. They often undergo stressful eye surgery under local or general anesthesia, and ophthalmologists need to be cognizant of these patients' risks of myocardial ischemia, myocardial infarction, CHF, and arrhythmias. Similarly, ophthalmologists need to be aware of the association between proliferative diabetic retinopathy and IHD. This information should be given to the primary medical care provider of patients with proliferative diabetic retinopathy but no diagnosis of IHD so that appropriate screening tests can be considered.

Cardiac complications of noncardiac surgery are a major cause of perioperative morbidity and mortality, MI being the most significant. Older age, preexisting CHD, and CHF are the principal risk factors for development of these complications.

ICDs are increasingly used for the management of cardiac arrhythmias. Although no cases of discharge of an ICD during ocular surgery have been reported, the ophthalmologist should discuss the status and possible perioperative disabling of the ICD with the cardiologist or anesthesiologist before ocular surgery to avoid surgical complications.

Finally, ophthalmologists should be aware of the potential ocular adverse effects associated with medications commonly used in treating CVD. Following are the medications of clinical relevance:

- *Amiodarone.* Corneal microdeposits occur in nearly all patients who use amiodarone for an extended period of time (years). The corneal epithelial whorl-like deposition is indistinguishable from that due to chloroquine. Visual changes are unusual; patients most often report hazy vision or colored halos around lights. Photosensitivity reactions from amiodarone may lead to discoloration (usually slate gray or blue) of periocular skin. A rare adverse effect is amiodarone optic neuropathy, which is characterized by an insidious onset, slow progression, bilateral vision loss, and protracted optic nerve head swelling that tends to stabilize within several months of discontinuing the medication. Patients on long-term amiodarone therapy should have a baseline ophthalmic examination, follow-up examinations every 6–12 months, and immediate evaluation of any new visual disturbances. Because of this drug's photosensitizing effects, UV-blocking spectacle lenses should be considered in selected cases of chronic eyelid disease or macular disease.
- *β-Blockers.* The use of some β-blockers can lead to a keratoconjunctivitis sicca–like syndrome, probably due to decreased lacrimation. They may also possibly enhance migraine ocular scotomata and may decrease intraocular pressure (IOP). Topical β-blockers, particularly timolol, may be less effective in lowering IOP in patients concurrently taking systemic β-blockers. Visual disturbances and vivid visual hallucinations may also be associated with the systemic use of β-blockers.
- *Digoxin.* Glare and disturbances of color vision are the most common and striking ocular adverse effects. They include decreased vision and problems with color vision, such as blue-yellow pattern defects; a yellow, green, blue, or red tinge to objects; and colored halos (mainly blue) around lights. Patients on digoxin may also describe yellow or green flickering vision, colored borders around objects, glare phenomena, light flashes, scintillating scotomata, a frosted appearance to objects, and formed visual hallucinations.
- *ACE inhibitors.* These agents may cause angioedema involving the eye and orbit. The presumed mechanism is the disruption of bradykinin metabolism.

American Academy of Ophthalmology website: www.aao.org.
American College of Cardiology website: www.acc.org.

American Heart Association website: www.heart.org.
Cheng HC, Yeh HJ, Huang N, et al. Amiodarone-associated optic neuropathy: a nationwide study. *Ophthalmology.* 2015;122(12):2553–2559.
European Society of Cardiology website: www.escardio.org.
Stoller GL. Ophthalmic surgery and the implantable cardioverter defibrillator. *Arch Ophthalmol.* 2006;124(1):123–125.
UpToDate: www.uptodate.com.

CHAPTER 6

Cerebrovascular Disease

Highlights

- "Time is brain." The most important factor in successful thrombolytic treatment in patients with acute ischemic stroke is *early* treatment.
- Intravenous recombinant tissue plasminogen activator (rtPA) is strongly recommended for carefully selected patients who can be treated within 3 hours of onset of ischemic stroke.
- For those patients who present with disabling symptoms, such as a complete hemianopia or visual extinction, rtPA is recommended regardless of the degree of initial improvement.
- Mechanical thrombectomy using second-generation stent retrievers is highly recommended in eligible patients after ischemic stroke involving large cerebral arteries of the anterior circulation, regardless of age, stroke severity, or whether they were treated with rtPA.
- Patients with acute ischemic stroke who received rtPA should be given aspirin (160–325 mg/day) 24–48 hours after symptom onset to prevent recurrent stroke, reduce stroke mortality, and decrease morbidity.
- Intensive treatment with statins after stroke reduces risk of recurrent ischemic stroke and other cardiovascular events.
- Carotid endarterectomy (CEA) may be considered in patients with greater than 70% stenosis, but the benefit of CEA versus best medical therapy is controversial.
- Flow diverting stents may supplant traditional endovascular coiling or clipping techniques in the general surgical management of intracranial aneurysms.

Introduction

Stroke is the third leading cause of death in developed countries, ranking behind heart disease and cancer. In the United States, it is the fifth leading cause of death. From 2000 to 2010, the relative rate of stroke death decreased by 35.8% in the United States, and the actual number of US stroke deaths declined by 22.8%; yet the number of strokes occurring annually in the United States remains approximately 795,000, of which 610,000 are first attacks. Each year, approximately 129,000 individuals die in the United States as a result of ischemic stroke. Better control of hypertension, cholesterol levels, and diabetes mellitus, as well as increases in smoking cessation, have contributed to this reduction in stroke mortality rates. The annual incidence of ischemic stroke has increased in Eastern Europe, China, and other nations where improved economic status is accompanied by a widespread adoption of unhealthful lifestyles. Stroke is the leading cause of long-term disability in the United States today.

There are 2 primary types of stroke: ischemic stroke and hemorrhagic stroke. Ischemic stroke accounts for about 87% of cerebrovascular accidents.

For more information on cerebrovascular disease, refer to BCSC Section 5, *Neuro-Ophthalmology.*

Cerebral Ischemia

Cerebral ischemia results from interference with blood circulation to the brain. The ischemic event can occur as a result of intrinsic vessel pathology that leads to thrombosis; embolic phenomena; or systemic hypoperfusion. Cerebral circulation is usually maintained by a very efficient collateral arterial system that includes the 2 carotid and the 2 vertebral arteries, anastomoses in the circle of Willis, and collateral circulation in the cerebral hemispheres. However, atheromas and congenital arteriovenous malformations (AVMs) can lead to a reduction in cerebral blood flow. This reduction may be generalized or localized. Interruptions in cerebral blood flow can result in permanent neurologic deficits, depending on the extent and duration of the cerebral ischemia.

Transient Cerebral Ischemia

Transient cerebral ischemia (TCI) is now defined as a transient episode of neurologic dysfunction caused by focal ischemia *without* infarction. The previous, time-based definition of TCI (formerly referred to as a transient ischemic attack), which described the episode as a sudden-onset focal loss of neurologic function, persisting for less than 24 hours, is inadequate; infarction can occur even after a brief period of ischemia, even if the presenting focal neurologic symptoms resolve in less than 1 hour. The new term TCI, with its tissue-based definition, more accurately reflects its pathophysiology and encourages the use of diagnostic testing to identify evidence of permanent tissue injury. The presence of acute infarction is a strong predictor of a recurrent ischemic stroke. The occurrence of TCI is not only an important prognostic indicator for a future stroke but is also associated with a rising mortality over time. Most TCIs last only a few minutes, and the symptoms are primarily associated with insufficiency of the internal carotid, middle cerebral, or vertebrobasilar arterial territories.

Ischemic Stroke

A *completed stroke* is an ischemic event that produces a stable, permanent neurologic disability. Most *ischemic strokes* consist of small regions of complete ischemia in conjunction with a larger area of incomplete ischemia. This ischemic but not infarcted area is called the *penumbra.* The penumbra is dynamic, resulting in changes to the previously passive treatment approach in patients with acute cerebral ischemia. Clinical manifestations of cerebral ischemia reflect the functions associated with the area of ischemia and include paresis, paresthesia, vision loss, language disturbances, vertigo, diplopia, ataxia, dysarthria, headache, nausea, and vomiting.

Emboli or thrombi caused by atherosclerosis, hypertension, or diabetes mellitus and located in large, medium, and small arteries account for most strokes. Strokes caused by emboli of cardiac origin account for 20% of total ischemic stroke incidence. Atrial fibrillation is the most common cause of cardioembolic strokes, occurring in up to 20% of these patients. Mural thrombi forming on the endocardium in conjunction with myocardial infarction (MI) account for 8%–10% of total stroke incidence worldwide. Other cardiac conditions associated with intracranial embolism include mitral stenosis and atrial myxoma. Cerebral autosomal dominant arteriopathy with subcortical infarcts and leukoencephalopathy (CADASIL), which is a rare genetic small-vessel vasculopathy, can mimic multiple sclerosis and cause ischemic stroke.

Nonarteriosclerotic causes of thrombotic occlusion leading to TCI and stroke include internal carotid dissection (causing the classic triad of Horner sign, neck pain/headache, and neurologic signs and symptoms) and inflammatory arteritis (eg, collagen vascular disease, giant cell arteritis, meningovascular syphilis, acute and chronic meningitis, and moyamoya disease).

Another cause of cerebral ischemia is increased viscosity of the blood due to pregnancy and the postpartum period, use of oral contraceptives, postoperative and posttraumatic states, hyperviscosity syndromes, polycythemia, and sickle cell disease. In addition, stroke may occur as a result of hypoxemia caused by conditions such as carbon monoxide poisoning, chronic obstructive pulmonary disease, profound anemia, and pulmonary emboli.

Diagnosis and Management

The differential diagnosis of ischemic stroke and TCIs includes diabetic and convulsive seizures, migraine, vertigo, and neoplasms. Although the presentation of stroke is usually characteristic, the diagnosis should be differentiated from that of other conditions that may mimic strokes, such as multiple sclerosis, subdural hematoma, cranial nerve palsy, encephalitis, hypoglycemia, seizures, brain tumor, hypertensive encephalopathy, syncope, migraine, and functional disorder.

Obtaining a detailed history from the patient, including the time and duration of onset, is important. Also, an assessment of risk factors is critical for treating a patient with suspected stroke. Nonmodifiable risk factors include age older than 60 years, male sex, and family history or prior history of stroke or TCIs. Modifiable risk factors include diabetes mellitus, hypertension, hyperlipidemia, cardiac arrhythmias, smoking, alcohol use, illicit drug use, migraine, and hypercoagulable states.

The clinical severity of a stroke can be determined using the US National Institutes of Health Stroke Scale (NIHSS), which assesses level of consciousness, gaze, visual fields, facial strength, motor function of the arms and legs, ataxia, sensation, language, dysarthria, and inattention, giving a specified number of points to each impairment found. A scale of 0–42 is used for the assessment, with *0* representing normal function and *42* representing the most severe functional impairment.

Patients presenting with TCI within 72 hours of the event should be hospitalized if they have a known source of embolic phenomena that is treatable, such as cardiac valvular disease, evidence of acute infarction on initial imaging, and significant concurrent morbidities. Individuals who are not hospitalized should be instructed to undergo diagnostic workup within 48 hours and warned to return to the emergency department if symptoms recur.

For practical purposes, diagnostic studies may be separated into those done in an acute care setting, such as in the emergency department, and those done in a more subacute setting, such as in a stable inpatient or stable outpatient clinic. Emergent testing assesses the patient's clinical stability and the possibility of conditions that mimic stroke or conditions that could contribute to stroke; the tests should include blood glucose, complete blood count, blood chemistry, coagulation studies such as PT/aPTT (prothrombin time/activated partial thromboplastin time), international normalized ratio, troponins, and electrocardiogram. Ideally, all suspected cases of stroke and TCI should be evaluated with urgent noncontrast *computed tomography (CT)* of the brain, because contrast and blood appear similar on CT, and this similarity can result in misinterpretation of the image. Noncontrast CT is very sensitive for the presence of intracranial hemorrhage and remains the imaging modality of choice for emergent initial evaluation of stroke. However, enhancement in CT imaging has also improved its diagnostic capability in the evaluation of early cerebral ischemia.

Investigation of the systemic arteries and the heart is essential in determining the cause of cerebral ischemia. Differences between upper limb pulse rates and blood pressure (BP) may indicate serious subclavian disease. Multiple bruits may suggest widespread arterial disease but may be present without significant occlusion. Evidence of a cardioembolic source should be pursued aggressively, especially in younger normotensive persons with cerebral ischemia and in older patients, for whom atrial fibrillation is included in the differential diagnosis. Electrocardiography and telemetry or Holter monitoring should be routinely performed to exclude cardiac dysrhythmia and occult MI. Echocardiography is often helpful in excluding intracardiac thrombi; transesophageal Doppler echocardiography is most sensitive in this regard. Lumbar puncture is required in the evaluation of stroke or TIA only in rare instances, for example, if meningovascular syphilis, meningitis, or subarachnoid hemorrhage is a serious consideration.

Imaging studies for evaluation of cerebral ischemia

Updates in imaging techniques have now provided numerous options for the clinician in assessing the presence or absence of tissue injury, tissue at risk, and the anatomy of the regional circulation.

Multimodal computed tomography In multimodal CT, 3 CT modes are combined: noncontrast CT, CT perfusion imaging, and CT angiography. This type of imaging can rule out hemorrhage, permit early detection of acute infarction, and allow assessment of the site of occlusion, infarct core, and salvageable brain tissue. In addition, the angiography mode can assess collateral circulation.

Magnetic resonance imaging and magnetic resonance angiography Magnetic resonance imaging (MRI) is more sensitive than noncontrast CT in detecting an evolving stroke within hours of its onset. *Diffusion-weighted imaging (DWI)* MRI with *apparent diffusion coefficient (ADC) mapping* is useful in the evaluation of early cerebral ischemia and regional blood flow to determine the presence or absence of acute infarction. MRI perfusion-weighted imaging (PWI) assesses transit time of the contrast agent. Magnetic resonance angiography (MRA) can be used to detect vascular stenosis and/or occlusion. Multimodal MRI, which combines DWI with PWI, is useful in predicting outcomes in patients with TCI. To date, DWI appears to be the imaging modality of choice in the evaluation of a TCI.

Helical computed tomography angiography This type of angiography can rapidly and noninvasively image the large cerebral arteries with very high specificity and sensitivity.

Carotid duplex ultrasonography This imaging modality may be used to evaluate the patency of the extracranial carotid arteries.

Transcranial doppler ultrasonography This type of ultrasonography is used for evaluation of the intracranial arteries (see more in the section Carotid Occlusive Disease).

Cerebral arteriography Although it is the gold standard for angiographic technique, cerebral arteriography has high morbidity and is usually required only if the cause of the TCI is unclear or if intra-arterial thrombolysis or surgical intervention is being strongly considered.

Treatment

The goals of treating ischemic stroke are to restore blood flow to the brain and to salvage ischemic brain tissue that has not already infarcted. Achieving these goals involves ensuring the patient's medical stability and determining whether the patient is eligible for thrombolytic therapy. There is a narrow window in which to accomplish these objectives, ideally within 3 hours of symptom onset.

Intravenous thrombolysis Thrombolytic and antithrombotic agents are the primary drugs used in the treatment of ischemic stroke, and recombinant tissue plasminogen activator (rtPA) is the fibrinolytic agent of choice. In the US National Institute of Neurological Diseases and Stroke (NINDS) rtPA Stroke Study, the administration of rtPA within 3 hours of acute ischemic stroke was associated with improved function at 3 months but not with earlier neurologic improvement or lower mortality. The European Cooperative Acute Stroke Study III (ECASS III) demonstrated the benefit of rtPA initiated up to 4½ hours after the onset of stroke. However, the exclusion criteria for patients treated 3–4½ hours from symptom onset (age older than 80 years, severe stroke, diabetes mellitus with a previous infarct, and any anticoagulant use) were more restrictive than for those treated at 3 hours or less. Most studies indicate that the sooner rtPA is initiated, the more likely it is to be beneficial. The most serious complication of administering rtPA is symptomatic intracranial hemorrhage, which occurs in 6.4% of treated patients and has a mortality rate of 50%.

Mechanical (endovascular) thrombectomy Unfortunately, patients with a large cerebral artery occlusion and a large clot burden are less likely to benefit from rtPA and are at high risk of a neurologically disabling outcome. More proximal occlusions are also more resistant to thrombolysis, as are those occlusions resulting from clots with less favorable composition. Furthermore, because some patients fail to meet the eligibility criteria for intravenous rtPA, thrombectomy techniques were developed with clot-retrieving devices to improve canalization of the artery and arrest the ischemic stroke. Therefore, as part of the initial imaging evaluation of acute ischemic stroke, noninvasive vascular study, such as CT angiography, should be performed to assess the patient's candidacy for endovascular intervention.

Mechanical thrombectomy (MT) performed with first-generation stent retrievers such as the Merci and Penumbra failed to show an improvement in patient outcomes. However, second-generation stent retrievers such as Solitaire and Trevo achieved significantly higher recanalization rates with correspondingly improved outcomes. Five clinical trials with second-generation stent retrieval devices (ESCAPE, EXTEND-IA, MR CLEAN, REVASCAT, and SWIFT PRIME) showed the efficacy of MT when compared with standard medical care in patients with acute ischemic stroke caused by occlusion of the large arteries of the proximal anterior circulation. Anatomic success with recanalization, functional independence, and major neurologic recovery was significantly better in those patients receiving MT. However, mortality at 90 days, risk of intracranial hemorrhage, and risk of parenchymal hematoma involving greater than 30% of the infarct territory did not differ between the 2 study populations. These data have resulted in a paradigm shift in the early treatment of ischemic stroke; mechanical thrombectomy with second-generation stent retrieving devices is now highly recommended in eligible patients. Mechanical thrombectomy should be performed at centers with surgeons skilled in the use of stent-retrieving devices, and initiation of MT should be within 6 hours of stroke onset.

Investigational reperfusion techniques Currently under investigation are other methods of reperfusion, such as intra-arterial thrombolysis (SYNTHESIS expansion trial), use of alternative fibrinolytic agents, combined intravenous and intra-arterial thrombolysis (IMS III trial), stenting, and combined use of fibrinolytics and glycoprotein IIb/IIIa antagonists, but none of these techniques have yet demonstrated improved outcomes.

Post-acute management

The cornerstone of stroke management is to prevent future events, especially because most stroke patients do not receive the acute care treatment previously discussed. In addition to thrombolytic drugs and mechanical thrombectomy, the management of stroke includes antithrombotic therapy with antiplatelet agents, initiation of statins, and control of BP after the acute phase is over.

Antithrombotic therapy Although aspirin, clopidogrel, and aspirin/extended-release dipyridamole combination are acceptable drug choices for secondary stroke prevention, aspirin is the only antiplatelet agent that is effective in the early treatment of ischemic stroke. Two large clinical trials showed a benefit of treatment with aspirin over placebo in short-term mortality and recurrent stroke risk when aspirin is initiated within 48 hours of ischemic stroke onset. Early use of combination antiplatelet agents such as aspirin with clopidogrel for acute ischemic stroke may be beneficial, but the available evidence is not consistent and is limited to the specific populations studied. Heparin and related agents are not effective in reduction of mortality or recurrent stroke in patients with cardioembolic or noncardioembolic stroke; in fact, they are associated with higher mortality and a worse outcome. However, use of heparin may be considered in the acute care setting for stroke resulting from postoperative atrial fibrillation in patients with mechanical heart valves or in those with cervicocephalic arterial dissections.

Statins Initiation or continuation of statins early after presentation is critically important. Studies have shown that long-term intensive use of statins after stroke reduces risk of recurrent ischemic stroke and other cardiovascular events. In addition, numerous reports support the beneficial effects of statin administration during the acute phase of ischemic stroke.

Blood pressure control Hypertension is the most important risk factor for stroke. Treatment with antihypertensives in the prevention of recurrent ischemic stroke is supported by data from multiple randomized clinical trials and from 2 meta-analyses of a total of 24 clinical trials with over 70,000 patients. Current guidelines from the 2021 American Heart Association/American Stroke Association (AHA/ASA) recommend continued treatment with antihypertensive drugs in patients with hypertension prior to the stroke event and initiation of antihypertensive treatment for patients with newly diagnosed hypertension. Antihypertensive therapy is *not* recommended in patients with blood pressures lower than 120/70 mm Hg as there may be risk of harm in individuals with systolic blood pressures lower than 120 mm Hg. Although blood pressure reduction is critical in preventing recurrent ischemic stroke and other ischemic cardiovascular events, care must be taken to maintain blood pressure at a level that will not compromise cerebral perfusion.

For further discussion of hypertension, see Chapter 3 in this volume.

Cappellari M, Bovi P, Moretto G, et al. The THRombolysis and STatins (THRaST) study. *Neurology.* 2013;80(7):655–661.

Goyal M, Menon BK, van Zwam WH, et al. Endovascular thrombectomy after large-vessel ischaemic stroke: a meta-analysis of individual patient data from five randomised trials. *Lancet.* 2016;387(10029):1723–1731.

Kernan WN, Ovbiagele B, Black HR, et al; American Heart Association Stroke Council, Council on Cardiovascular and Stroke Nursing, Council on Clinical Cardiology, Council on Peripheral Vascular Disease. Guidelines for the prevention of stroke in patients with stroke and transient ischemic attack: a guideline for healthcare professionals from the American Heart Association/American Stroke Association. *Stroke.* 2014;45(7):2160–2236.

Powers WJ, Derdeyn CP, Biller J, et al; American Heart Association Stroke Council. 2015 American Heart Association Guidelines for the early management of patients with acute ischemic stroke regarding endovascular treatment: a guideline for healthcare professionals from the American Heart Association/American Stroke Association. *Stroke.* 2015;46(10):3020–3025.

Powers WJ, Rabinstein AA, Ackerson T, et al; American Heart Association Stroke Council. 2018 Guidelines for the early management of patients with acute ischemic stroke: a guideline for healthcare professionals from the American Heart Association/American Stroke Association. *Stroke.* 2018;49(3):e46–e110.

Carotid Occlusive Disease

Carotid atherosclerosis occurs most frequently in the proximal internal carotid artery (origin) and at the carotid bifurcation. The progression of luminal narrowing and ulceration leads to ischemic stroke or TCI from embolization, thrombosis, or hemodynamic compromise.

Diagnostic Evaluation

This section describes the 4 main diagnostic techniques currently used to identify the degree of carotid stenosis.

Carotid duplex ultrasonography

Carotid duplex ultrasonography is relatively inexpensive, quick, and noninvasive, with high sensitivity and high specificity for diagnosing high-grade carotid stenosis. However, ultrasonography may overestimate the degree of stenosis and is less accurate in individuals with less than 69% stenosis. The accuracy of the results is also very much operator-dependent, resulting in high variability among different ultrasound laboratories. If the ultrasonography findings suggest the need for surgical intervention, it may be prudent to confirm with a second imaging modality.

Magnetic resonance angiography

MRA is more expensive than carotid ultrasonography and cannot be done in patients who are unable to assume a supine position or in those who have ferromagnetic implants and/or pacemakers. However, the 3-dimensional image of the carotid artery produced by MRA is useful in diagnosing high-grade carotid stenosis and provides an anatomic complement to carotid ultrasonography. The use of advanced MRI techniques is being studied to help physicians identify changes in plaque composition that may be useful for prognosticating risk of rupture and stroke.

Computed tomography angiography

Computed tomography angiography (CTA) is superior to carotid ultrasonography for differentiating high-grade carotid stenosis from total occlusion and effectively excludes carotid stenosis that is greater than 70%, making CTA useful as a screening test. If there is disagreement between MRA and carotid ultrasonography results, CTA is useful in adjudicating the findings.

Cerebral angiography

Cerebral angiography remains the gold standard imaging modality for patients with suspected carotid occlusive disease, but its invasive nature and associated morbidity and mortality risk limits its applicability.

Transcranial doppler ultrasonography

Transcranial doppler ultrasonography (TCD) is a useful adjunct to carotid ultrasonography because it gives physicians the ability to evaluate the flow characteristics of intracerebral vessels. This ability enables the identification of high-grade internal carotid stenosis via the examination of the flow patterns of collateral vessels, including the reversal of ophthalmic artery flow.

Management of Carotid Stenosis

Asymptomatic carotid stenosis

Asymptomatic carotid bruits occur in 4% of the US population older than 40 years, and the annual stroke rate in these individuals is 1.5%.

This same population has an annual mortality rate of 4%, primarily from complications of heart disease. The presence of a carotid bruit is, therefore, a better predictor of arteriosclerotic disease than of stroke. As of 2014 the current AHA/ASA guidelines for management of asymptomatic carotid stenosis include the following:

- Patients with asymptomatic carotid stenosis should be prescribed a statin and aspirin. They should also be screened for conditions that are risk factors for stroke, with appropriate institution of medical therapy and lifestyle modifications.
- Individuals with greater than 50% stenosis should undergo serial annual ultrasonography to identify progression.
- It is reasonable to consider CEA in patients with greater than 70% stenosis if the perioperative complication risk for stroke, myocardial infarction, and death is less than 3%. However, the benefit of CEA over best medical therapy is controversial.
- For patients undergoing CEA, aspirin is recommended perioperatively and postoperatively, unless contraindicated.
- Prophylactic carotid artery stenting (CAS) might be considered in select patients with stenosis that is greater than or equal to 60% on angiography or stenosis that is greater than or equal to 70% on ultrasonography, but the benefit of CAS over best medical therapy is not proven.
- In patients at high risk for complications related to revascularization that might result from either CEA or CAS, the effectiveness of revascularization versus medical therapy is not well established.

Contemporary intensive medical management (also called best medical therapy), which includes the more widespread and aggressive use of statins, newer antiplatelet agents, and lifestyle modifications (eg, cessation of smoking), as well as improvements in pharmacologic therapy for treatment of diabetes and hypertension, seems to have altered the prognosis in those assigned to medical therapy, which may now be equivalent or superior to outcomes from revascularization procedures. Furthermore, because most ischemic strokes due to carotid stenosis are preceded by a TCI, some experts feel that medical management should be the preferred treatment, and that physicians should wait until symptoms occur in the patient before subjecting a patient to the risks associated with revascularization. The Carotid Revascularization Endarterectomy Versus Stenting Trial-2 (CREST-2) study is now under way; it will compare outcomes in patients treated with best medical therapy versus those who undergo CEA.

Symptomatic carotid stenosis

Patients with TCI, transient monocular visual loss (TMVL), or previous stroke resulting from carotid stenosis are considered symptomatic. The risk of stroke within 1 year of onset of symptoms is 8% in patients with TCI; the risk thereafter is approximately 6% per year, with a 5-year risk of 35%–50%. Current AHA/ASA guidelines for management of symptomatic carotid stenosis are as follows:

- For patients with recent (within the past 6 months) TCI or ischemic stroke and severe (70%–99%) ipsilateral carotid artery stenosis, CEA is recommended if the perioperative morbidity and mortality risk is less than 6% and the patient's life expectancy is greater than 5 years.

- For patients with recent cerebrovascular events and moderate ipsilateral stenosis (50%–69%), CEA is recommended, depending on patient-specific factors such as age, sex, and other comorbidities.
- There is no benefit of CEA or CAS in a patient with stenosis of less than 50%.
- Surgery may be performed within 2 weeks of a TCI or stroke.
- CAS can be considered as an alternative to CEA in symptomatic patients when the patient is at low risk for endovascular intervention *and* an internal carotid artery stenosis of greater than 70% is indicated by noninvasive imaging or an internal carotid artery stenosis of greater than 50% is indicated by catheter angiography. CAS may also be considered in other selected patients.

Carotid artery stenting versus carotid endarterectomy

The first CREST study randomly assigned patients with asymptomatic or symptomatic carotid disease to CEA or CAS. The primary endpoint of the trial—a composite of any stroke, MI, or death within 30 days of the procedure and ipsilateral stroke during long-term follow-up—was similar in both groups, including the rate of ipsilateral stroke at 31 days to up to 4 years after the procedure. The study showed that:

- Endarterectomy had a greater benefit in older patients (≥70 years).
- Stenting was more beneficial in patients in younger age groups (<60 years).
- There was a greater incidence of stroke and death at 30 days in the stenting group versus the endarterectomy group, but the incidence of MI was significantly lower in the CAS group.
- Despite the higher rate of stroke associated with stenting, at 1-year follow-up there were no significant differences in any quality-of-life measure between the CEA and CAS groups.

Transient monocular visual loss and cardioaortic causes of ischemic stroke

In addition to cerebral conditions, ocular conditions such as TMVL and retinal TCIs can be associated with carotid stenosis. The ophthalmologist is often the first physician to see a patient with TMVL; the TMVL is usually embolic, with either a carotid or a cardiac source. The annual stroke rate among patients with isolated TMVL, retinal infarcts, or TCIs is approximately 2%, 3%, and 8%, respectively. Untreated individuals with TMVL, retinal infarcts, or TCIs have a 30% risk of MI and an 18% risk of death over a 5-year period. A cardiac source of embolization should be excluded for all patients presenting with isolated TMVL. Transthoracic echocardiography (TTE) can identify multiple potential cardiac causes for embolism and, as expected, the diagnostic yield is highest if the clinical history and physical examination suggest a cardiac source such as atrial fibrillation, rheumatic mitral stenosis, diffuse atherosclerosis, left ventricular aneurysm, or clinical endocarditis. Transesophageal echocardiography (TEE) is superior to transthoracic echocardiography in diagnosing a cardioembolic source, except for a left ventricular thrombus, which is better seen on TTE. Because TEE is invasive and uncomfortable and may not be tolerated well by the patient, TTE is recommended first in the evaluation of a potential cardioaortic source of stroke. If the results from TTE imaging are negative, the use of TEE would then be indicated. TEE is the best imaging modality to use to rule out atheromatous plaques in the ascending aorta, a patent foramen ovale, a left atrial appendage clot, or other causes of "cryptogenic" stroke. TEE is also superior for identifying certain anatomic abnormalities, but the identification of intracardiac thrombi or tumors with TEE is rare (<3%). Therefore, whether the use of TEE will become routine in the evaluation of cryptogenic stroke remains to be seen. Other modalities used in the diagnosis of cardioembolic sources of stroke include inpatient telemetry, ambulatory Holter monitoring, loop recorders, and surgically implantable cardiac monitors.

If evidence suggests that a carotid lesion is the cause of the TMVL, or if venous stasis retinopathy is present, duplex ultrasonography should be performed to determine whether vessel wall disease or carotid stenosis is present.

The following approach should be considered for a patient presenting with a cerebral or retinal transient ischemic attack (TIA):

- emergency department or urgent outpatient evaluation or hospital admission if the event occurred within the previous 48 hours
- patient evaluation for the presence of risk factors associated with atherogenesis: hypertension, diabetes mellitus, obesity, hyperlipidemia, and smoking
- institution of appropriate medical therapy
- evaluation by appropriate testing for the presence of a cardiac source of emboli
- determination using duplex ultrasonography of the possibility of carotid stenosis

If ipsilateral carotid stenosis exceeds 70%, if bilateral carotid stenosis greater than 50% is present, or if long-term evidence indicates progressive disease, CEA should be considered—but only if the surgeon's perioperative stroke and death rate is less than 6%. Otherwise, antiplatelet therapy with aspirin (325 mg/day), aspirin/extended-release dipyridamole combination, or clopidogrel should be initiated. A patient presenting with TIA symptoms who has previously undergone CEA should be evaluated and treated similarly. Special attention should be paid to evaluating patients for the presence of early restenosis and thrombosis.

For further discussion of TIA and TMVL, see BCSC Section 5, *Neuro-Ophthalmology.*

Ophthalmic considerations Giant cell arteritis (GCA), which may present as TMVL, should always be considered in the differential diagnosis of TMVL and may warrant further laboratory investigation depending on age (>50 years). For more on GCA and TMVL, see BCSC Section 5, *Neuro-Ophthalmology.*

Katsanos AH, Giannopoulos S, Frogoudaki A, et al. The diagnostic yield of transesophageal echocardiography in patients with cryptogenic cerebral ischaemia: a meta-analysis. *Eur J Neurol.* 2016;23(3):569–579.

Meschia JF, Bushnell C, Boden-Albala B, et al; American Heart Association Stroke Council, Council on Cardiovascular and Stroke Nursing, Council on Clinical Cardiology, Council on Functional Genomics and Translational Biology, Council on Hypertension. Guidelines for the primary prevention of stroke: a statement for health care professionals from the American Heart Association/American Stroke Association. *Stroke.* 2014;45(12):3754–3832.

Safian RD. Asymptomatic carotid stenosis: revascularization. *Prog Cardiovasc Dis.* 2017;59(6):591–600.

Intracranial Hemorrhage

In the United States, intracranial hemorrhage constitutes approximately 13%–15% of acute cerebrovascular disorders. The most common causes of intracranial hemorrhage are bleeding from aneurysms of the arteries that compose the circle of Willis, bleeding from arterioles damaged by hypertension or arteriosclerosis, and trauma. Although intracranial hemorrhage has many causes, the anatomical location of the bleeding greatly influences the clinical picture. By location, hemorrhages can be broadly categorized as intracerebral, intraventricular, or subarachnoid.

Intracerebral Hemorrhage

Hypertension is the most common cause of nontraumatic intracranial hemorrhage. Cerebral amyloid angiopathy is the most common cause of nontraumatic intracranial hemorrhage in elderly individuals, whereas AVMs are the most common cause in children. Infections resulting from septic emboli, hemorrhagic infarction, brain tumors, coagulopathies, and intrinsic vascular conditions such as moyamoya disease and vasculitis are all associated with intracerebral bleeding.

The pathophysiology of intracerebral bleeding secondary to hypertension appears to be intimal hyperplasia with hyalinosis that results in focal necrosis with pseudoaneurysm formation. When the vessel is exposed to high pressure that cannot be compensated for by the clotting cascade, small leaks lead to massive hemorrhage. Direct pressure to the brain parenchyma by the expanding clot and from cytotoxic perilesional edema results in direct tissue injury. As the clot expands, the ischemia increases and the cytotoxic edema develops further, raising intracranial pressure; if severe enough, this pressure may lead to herniation. Expansion of the hemorrhage into the intraventricular space occurs in 40%–60% of patients worldwide, greatly increasing morbidity and mortality.

In addition to hypertension, a prospective study showed that age, high alcohol intake, African American race, and, oddly, low levels of low-density lipoprotein and triglycerides are associated with increased risk of intracerebral hemorrhage. Most hypertensive hemorrhages occur during routine activity, but some may occur with exertion or intense emotional stress. Symptoms increase gradually over a few minutes to hours. Headache and vomiting occur in about 50% of cases. When intraventricular blood is involved, meningismus with stiff neck and nuchal rigidity occur.

Intraventricular Hemorrhage

Worldwide, intraventricular hemorrhage (IVH) accounts for only 3% of intracranial bleeding. IVH typically occurs as a secondary phenomenon when an intracerebral or subarachnoid hemorrhage extends into the ventricles. Thus, hypertension is also found in nearly half of individuals with IVH. Primary IVH is uncommon and is usually due to vascular malformations. Patients with IVH typically present with abrupt onset headache, nausea, vomiting, and varying degrees of impaired consciousness. Focal neurologic findings are uncommon. The diagnostic test of choice for IVH is a noncontrast head CT. After the CT, MRI or MRA can be used to identify the anatomical cause of the hemorrhage.

Treatment is aimed at cessation of the bleeding, reducing hydrocephalus, and managing raised intracranial pressure. Gradual lowering of blood pressure, placement of an intraventricular drain, and treating the specific cause (eg, repair of the aneurysm or obliteration of the AVM) should be undertaken.

Subarachnoid Hemorrhage

Subarachnoid hemorrhage (SAH) accounts for nearly 50% of cases of intracranial hemorrhage. Its incidence increases with age, and it is more common in women. African American and Hispanic individuals have a higher incidence of SAH when compared with White individuals. Most SAHs result from saccular, or "berry," aneurysms. Only a minority of cases of SAH are nonaneurysmal in etiology. Approximately 85% of congenital saccular, or "berry," aneurysms develop in the anterior part of the circle of Willis. The origin of the posterior communicating artery from the internal carotid artery is the most common site. Such an aneurysm typically presents with headache and third cranial nerve palsy involving the pupil. Vascular malformations within and on the surface of the brain parenchyma constitute approximately 7% of cases of subarachnoid hemorrhage and arise from capillary telangiectasias, cavernous hemangiomas, venous angiomas, or AVMs.

Capillary telangiectasias and both types of angiomas typically have a low bleeding risk (<0.5%/year). Findings that suggest an AVM as the cause of subarachnoid hemorrhage include a history of previous focal seizures, slow stepwise progression of focal neurologic signs, and, occasionally, recurrent unilateral throbbing headache resembling migraine. A bruit may be present over the orbit or skull in approximately 40% of patients. SAH usually presents with abrupt onset severe headache that is typically described by patients as the "worst headache of my life." The headache occurs in 97% of cases; 30% have symptoms lateralized to the side of the hemorrhage. The combination of vitreous hemorrhage and subarachnoid hemorrhage *(Terson syndrome)* portends a worse prognosis. Maintaining a high index of suspicion and evaluating the patient with noncontrast CT, followed by mandatory lumbar puncture if CT results are negative, are essential in making the diagnosis. Digital subtraction angiography is superior to CT or MRA for the detection of SAH due to aneurysm.

Prognosis and treatment

Aneurysmal SAH carries a high mortality rate; 10% of individuals with an aneurysmal SAH die before they reach the hospital, 25% die within 24 hours, and 45% within 30 days. Prognostic factors include the patient's level of consciousness and neurologic grade on hospital admission, the patient's age, and the amount of blood hemorrhaged, as discovered via the initial head CT. Initial clinical severity may be assessed by a validated scale such as the Hunt and Hess scale because it is the most useful indicator of outcome after acute subarachnoid hemorrhage.

Control and maintenance of BP are mandatory in the treatment of ruptured aneurysms. Surgical intervention is ideally accomplished within 24–72 hours because the likelihood of early rebleeding is high and is associated with a poor outcome. The 2 traditional methods of interventional management are (1) placing a small clip or ligature (clipping) across the neck of the sac and (2) endovascular coiling. If an aneurysm is judged to be suitable for either technique, results of an analysis of 3 randomized trials favor endovascular coiling over clipping in the surgical management of intracranial aneurysms. Patients with large intraparenchymal hematomas or middle cerebral artery aneurysms may have better outcomes with clipping. Complete obliteration of the aneurysm is recommended, and patients who undergo either surgical intervention should undergo immediate angiography after the surgery to identify any remnants that may require retreatment. If the aneurysm cannot be directly obliterated, surgical ligation of a proximal vessel may be necessary. Complex aneurysms can also be treated with flow-diverting stents, which shunt blood flow from the aneurysmal vessel, thereby activating the coagulation cascade to stimulate gradual thrombosis of the aneurysm. Flow-diverting stents may result in a paradigm shift in treatment of aneurysms usually treated by traditional endovascular or microsurgical intervention, but long-term comparative data are not yet available.

The current gold standard of treatment is the surgical excision of a symptomatic AVM. Stereotactic radiosurgery and hypofractionated stereotactic radiotherapy are valuable treatment options in patients with symptomatic AVMs deemed at a high risk for surgical excision; these methods are associated with low morbidity and mortality, with good occlusion rate. At present, medical therapy is preferred over surgery in patients with unruptured AVMs.

Al-Mufti F, Amuluru K, Ghandi CD, Prestigiacomo CJ. Flow-diversion for intracranial aneurysm management: a new standard of care. *Neurotherapeutics.* 2016;13(3):582–589.

Connolly ES Jr, Rabinstein AA, Carhuapoma JR, et al; American Heart Association Stroke Council, Council on Cardiovascular Radiology and Intervention, Council on Cardiovascular Nursing, Council on Cardiovascular Surgery and Anesthesia, Council on Clinical Cardiology. Guidelines for the management of aneurysmal subarachnoid hemorrhage: a guideline for healthcare professionals from the American Heart Association/American Stroke Association. *Stroke.* 2012;43(6):1711–1737.

Lu L, Zhang LJ, Poon CS, et al. Digital subtraction CT angiography for detection of intracranial aneurysms: comparison with three-dimensional digital subtraction angiography. *Radiology.* 2012;262(2):605–612.

CHAPTER 7

Pulmonary Diseases

Highlights

- Untreated obstructive sleep apnea is associated with coronary artery disease, congestive heart failure, arrhythmias, refractory hypertension, and type 2 diabetes mellitus. It is also strongly associated with various ocular conditions.
- Smoking cessation is the single most efficacious and cost-effective intervention in reducing the risk of COPD, heart disease, and stroke. Ophthalmologists should obtain a smoking history from their patients and encourage smoking cessation.

Introduction

The lungs can be affected by numerous pathologic processes, including inflammation (allergic, infectious, autoimmune, toxic), vascular insults, fibrosis, carcinoma, and changes resulting from cardiac or musculoskeletal problems. The functional consequences of the pathology can be divided into *obstructive* ventilatory functions and *restrictive* ventilatory functions.

Symptoms of lung disease include dyspnea, cough, and wheezing. *Dyspnea* develops when the demand for gas exchange exceeds the capacity of the respiratory system, as in hypoxemia or hypercapnia. Dyspnea may also reflect the increased work of breathing, as occurs in cases of airway obstruction or reduced compliance of the lungs or chest. *Cough* develops when mucus, inflammatory debris, or irritants stimulate the bronchi, causing reflex clearing expectoration, or when the lung parenchyma is infiltrated with fluid, cells, or fibrosis. *Wheezing* occurs when bronchospasm narrows the large airways and exhaled air is forced through narrowed passages.

Obstructive Lung Diseases

In patients with obstructive lung disease, changes in the bronchi, bronchioles, and lung parenchyma can cause airway obstruction. Obstructive lung diseases can be categorized as reversible or irreversible, although many cases may have some degree of both reversible and irreversible obstruction.

Reversible obstructive diseases are grouped under the term *asthma.* In patients with asthma, the airways are hyperresponsive and develop an inflammatory response with bronchospasm to various stimuli; the specific cause and duration of the bronchospasm can vary.

In some persons, allergic immunoglobulin E (IgE)–mediated reactions to defined antigens cause bronchospasm. In many individuals with asthma, however, the cause of abnormal airway reactivity remains unknown. Precipitating factors may include exercise, aspirin, sulfites, tartrazine dye, emotional stress, cold air, environmental pollutants, or viral infection. Bronchial smooth muscle constriction, mucosal edema, excess mucus accumulation, and epithelial cell shedding all contribute to airway obstruction. This obstruction may be reversible, either spontaneously or with treatment. One marker of eosinophilic airway inflammation is an increase in exhaled nitric oxide; identifying this increase may be important in measuring an individual's responsiveness to therapeutic intervention. Mepolizumab, a monoclonal antibody, is approved for use in cases of severe eosinophilic asthma.

Irreversible obstructive disease (sometimes known as *chronic obstructive pulmonary disease [COPD]*) comprises a group of conditions in which forced expiratory flow is reduced in either a constant or a slowly progressive manner over months or years. COPD is the third leading cause of death in the United States. The Global Initiative for Chronic Obstructive Lung Disease (GOLD), an international consortium working to improve prevention and treatment of COPD, publishes a guide on the diagnosis, classification, and management of this condition. The guide, which is updated regularly, can be downloaded from the GOLD website (www.goldcopd.org). GOLD offers a framework for the management of COPD. Some conditions, such as *cystic fibrosis* or *bronchiectasis,* which are either secondary to recurrent necrotizing bacterial infections or which occur as part of Kartagener syndrome, have an identifiable cause. However, most irreversible obstructive diseases, such as *emphysema, chronic bronchitis,* and *peripheral airway disease,* cannot be ascribed to specific conditions; rather, they represent an individual response to cigarette smoking and various airborne pollutants. For example, such responses occur in patients with either α_1-antitrypsin deficiency (associated with certain forms of emphysema) or airway hyperactivity and mucus hypersecretion (as in bronchitis). The pathologic consequences of the abnormal response result in specific damage to lung tissue. Emphysema is characterized by pathologic enlargement of the terminal bronchiole air spaces and by destruction of the alveolar connective tissue septa. Bronchitis is characterized by hypertrophied mucous glands in the bronchi; in peripheral airway disease, only the small airways demonstrate fibrosis, inflammation, and tortuosity.

Obstructive sleep apnea (OSA) has similar pathophysiologic processes to COPD: compromised gas exchange that leads to hypoxia and hypercapnia. OSA is a breathing disorder characterized by the narrowing of the upper airway, which impairs normal ventilation during sleep. This physical disruption of the upper airway distinguishes OSA from central sleep apnea, which occurs as a result of the brain temporarily not transmitting signals to the muscles that control breathing, leading to insufficient ventilation and compromised gas exchange. The current prevalence of OSA in the United States is estimated at 14% for men and 5% for women. The prevalence of OSA is much higher in patients with coronary artery disease, congestive heart failure, arrhythmias, refractory hypertension, type 2 diabetes mellitus, and polycystic ovary disease. The fragmented sleep experienced by individuals with untreated OSA can lead to many negative consequences, including daytime sleepiness, cognitive disfunction, and decreased quality of life. Untreated OSA is also associated with an increased risk of developing cardiovascular disease, resistant hypertension, coronary artery disease, congestive heart failure, arrhythmias, stroke, and metabolic dysregulation that affects glucose control. In order for OSA to be diagnosed and evaluated, a patient must undergo polysomnography, a type of sleep study that records the many biophysical changes that occur during sleep, including respiratory functions. Treatment of OSA has been shown to improve the individual's quality of life, decrease motor vehicle collisions, and reduce the chronic health consequences associated with untreated OSA.

Global Initiative for Chronic Obstructive Lung Disease. Global strategy for the diagnosis, management, and prevention of chronic obstructive pulmonary disease (updated 2020). www.goldcopd.org/gold-reports. Accessed September 10, 2021.

Song WJ, Kim HJ, Shim JS, et al. Diagnostic accuracy of fractional exhaled nitric oxide measurement in predicting cough-variant asthma and eosinophilic bronchitis in adults with chronic cough: a systematic review and meta-analysis. *J Allergy Clin Immunol.* 2017;140(3):701–709.

Restrictive Lung Diseases

The restrictive lung diseases encompass a diverse group of conditions that cause diffuse parenchymal damage. The physiologic consequences of this damage include a reduction in total lung volume, diffusion capacity, and vital capacity. Occasionally, patients without parenchymal involvement who have diseases of the chest wall, respiratory muscles, pleura, or spine may have similarly restricted lung volumes. A *fibrotic* parenchymal response can result from occupational exposure to various substances, including asbestos, silica dust, graphite, talc, coal, and tungsten. A *granulomatous* hypersensitivity reaction can develop in response to moldy hay, grains, birds, humidifiers, and cooling systems. Endogenous pulmonary disease can result from collagen vascular diseases, sarcoidosis, eosinophilic granuloma, granulomatosis with polyangiitis (formerly known as Wegener granulomatosis), Goodpasture syndrome, alveolar proteinosis, idiopathic pulmonary hemosiderosis, idiopathic pulmonary fibrosis, and other idiopathic parenchymal diseases. Therapeutic agents such as phenytoin, penicillin, gold, methotrexate, and radiation can also cause pulmonary disease.

Evaluation

Although all patients with respiratory problems should be under the care of a capable internist or pulmonologist, ophthalmologists and other physicians should be aware of the key components in the diagnosis and evaluation of patients with pulmonary diseases. The following should be considered:

- *Symptoms:* Dyspnea, orthopnea, chronic cough, and chronic sputum production.
- *History:* Occupational exposure to various toxins and irritants, family history, cigarette use.
- *Signs:* Audible wheezing, cyanosis, finger clubbing, forced expiratory time greater than 4 seconds, increased anteroposterior diameter of the chest.

- *Laboratory studies:* Elevated hematocrit level and hypoxia or hypercapnia on arterial blood gas measurement.
- *Chest radiography:* Parenchymal disease, hyperinflation, diaphragmatic flattening, increased retrosternal lucency, and pleural abnormalities.
- *Computed tomography* of the chest: Can detect many abnormalities not seen on chest radiographs, such as small areas of adenopathy, pulmonary embolus, small nodules, infiltrative lung disease, and bronchiectasis.
- *Bronchoscopy, transbronchial biopsy,* and *bronchial lavage:* Used to obtain culture material, cytology material, and pathologic specimens for analysis.
- *Pulmonary function tests:* Measure the mechanical and gas exchange functions of the lungs. The *forced expiratory volume over 1 second* (FEV_1) represents the volume exhaled in the first second of exhalation; the *forced vital capacity (FVC)* represents the total volume that the patient can exhale. Both parameters and their serial rate of decline in a patient are objective measures of lung function as well as predictors of comorbidity and mortality from lung cancer and cardiovascular disease. An FEV_1/FVC ratio less than 70% of predicted reference values suggests obstructive disease; total lung capacity less than 70% of predicted values suggests restrictive disease.

Treatment

There are 2 major goals in the treatment of pulmonary disease. The first goal is to favorably alter the natural history of the disease. The second is to improve the patient's symptoms and functional status and minimize associated problems.

Nonpharmacologic Treatment

Smoking cessation is the single most efficacious and cost-effective intervention in reducing the risk of COPD and slowing its progression. Ophthalmologists should not underestimate the power of even a brief discussion with a patient about the impact of smoking and the beneficial effects of smoking cessation.

Similarly, *avoiding precipitants* of airway obstruction is important in ameliorating asthmatic conditions. In patients with severe pulmonary hypertension and cor pulmonale, use of supplemental oxygen to maintain an arterial oxygen pressure above 60 mm Hg confers a modest reduction in pulmonary hypertension and improved survival rates. However, a patient receiving supplemental oxygen must be carefully monitored because such treatment may decrease the body's respiratory drive to eliminate carbon dioxide, aggravating respiratory acidosis and possibly leading to carbon dioxide narcosis. *Breathing exercises* and *postoperative chest physiotherapy* have demonstrable short-term effects in improving respiratory function.

Noninvasive pressure support ventilation can be used to deliver increased airway pressure. Continuous positive airway pressure (CPAP) throughout the ventilation cycle improves alveolar oxygen exchange. In CPAP therapy, a tight, well-fitting mask is placed either over the patient's mouth and nose or just over the nose. Noninvasive pressure support ventilation is recommended for patients with respiratory failure who are expected to quickly respond to medical therapy. Intubation and standard ventilation are preferred for patients who require total ventilatory support, because the mask may slip, and effective ventilation may cease.

Currently, the most effective treatment for OSA is CPAP; the positive pressure acts as a pneumatic splint to maintain airway patency. Treatment of OSA with CPAP therapy has been shown to improve daytime sleepiness, health-related quality of life, and mood and attendance at work, as well as reduce the risk of developing cardiovascular disease, refractory hypertension, coronary artery disease, congestive heart failure, arrhythmias, and stroke. Despite these proven benefits, a recent meta-analysis found that CPAP therapy did not reduce the risk of major cardiovascular events (acute coronary events, stroke, or vascular death) or all-cause mortality. In addition, although there are now over 100 different mask options to help optimize patient comfort and adherence to mask use, patient adherence to this treatment option is low due to discomfort; some patients still find the mask cumbersome to wear.

McEvoy RD, Antic NA, Heeley E, et al; SAVE Investigators and Coordinators. CPAP for prevention of cardiovascular events in obstructive sleep apnea. *N Engl J Med.* 2016;375(10):919–931.

Park JG, Ramar K, Olson EJ. Updates on definition, consequences, and management of obstructive sleep apnea. *Mayo Clin Proc.* 2011;86(6):549–554.

Yu J, Zhou Z, McEvoy RD, Anderson CS, Rodgers A, Perkovic V, Neal B. Association of positive airway pressure with cardiovascular events and deaths in adults with sleep apnea: a systematic review and meta-analysis. *JAMA.* 2017;318(2):156–166.

Ophthalmic considerations Several ocular conditions are associated with OSA, including dry eye syndrome, floppy eyelid syndrome, normal-tension glaucoma, papilledema, central serous chorioretinopathy, and nonarteritic anterior ischemic optic neuropathy (NAION). Recently, untreated OSA was shown to hinder the response of exudative AMD to intravitreal bevacizumab. Patients with OSA undergoing CPAP treatment have improved AMD response to anti-VEGF treatment and require significantly fewer injections.

Santos M, Hofmann RJ. Ocular manifestations of obstructive sleep apnea. *J Clin Sleep Med.* 2017;13(11):1345–1348.

Schaal S, Sherman MP, Nesmith B, Barak Y. Untreated obstructive sleep apnea hinders response to bevacizumab in age-related macular degeneration. *Retina.* 2016;36(4):791–797.

Pharmacologic Treatment

Pharmacologic approaches to pulmonary disease include medications that are specific for the particular condition and medications that improve the patient's symptoms and functional status. *Specific medications* directly alter the pathophysiologic mechanisms underlying pulmonary disease. Some examples include cyclophosphamide for granulomatosis with polyangiitis, corticosteroids for sarcoidosis, and plasmapheresis in combination with immunosuppressive drug therapy for Goodpasture syndrome.

Symptomatic medications are designed to reduce the obstructive or restrictive components affecting the patient's lung function. Medications used to treat symptomatic bronchospastic airway obstruction include bronchodilators and inhibitors of inflammation (Fig 7-1), as well as antibiotics for infection-precipitated airway closures.

Bronchodilators, which include theophylline, β-adrenergic agonists, and anticholinergics, act primarily by relaxing the tracheobronchial smooth muscle. *β-Adrenergic agonists* activate bronchial smooth muscle, resulting in bronchodilation. The selective β_2-adrenergics, which have greater bronchodilatory effect and less cardiostimulatory effect, are commonly used, often in metered-dose inhalers (they can also be administered orally or parenterally). These drugs have replaced the nonselective β-adrenergic agents such as isoproterenol. The short-acting β_2-agonists include fenoterol, salbutamol, and isoetharine. These drugs differ in time of onset of action and duration of action. For example, the onset of action of isoetharine is within 1–3 minutes, and its duration is 60–90 minutes. Common long-acting β_2-agonists include formoterol and salmeterol. Salmeterol, a particularly long-acting β_2-adrenergic, is helpful in maintenance treatment of asthma; it should not be used for acute exacerbations. Although epinephrine causes predominantly β-adrenergic stimulation in the lungs, it also causes peripheral α-adrenergic stimulation, resulting in vasoconstrictive hypertension and tachycardia. Epinephrine is most often administered subcutaneously to help control an acute asthma attack.

Anticholinergic agents directly relax smooth muscle by competing for acetylcholine at muscarinic receptors. Atropine and similar agents have been replaced by poorly absorbing atropinic congeners such as ipratropium bromide, oxitropium bromide, and tiotropium bromide. These inhalation agents have few systemic and minimal cardiac effects. They have an additive bronchodilator effect when combined with submaximal doses of β-adrenergic agonists.

Inhibitors of inflammation include corticosteroids, leukotriene inhibitors, mast-cell stabilizers (cromolyn), and immunosuppressive agents. *Corticosteroids* not only suppress inflammation of the bronchioles but also potentiate the bronchodilator response to β-adrenergic receptors. Inhaled corticosteroids can be used for an extended period to reduce bronchial hyperreactivity; they are not used to manage acute attacks. Systemic corticosteroids are highly effective in managing acute episodes, but because of the potential adverse effects associated with their use, they should be used only when necessary for serious flare-ups. *Leukotriene inhibitors* suppress the effects of inflammatory mediators. They are especially useful for prophylaxis and long-term maintenance therapy in asthma. *Cromolyn* prevents the release of chemical mediators from mast cells in the presence of IgE antibody and the specific antigen. *Immunotherapy* has been shown to be helpful for asthma triggered by a defined antigen.

Asthma treatment should be tailored to disease severity. Medication doses should be adequate to control symptoms rapidly and should later be reduced to the minimal level required to maintain control. The goals of therapy should include prevention of symptoms, reduction in frequency and severity of exacerbations, maintenance of normal (or near-normal) pulmonary function, maintenance of normal activity levels, and minimization of medication adverse effects. Maintenance medications include inhaled corticosteroids, cromolyns, leukotriene inhibitors, long-acting β_2-agonists, anticholinergic agents, and oral

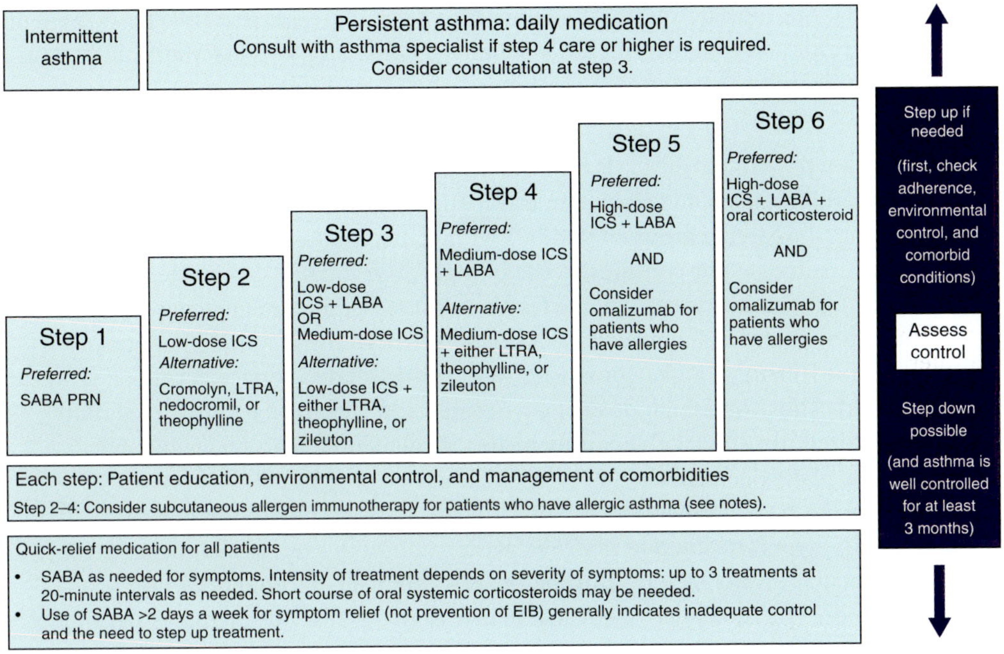

Figure 7-1 Stepwise approach for managing asthma in adults and in youths ≥ 12 years of age. Alphabetical order is used when more than one treatment option is listed within either preferred or alternative therapy. EIB = exercise-induced bronchospasm, ICS = inhaled corticosteroid, LABA = long-acting inhaled β_2-agonist, LTRA = leukotriene receptor antagonist, SABA = (inhaled) short-acting β_2-agonist.

Notes:

- The stepwise approach is meant to assist, not replace, the clinical decision-making required to meet individual patient needs.
- If alternative treatment is used and response is inadequate, discontinue it and use the preferred treatment before stepping up.
- Zileuton is a less desirable alternative due to limited studies as adjunctive therapy and the need to monitor liver function. Theophylline requires monitoring of serum concentration levels.
- In step 6, before oral systemic corticosteroids are introduced, a trial of high-dose ICS + LABA + either LTRA, theophylline, or zileuton may be considered, although this approach has not been studied in clinical trials.
- Steps 1, 2, and 3 preferred therapies are based on Evidence A; step 3 alternative therapy is based on Evidence A for LTRA, Evidence B for theophylline, and Evidence D for zileuton. Step 4 preferred therapy is based on Evidence B, and alternative therapy is based on Evidence B for LTRA and theophylline and Evidence D for zileuton. Step 5 preferred therapy is based on Evidence B. Step 6 preferred therapy is based on *Expert Panel Report 2: Guidelines for the Diagnosis and Management of Asthma* (EPR—2 1997) and Evidence B for omalizumab.
- Immunotherapy for steps 2–4 is based on Evidence B for house-dust mites, animal danders, and pollens; evidence is weak or lacking for molds and cockroaches. Evidence is strongest for immunotherapy with single allergens. The role of allergy in asthma is greater in children than in adults.
- Clinicians who administer immunotherapy or omalizumab should be prepared and equipped to identify and treat anaphylaxis that may occur.

(Modified with permission from National Heart, Lung, and Blood Institute; National Asthma Education and Prevention Program. Expert Panel Report 3: Guidelines for the Diagnosis and Management of Asthma. Full Report 2007. *Bethesda, MD: National Institutes of Health, US Dept of Health and Human Services; 2007.)*

corticosteroids. Appropriately used supplemental oxygen increases survival among patients with chronic respiratory failure and has a beneficial effect on pulmonary arterial pressure, polycythemia, exercise capacity, lung mechanics, and mental state.

Ophthalmic considerations It remains unclear whether the use of inhaled corticosteroids causes an increase in intraocular pressure. In a case-control study that compared a group of patients with glaucoma to a control group, neither current use nor continuous use of high-dose inhaled corticosteroids for 3 or more months was associated with an increased risk of glaucoma. An earlier study found an increased risk of ocular hypertension among patients with a family history of glaucoma who were using inhaled corticosteroids, particularly those on a high dose of corticosteroids. Intraocular pressure should be monitored in adults with a family history of glaucoma who are using high-dose inhaled corticosteroids.

The FDA has approved the use of sildenafil to slow the progression of pulmonary hypertension and improve patient ability to exercise. Associated adverse ocular events include chromatopsia, cyanopsia, photophobia, and visual disturbance. The incidence of adverse ocular events is low but increases with increased medication dosing.

Gonzalez AV, Li G, Suissa S, Ernst P. Risk of glaucoma in elderly patients treated with inhaled corticosteroids for chronic airflow obstruction. *Pulm Pharmacol Ther.* 2010;23(2):65–70.

Mitchell P, Cumming RG, Mackay DA. Inhaled corticosteroids, family history, and risk of glaucoma. *Ophthalmology.* 1999;106(12):2301–2306.

Morales DR, Dreischulte T, Lipworth BJ, Donnan PT, Jackson C, Guthrie B. Respiratory effect of beta-blocker eye drops in asthma: population-based study and meta-analysis of clinical trials. *Br J Clin Pharmacol.* 2016;82(3):814–822.

Wirostko BM, Tressler C, Hwang, LJ, Burgess G, Laties AM. Ocular safety of sildenafil citrate when administered chronically for pulmonary arterial hypertension: results from phase III, randomised, double masked, placebo controlled trial and open label extension. *BMJ.* 2012; 344:e554.

CHAPTER 8

Hematologic Disorders

Highlights

- Alternate-day dosing of iron may yield greater absorption with fewer gastrointestinal adverse effects than a daily regimen in patients with iron deficiency anemia.
- Allogeneic hematopoietic cell transplantation (HCT) is potentially curative in sickle cell disease and is strongly recommended for selected pediatric patients.
- HCT may have a better than 90% cure rate for β-thalassemia when performed in a child with an HLA-identical sibling donor.
- Rivaroxaban, apixaban, and edosaban are 3 factor Xa inhibitors recently approved for clinical use.
- Idarucizumab is now available as an antidote for the thrombin inhibitor dabigatran; andexanet alfa has also been approved for reversal of rivaroxaban and apixaban.
- Fostamatinib has received FDA approval for treatment of chronic idiopathic thrombocytopenic purpura (ITP).

Blood Composition

Formed elements—erythrocytes (red blood cells, or RBCs), leukocytes (white blood cells), and platelets—constitute approximately 45% of the total blood volume. The fluid portion, *plasma,* is about 90% water. The remaining 10% of the plasma consists of proteins (albumin, globulin, fibrinogen, and enzymes), lipids, carbohydrates, hormones, vitamins, and salts. If a blood specimen is allowed to clot, the fibrinogen is consumed, and the resultant fluid portion is called *serum.*

Erythropoiesis

All blood cells originate from the uncommitted pluripotent stem cells, which give rise to lymphoid stem cells and myeloid stem cells. *Myeloid stem cells* are the precursors of RBCs, granulocytes, monocytes, and platelets. Hormones such as erythropoietin, thrombopoietin, and granulocyte colony-stimulating factor initiate the differentiation of the various cellular elements. The life span of a circulating RBC is 120 days.

Anemia

Anemia is the result of an insufficient quantity of erythrocytes to carry oxygen to the peripheral tissues. It can be classified according to 3 pathophysiologic states: (1) blood loss or nutritional deficiency, (2) underproduction of erythrocytes, and (3) premature destruction of erythrocytes (hemolysis). The normal hemoglobin level in men ranges from 14 to 17 g/dL, while the normal hemoglobin level in women is lower (12–16 g/dL). The higher level in men is due to the erythropoietic effects of androgens.

In the evaluation of a patient with anemia, it is important for the clinician to classify the disorder by reviewing the RBC indexes, including complete blood count, hemoglobin concentration, and erythrocyte count, as well as indexes specifically indicative of RBC size: the mean corpuscular volume (MCV) of erythrocytes and their size distribution (red cell distribution width [RDW]). Reviewing these indexes and observing the morphology on a peripheral blood smear help the clinician determine whether the anemia is *microcytic* (MCV <80 femtoliter [fL]), *normocytic* (MCV 80–100 fL), or *macrocytic* (MCV >100 fL). In addition to the peripheral blood smear, the reticulocyte count gives an indication of erythrocyte production. Patients with normal bone marrow who have lost blood or undergone hemolysis have increased reticulocyte counts, whereas patients with underproduction anemia have low reticulocyte counts for their degree of anemia.

Anemia Due to Blood Loss or Nutritional Deficiency

Iron deficiency anemia

By far, the most common type of anemia, affecting nearly 1 billion persons worldwide, is *iron deficiency anemia*. It is also the most common nutritional deficiency in the world. Iron deficiency anemia is diagnosed when the serum ferritin concentration is less than 15 µg/L or when transferrin saturation is less than 16%; the gold standard for diagnosis is the absence of stainable iron in the bone marrow.

In developing countries, iron deficiency is typically caused by poor intake and/or parasitic infections, whereas in high-income countries, chronic blood loss, vegetarian or vegan diet, and poor absorption are the more common causes. Absorption can be affected by inflammatory bowel disease, celiac sprue, and *Helicobacter pylori* infection. Bariatric surgery is an increasingly common cause of iron deficiency.

Iron deficiency anemia is also characterized by low hepcidin levels. *Hepcidin,* a peptide hormone produced by the liver, inhibits iron transport across the intestinal mucosa, thereby preventing excess iron absorption and maintaining normal iron levels within the body. Hepcidin also inhibits the transport of iron out of macrophages and enterocytes, that is, the site of iron storage and transport. Every adult with iron deficiency anemia should be suspected to be bleeding until proven otherwise. Menstrual blood loss in women plays a major role, as does gastrointestinal bleeding in both men and women. Aspirin can cause gastrointestinal bleeding.

Patients with mild iron deficiency anemia may experience fatigue, malaise, irritability, decreased exercise tolerance, restless legs syndrome, and headaches before symptoms of overt anemia occur. Patients with iron deficiency anemia typically have normal findings on physical examination. However, in severe cases, abnormal findings such as facial pallor, glossitis, stomatitis, koilonychia (spoon nails), and conjunctival pallor may be present. Occasionally, patients with severe iron deficiency anemia exhibit pica, a tendency to eat ice, clay, starch, paper, or crunchy materials.

Once the etiology of iron deficiency anemia has been identified, it may be treated with oral ferrous sulfate, which is the least expensive preparation for treating this disorder. It is typically administered at a dosage of 325 mg 3 times daily, although recent data suggest that an alternate-day dosing regimen may yield greater absorption of iron due to its favorable effect on hepcidin levels, with fewer gastrointestinal adverse effects. Parenteral iron preparations are indicated for patients who are unable to absorb oral iron, are intolerant of its adverse effects, are on dialysis, or have iron deficiency due to blood loss from inflammatory bowel disease.

Stoffel NU, Cercamondi CI, Brittenham G, et al. Iron absorption from oral iron supplements given on consecutive versus alternate days and as single morning doses versus twice-daily split dosing in iron-depleted women: two open-label randomised controlled trials. *Lancet Haematol.* 2017;4(11):e524–e533.

Vitamin B_{12} deficiency

Vitamin B_{12} comes from the diet and is available in all foods of animal origin. Absorption of vitamin B_{12} requires an intrinsic factor produced by the gastroparietal cells. This complex is absorbed in the terminal ileum and stored in the liver. It takes 3 years to deplete the reserves of vitamin B_{12} in the liver. Strict vegetarians (vegans), patients with a history of abdominal surgery or gastrectomy/bariatric surgery, and individuals with parasitic (tapeworm) or pancreatic disease are at increased risk for vitamin B_{12} deficiency. *Pernicious anemia* is an autoimmune disease in which atrophic gastritis and subsequent intrinsic factor deficiency lead to impaired vitamin B_{12} absorption. *Megaloblastic anemia* is a type of macrocytic anemia resulting from inhibition of DNA synthesis in RBC precursors in the marrow, leading to reduced cell division. When B_{12} levels are in the low normal range, the physician should examine levels of serum cobalamin B_{12}, folate, homocysteine, and methylmalonic acid (a more sensitive and specific test for diagnosing vitamin B_{12} deficiency). Often, leukopenia and thrombocytopenia accompany the anemia. Even in the absence of hematologic changes, vitamin B_{12} deficiency can cause a neurologic syndrome; peripheral nerves are affected first, while balance problems and alteration of cerebral function (eg, dementia, neuropsychiatric changes) occur in more severe cases. Parenteral B_{12} is used for treatment of pernicious anemia; otherwise, daily oral B_{12} is effective, less expensive, and less cumbersome than parenteral B_{12}.

Ophthalmic considerations Vitamin B_{12} deficiency may cause bilateral optic neuropathy presenting with central acuity loss and cecocentral scotomata on visual field testing.

Folate deficiency

Folate deficiency (also called folic acid deficiency) is another etiology of megaloblastic, or macrocytic, anemia. The most common etiology of the deficiency is inadequate dietary intake of folate due to generalized malnutrition or poor nutrition associated with alcohol dependence. Other causes of folate deficiency include

- malabsorption (celiac disease or tropical sprue, zinc deficiency)
- impaired metabolism (alcoholism, folate inhibitor drugs such as methotrexate and trimethoprim)
- increased requirements (hemolytic anemia, pregnancy, lactation, infection, malignancy)
- increased excretion (dialysis, subsequent to vitamin B_{12} deficiency)

It is important to exclude vitamin B_{12} deficiency in patients with presumed folate deficiency; although treatment with folic acid can correct anemia in patients with vitamin B_{12} deficiency, it does not reverse the neuropsychiatric symptoms that can occur in severe B_{12} deficiency. Patients with folate deficiency may also develop neuropsychiatric symptoms that overlap with vitamin B_{12} deficiency. Once vitamin B_{12} deficiency is excluded, a therapeutic trial of folic acid in patients with presumed folate deficiency may be the most cost-effective way of establishing the diagnosis.

Anemia Due to Defective Hemoglobin Synthesis (Hemoglobinopathies)

Thalassemia

The thalassemias are a group of hereditary anemias characterized by a reduced rate of synthesis of hemoglobin polypeptide chains alpha or beta. This decreased synthesis leads, in turn, to reduced hemoglobin and a hypochromic microcytic anemia. *α-Thalassemia* is due to a gene deletion that reduces synthesis of alpha hemoglobin chains. Homozygous α-thalassemia leads to hydrops fetalis, which usually results in intrauterine or perinatal death. *β-Thalassemia* is caused by a point mutation rather than a deletion. In the absence of beta chains, the excess of alpha chains leads to instability in the RBC and hemolysis. The bone marrow becomes hyperplastic, which may lead to bone deformities and fractures in severe cases.

Management includes transfusion and iron chelation to minimize iron overload. Advances in transfusion and institution of regular chelation therapy with better-tolerated iron-chelating agents—as well as earlier recognition and treatment of iron-induced organ injury—have markedly improved survival rates. *Allogeneic hematopoietic stem cell transplantation (HCT)* is the only cure available for thalassemia. At present, there are no randomized trials comparing HCT with medical therapy, and refinements in treatment have improved both modalities. Prognostic factors associated with a good outcome for HCT are young age of patient, availability of an HLA-identical sibling donor without thalassemia, and matched sibling bone marrow—or umbilical cord blood–derived transplant stem cells. The prognosis for HCT is also correlated with the severity and duration of iron overload. Thus, the importance of iron chelation performed on a regular basis cannot be overemphasized. The likelihood of cure in optimal patients exceeds 90%, with a 4% risk of transplant-related mortality. Splenectomy is an option for some patients with hypersplenism and splenic complications such as splenic infarction or splenic vein thrombosis and may reduce the need for transfusions. The effect of splenectomy, however, may be transient, and its benefits must be weighed against the risk of infection after the procedure.

Jagannath VA, Fedorowicz Z, Al Hajeri A, Sharma A. Hematopoietic stem cell transplantation for people with β-thalassemia major. *Cochrane Database Syst Rev.* 2016;11:CD008708.

Sickle cell disease

Sickle cell disease (SCD), or *sickle cell anemia*, is an autosomal recessive disorder caused by an amino acid substitution on the beta chain, which produces an abnormal form of hemoglobin (*hemoglobin* S) that leads, in turn, to chronic hemolytic anemia. Hemoglobin S, which appears several months after birth, damages the RBC membrane, resulting in malformed sickle-shaped cells. Couples at risk of having a child with SCD can be tested for sickle cell trait, and genetic counseling should be made available to them. SCD is on the list for disorders that newborns are screened for at time of birth. One out of 400 Black persons born in the United States, 1 out of 250 Black persons born in the West Indies, and 1 out of 4000 born in France have SCD. Chronic hemolytic anemia can result in jaundice, gallstones, poorly healing ulcers over the lower tibia, and splenomegaly (which disappears after a few years because of repeated splenic infarction).

In addition to causing hemolytic anemia, SCD has systemic, multiorgan manifestations. It is characterized by acute, painful episodes caused by the sickling of the RBCs (*vaso-occlusive crisis*); these episodes can be precipitated by infection, dehydration, and/or hypoxia. Vascular occlusion can lead to necrosis of bone and to infection. Hematuria can be caused by infarction of the renal papillae. Sickle cell retinopathy can lead to vision loss in severe cases.

With improved supportive care, an affected person now has an average life expectancy into the 50s or 60s. Diagnosis is made with a screening test for sickle cell hemoglobin and confirmed by hemoglobin electrophoresis. SCD requires lifelong routine medical care, which includes regular updating of vaccinations; annual ophthalmologic examinations; and screening for hypertension, proteinuria, and pulmonary hypertension. Patients should be given folic acid supplements and, if infections arise, specific antibiotic treatment. Routine oxygen is no longer used in uncomplicated crises and without pulmonary symptoms. *Hydroxyurea*, the only disease-modifying drug in SCD, has resulted in decreased mortality. *Crizanlizumab*, a novel, investigational monoclonal antibody against P-selectin adhesion molecule, has been shown to reduce episodes of painful vaso-occlusive crisis. Clinical trials are currently under way.

Hematopoietic cell transplantation from an HLA-identical sibling is a potentially curative option in the treatment of SCD. When and for whom HCT should be pursued are controversial. Current data from the Center for International Blood and Bone Marrow Transplant Research and from European Blood and Marrow Transplant registries show an overall survival of 91% and 95%, respectively, after HCT, as well as improved quality of life. However, the possible consequences of HCT must also be considered, including the risk of mortality, debilitating chronic graft-vs-host disease, and infertility. If an HLA-matched sibling donor is available, HCT is recommended for persons under 17 years of age with severe symptoms of SCD that are unresponsive to transfusions and hydroxyurea. Recently, gene editing therapies have shown promise in treating both SCD and β-thalassemia.

Azar S, Wong TE. Sickle cell disease: a brief update. *Med Clin North Am.* 2017;101(2):375–393.

Anemia Due to Destruction of Red Blood Cells

Hemolytic anemia is defined as a condition in which the life span of RBCs is shortened by premature destruction. In response to hemolysis, the kidneys increase synthesis of erythropoietin, stimulating production of RBC precursors and a subsequent rise in reticulocyte count. Peripheral blood smear evaluation may show a pattern of red cell destruction (evidenced by schistocytes or helmet cells) that reveals a potentially life-threatening disease process such as thrombotic microangiopathy associated with thrombotic thrombocytopenic purpura (TTP) or hemolytic-uremic syndrome (HUS).

The causes of hemolytic anemia are numerous and include acquired conditions as well as genetic conditions. Hemolytic anemia may be severe and life-threatening or mild and chronic. Given the numerous etiologies, it is useful to conceptualize the mechanisms of hemolysis as being either *intracorpuscular* (intrinsic defects of the red blood cell that lead to premature destruction) or *extracorpuscular* (in which the red blood cell is rendered susceptible to lysis by extrinsic factors).

Intracorpuscular defects

Intracorpuscular defects may be caused by hemoglobinopathies, genetic membrane or cytoskeletal defects, acquired membrane disorders, or intrinsic metabolic abnormalities, such as the following:

- *Hereditary membrane disorders.* Hereditary spherocytosis is the most common type.
- *Acquired membrane disorders.* Paroxysmal nocturnal hemoglobinuria (PNH) manifests clinically with intravascular hemolysis, nocturnal pink or red urine, and a variable degree of jaundice and fatigue. Diagnosis of PNH is made by flow cytometry, which may incorporate fluorescent aerolysin (FLAER) assay.
- *Metabolic disorders.* Glucose-6-phosphate dehydrogenase (G6PD) deficiency (X-linked inheritance) and pyruvate kinase deficiency increase the susceptibility of red blood cells to oxidative stress and damage.

Extracorpuscular causes

Antibody-mediated destruction leading to anemia (*Coombs-positive hemolytic anemia*) is caused by autoantibodies directed at RBC surface antigens. The condition may be assessed by direct antiglobulin testing (direct Coombs testing) for the presence of anti-IgG or anti-C3d. Other causes of antibody-mediated destruction include drug-induced autoimmune hemolytic anemia, autoimmune disease (systemic lupus erythematosus [SLE]), lymphoproliferative disorders, and transfusion-related hemolysis.

Other extracorpuscular factors leading to accelerated RBC destruction include hypersplenism with increased trapping; red blood cell pathogens like malaria, babesiosis, bartonellosis, and clostridial sepsis; mechanical heart valves; platelet microthrombi, as in TTP or HUS; or fibrin strands in blood vessels that shear the RBCs, as in disseminated intravascular coagulation. In addition, exposure to drugs that cause nonimmune (oxidative stress) destruction; trauma; and, less commonly, toxins such as snake venom, insect bites, and copper poisoning in Wilson disease are extrinsic causes of hemolytic anemia.

Evaluation and management

Hemolytic anemia may be suspected in a patient who has rapid-onset anemia in the absence of blood loss, dark urine, and jaundice, along with laboratory confirmation of hemolysis. A systematic approach to identifying the specific cause of hemolysis includes obtaining a detailed history that may, for example, reveal a recent transfusion, initiation of a new drug, or a family history of a hemoglobinopathy or other genetic disorder. Examination of the peripheral smear and flow cytometry may provide the diagnosis. Treatment of hemolytic anemia depends upon the underlying etiology, but regardless of cause, folic acid supplementation is necessary.

Robertson JJ, Brem E, Koyfman A. The acute hemolytic anemias: the importance of early diagnosis and management. *J Emerg Med.* 2017;53(2):202–211.

Anemia Due to Inflammation and Chronic Disease

Inflammatory anemia can occur in chronic conditions such as chronic infections (eg, tuberculosis, osteomyelitis), malignancies, collagen-vascular diseases, and liver disease. Chronic renal failure can also cause a more severe type of anemia, primarily due to the decrease in erythropoietin production.

Anemia Due to Bone Marrow Disorders

Aplastic anemia

Aplastic anemia refers to anemia with pancytopenia associated with varying degrees of bone marrow hypoplasia/aplasia. The causes are diverse, and the condition has a very high mortality if left untreated. The loss of hematopoietic stem cells in aplastic anemia may be caused by direct toxic injury by drugs, chemicals, ionizing radiation, autoimmune processes, or infectious agents, as well as by clonal and genetic abnormalities. Bone marrow aspiration and biopsy is required to confirm the diagnosis and exclude other conditions that cause pancytopenia such as megaloblastic anemia and bone marrow infiltration.

Sideroblastic anemia

If the incorporation of iron into the heme molecule is defective, hemoglobin synthesis is reduced; this condition is called *sideroblastic anemia (SA)*. Diagnosis of SA is made primarily on the basis of bone marrow examination with Prussian blue stain. A normal sideroblast is an erythroblast with few granules of hemosiderin in the cytoplasm; but in SA, iron accumulation, particularly in the mitochondria, leads to development of the "ring sideroblast." Sideroblastic anemia may be caused by a genetic disorder, or it may develop indirectly as part of a myelodysplastic syndrome (refractory anemia with ring sideroblasts) that can progress to acute myelogenous leukemia or other hematologic malignancies. Other causes of SA are usually acquired and include chronic alcoholism and lead poisoning.

Disorders of Hemostasis

Disorders of hemostasis may be due to defects in platelet number or function or to problems in formation of a fibrin clot (coagulation). A basic understanding of the hemostatic process and the manifestations associated with specific abnormalities helps the ophthalmologist with both medical and surgical management. (See Fig 8-1 for a diagram of blood-clotting pathways.) For the purpose of laboratory test interpretation, the coagulation cascade can be divided into *intrinsic* and *extrinsic* pathways. However, it is now understood that this is an oversimplification. For example, factor IX (an intrinsic factor) can be activated by factor VII (an extrinsic factor).

Hemostasis is initiated by damage to a blood vessel wall. This event triggers constriction of the vessel, followed by accumulation and adherence of platelets at the site of injury. Coagulation factors in the blood are activated, leading to formation of a fibrin clot. Slow fibrinolysis ensues, dissolving the clot while the damage is repaired. Circulating inhibitors are also present, modulating the process by inactivating coagulation factors to prevent widespread clotting. Normal endothelium plays a critical role in naturally anticoagulating

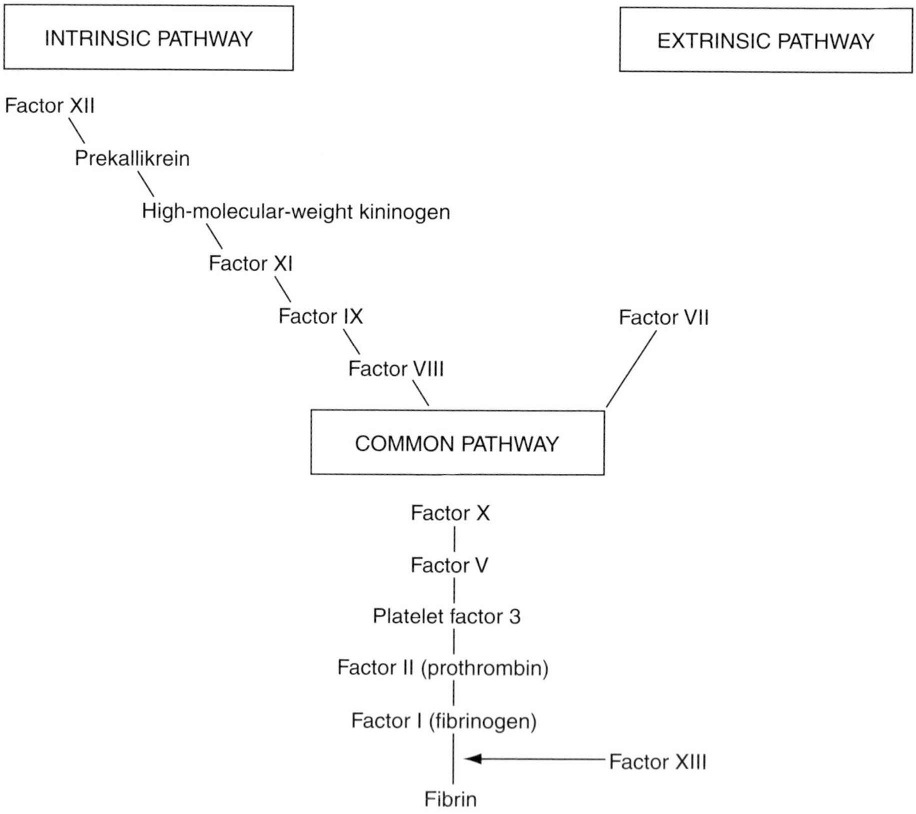

Figure 8-1 Blood-clotting pathways.

blood by preventing fibrin accumulation. The following physiologic antithrombotic components can produce this effect:

- antithrombin
- protein C and/or protein S
- tissue factor pathway inhibitor
- the fibrinolytic system

Antithrombin (formerly AT III) inactivates thrombin. Activated protein C (APC), with its cofactor protein S, functions as a natural anticoagulant by destroying factors Va and VIIa. Thrombin itself activates protein C. Although inherited deficiencies of antithrombin, protein C, or protein S are associated with a lifelong thrombotic tendency, tissue factor pathway inhibitor deficiency has not yet been related to the hypercoagulable state (see the section "Thrombotic disorders" later in this chapter).

Laboratory Evaluation of Hemostasis and Blood Coagulation

Various techniques are used to assess the status of a patient's hemostatic mechanisms. Following are some of the most common tests:

- *Platelet count.* Minor bleeding may occur at platelet counts below 50,000/μL. Abnormal bleeding at higher platelet counts suggests abnormal platelet function. Below 20,000/μL, spontaneous bleeding may be serious.
- *Tests of platelet function.*
  - *Bleeding time.* This was the first test of in vivo platelet function. However, because it is operator-dependent, insensitive, time-consuming, and poorly reproducible, it will likely be phased out.
  - *Platelet function analyzer.* This rapid and simple test measures the ability of activated platelets in a high-shear environment to occlude an aperture; it replaces in vivo bleeding time.
  - *Platelet aggregometry.* Various techniques include impedance whole blood, light transmission, and the VerifyNow assay. Light transmission aggregometry is the current gold standard test for measuring platelet function and inhibition.
  - *Activated partial thromboplastin time (aPTT).* The aPTT test incorporates factors I, II, V, VIII, IX, X, XI, and XII; prekallikrein; and high-molecular-weight kininogen. The aPTT test is most commonly used to measure the effect of heparin therapy. Platelet abnormalities do not affect the result of this test.
  - *Prothrombin time (PT).* The PT test measures the integrity of factors I, II, V, VII, and X. It requires a 30% concentration of the vitamin K–dependent factors II, VII, and X (but not factor IX, a part of the intrinsic pathway) and therefore is prolonged in conditions affecting these factors (see Disorders of Blood Coagulation later in this chapter). The PT test is most commonly used to monitor anticoagulant therapy. The action of heparin may slightly prolong PT.

Efforts have been made to tailor anticoagulation therapy to the problem being treated. For example, treatment or prevention of deep venous thrombosis is thought to require less oral anticoagulation therapy than treatment of endocardial mural thrombi or cardiac replacement valves. However, because of variation in test results among and within laboratories, the international normalized ratio (INR) was developed. The INR modifies the standard PT ratio (patient PT to control PT) to reflect the particular thromboplastin reagent used by a laboratory. The resulting reported INR value is an expression of the ratio of the patient's PT to the laboratory's mean normal PT. Thus, for prevention or treatment of deep venous thrombosis, the recommended INR value (comparable to subsequent values measured over time or across laboratories) is 2.0–3.0; for tissue replacement valves, 2.0–3.0; and for mechanical replacement valves, 2.5–3.5.

Genetic testing in the form of a DNA assay is also available to determine the correct warfarin dose for an individual patient, especially in cases in which resistance to the drug is suspected. This knowledge has substantially reduced the risk of bleeding and clotting events.

Clinical Manifestations of Hemostatic Abnormalities

Hemorrhage resulting from hemostatic derangement must be differentiated from hemorrhage caused by localized processes. The presence of generalized or recurrent bleeding suggests abnormal hemostasis. *Petechiae* (small capillary hemorrhages of the skin and mucous membranes) and *purpura* (ecchymoses) are typical of platelet disorders and vasculitis. Subcutaneous hematomas and hemarthroses characterize coagulation abnormalities. Bleeding due to trauma may be massive and life-threatening in coagulation disorders, whereas bleeding is more likely to be slow and prolonged when platelet function is impaired.

Vascular Disorders

A number of inherited and acquired disorders of blood vessels and their supporting connective tissues result in pathologic bleeding. *Hereditary hemorrhagic telangiectasia* (Rendu-Osler-Weber disease) is an autosomal dominant condition characterized by localized dilation of capillaries and venulae of the skin and mucous membranes. The lesions increase in size and number over a period of decades, often leading to profuse bleeding.

Several inherited vascular disorders are associated with hemorrhage. *Ehlers-Danlos syndrome* is characterized by hyperplastic fragile skin and hyperextensible joints; it is dominantly inherited. In *osteogenesis imperfecta,* also a dominant disorder, bone fractures and otosclerosis (leading to deafness) are common. In both conditions, easy bruising and hematomas are common. *Pseudoxanthoma elasticum,* a recessive disorder, is much rarer but is often complicated by gastrointestinal hemorrhage. *Marfan syndrome* is sometimes associated with mild bleeding as well as with aortic dissection.

Scurvy, the result of severe ascorbic acid deficiency, is associated with marked vascular fragility and hemorrhagic manifestations resulting from abnormal synthesis of collagen. In addition to the classic findings of perifollicular petechiae and gingival bleeding, intradermal, intramuscular, and subperiosteal hemorrhages are common. *Amyloidosis* is another acquired disorder in which petechiae and purpura are common.

Ophthalmic considerations All of the inherited vascular disorders have associated ocular findings. Conjunctival lesions occur in hereditary hemorrhagic telangiectasia. Blue sclerae are typical of osteogenesis imperfecta.

Ocular manifestations of Ehlers-Danlos syndrome include microcornea, myopia, and angioid streaks; retinal detachment and ectopia lentis have also been reported. Angioid streaks also occur in patients with pseudoxanthoma elasticum. Fifty percent of patients with Marfan syndrome have ectopia lentis; severe myopia and retinal detachment are common.

Platelet Disorders

By far the most common cause of abnormal bleeding, platelet disorders may result from an insufficient number of platelets, inadequate functioning, or both. Mild derangement of platelet function may be asymptomatic or may cause minor bruising, menorrhagia, or bleeding after surgery. More severe dysfunction leads to petechiae, purpura, and gastrointestinal bleeding and other types of serious bleeding.

Thrombocytopenia

The number of platelets may be reduced by decreased production, increased destruction, or abnormal distribution. Production may be suppressed by many factors, including radiation, drugs, chemotherapy, alcohol use, malignant invasion of the bone marrow, aplastic anemia, and vitamin B_{12} or folic acid deficiency.

Thrombocytopenia due to immune destruction *Idiopathic thrombocytopenic purpura (ITP)* is the result of platelet injury by antiplatelet antibodies. The International Working Group on ITP classifies it into 3 categories: primary ITP; secondary ITP associated with other conditions such as SLE, HIV infection, malignancy, and hepatitis C; and drug-induced thrombocytopenia. The acute form of ITP usually occurs in children and young adults, often following a viral illness, and commonly undergoes spontaneous remission. Chronic ITP is more common in adults and is characterized by mild manifestations; spontaneous remission is uncommon. Initial treatment consists of corticosteroid therapy. Patients with ITP who do not respond to corticosteroid therapy, who are bleeding and require rapid increase in platelet count, or who require surgical intervention should receive intravenous immunoglobulin. Alternatively, anti-D immunoglobulin may be administered in those who are Rh positive. Rituximab or splenectomy is recommended for ITP refractory to corticosteroids and intravenous immunoglobulin. Because spontaneous remission may occur, clinicians often delay splenectomy for at least 6 months. Thrombopoietin receptor agonists (TPO-RAs) such as eltrombopag, avatrombopag, or romiplostim, or immunosuppressive agents such as azathioprine, cyclosporine, or mycophenolate mofetil may also be of benefit. Fostamatinib has also recently received FDA approval for treatment of chronic ITP. Splenectomy, however, has been reported to provide the highest durable remission rate and, in balance, still appears to be the favored second-line treatment over rituximab and TPO-RAs, except in poor surgical candidates or those who prefer a nonsurgical approach.

A neonatal form of the disorder occurs in babies born to women with ITP; this form results from transplacental passage of antiplatelet antibodies. Recovery follows physiologic clearance of the antibodies from the child's circulation.

Many drugs and other substances, including quinine, quinidine, digitalis, procainamide, thiazide-type diuretics, sulfonamides, phenytoin, aspirin, penicillin, heparin, and gold compounds, have been implicated as causes of immunologic platelet destruction. Drug-induced thrombocytopenia is common, and discontinuation of the offending drug should result in platelet recovery.

Nonimmunologic thrombocytopenia Types of nonimmunologic thrombocytopenia include *thrombotic thrombocytopenic purpura (TTP), hemolytic-uremic syndrome (HUS),* and the syndromes of *disseminated intravascular coagulation* (see the section "Disseminated intravascular coagulation" later in the chapter). TTP is caused by an inherited or acquired deficiency of the von Willebrand factor–cleaving protease ADAMTS13. It is characterized by thrombotic microangiopathy and hemolytic anemia. Fever, neurologic symptoms, microangiopathic hemolytic anemia (MAHA), thrombocytopenia, and renal dysfunction occur, often with subacute onset. Death occurs in days to weeks in the majority of untreated cases. However, early treatment with exchange plasmapheresis has improved the survival rate to over 80%, especially when rituximab is given as part of initial therapy. Despite significant thrombocytopenia, bleeding is relatively uncommon. Therefore, platelet transfusions are usually unnecessary because plasma exchange abates the consumption process. However, platelet transfusion may be indicated in patients with severe bleeding or in those who will undergo an invasive procedure. Refractory cases may be treated with antiplatelet drugs, corticosteroids, and immunosuppressive agents. Eculizumab is recommended in complement-mediated TTP.

Hemolytic-uremic syndrome is similar in pathophysiology to TTP in that both are associated with MAHA, thrombocytopenia, and renal involvement. The most common cause of HUS, especially among children, is Shiga toxin–producing *Escherichia coli* (STEC), which accounts for 90% of cases of HUS. TTP and HUS are similar in clinical appearance, and laboratory confirmation of low ADAMTS13 activity (<10% in patients with TTP) may take several days; these factors complicate the decision whether to initiate plasma exchange or anticomplement therapy emergently. The abnormal distribution of platelets is most commonly caused by splenic sequestration. The usual clinical setting is hepatic cirrhosis, and the level of thrombocytopenia is mild. Patients with severely depressed platelet counts probably also have accelerated platelet destruction in the spleen.

Thrombocytosis and essential thrombocythemia

Thrombocytosis is defined as a platelet count exceeding 450,000. *Essential thrombocythemia (ET)* refers to an excess of platelets due to a primary bone marrow clonal disorder. *Reactive thrombocytosis* is secondary to other conditions such as inflammatory disorders. Management of reactive thrombocytosis is aimed at treating the underlying cause such as infection, inflammation (eg, giant cell arteritis), trauma, iron deficiency, congestive heart failure, renal failure, and pancreatitis. In contrast, ET is a clonal myeloproliferative disorder akin to neoplastic disease. Severe autonomous increase in platelet counts may also be caused by other myeloproliferative disorders such as polycythemia vera, primary myelofibrosis with myeloid metaplasia, chronic myeloid leukemia (CML), and myelodysplastic syndromes.

Epidemiologic studies have determined a prevalence rate of ET of 30/100,000 in the general population worldwide with a nearly 2:1 ratio between men and women. Regardless of etiology, severe thrombocytosis can cause both thrombotic and hemorrhagic events. However, thrombohemorrhagic complications are much more common in ET and in other clonal myeloproliferative disorders and include arterial and venous thromboses, cerebrovascular accident, myocardial infarction, and deep venous thrombosis. Hemorrhagic events include ecchymoses, subcutaneous hematomas, epistaxis, and gum bleeding. About 36% of patients, however, are asymptomatic. There is a 2%–5% long-term risk of leukemic transformation into acute myeloid leukemia. Treatment is centered on inhibition of platelet aggregation, especially in patients at high risk of thrombotic events, as well as cytoreduction. Aspirin and other antiplatelet agents such as ticlopidine and clopidogrel inhibit aggregation. Hydroxyurea and interferon alfa reduce platelet counts by bone marrow inhibition. Anagrelide, a phosphodiesterase inhibitor, has both platelet antiaggregating and cytoreductive properties.

Birgegård G. Advances and challenges in the management of essential thrombocythemia. *Ther Adv Hematol.* 2015; 6(3):142–156.

Geyer HL, Kosiorek H, Dueck AC, et al. Associations between gender, disease features and symptom burden in patients with myeloproliferative neoplasms: an analysis by the MPN QOL International Working Group. *Haematologica.* 2017;102(1):85–93.

Ophthalmic considerations Reported ocular manifestations of ET include ischemic optic neuropathy and retinal vein occlusion. For more information on these conditions, see BCSC Section 5, *Neuro-Ophthalmology,* and Section 12, *Retina and Vitreous.*

Platelet dysfunction

Patients with platelet dysfunction usually come to the physician's attention because of easy bruising, epistaxis, menorrhagia, or excessive bleeding after surgery or dental work. Unlike patients with marked thrombocytopenia, patients with platelet dysfunction rarely have petechiae.

Hereditary disorders of platelet function are rare. Much more important clinically are the acquired forms, of which drug ingestion is the most common cause. As with drugs causing antiplatelet antibodies, the list of causative agents is very long. A single aspirin tablet taken orally irreversibly inhibits platelet aggregation for the life span of the circulating platelets present, causing a modest prolongation of bleeding time for at least 48–72 hours following ingestion. This reaction has remarkably little effect in otherwise healthy individuals, although intraoperative blood loss may be slightly increased. However, bleeding may be significant in patients with hemophilia, severe thrombocytopenia, or uremia and in those on warfarin or heparin therapy.

Nonsteroidal anti-inflammatory drugs cause reversible inhibition of platelet function in the presence of the drug; the effect disappears as the drug is cleared from the blood. Other commonly used drugs that may affect platelet function include ethanol, tricyclic antidepressants, and antihistamines.

In addition to uremia, clinical conditions associated with abnormal platelet function include liver disease, multiple myeloma, SLE, chronic lymphocytic leukemia, and Hermansky-Pudlak syndrome (an autosomal recessive form of oculocutaneous albinism).

Disorders of Blood Coagulation

Hereditary coagulation disorders

Inherited coagulation abnormalities involve all of the coagulation factors except factors III and IV. The most common and most severe of these abnormalities is factor VIII deficiency, called *hemophilia A,* or *classical hemophilia.* Factor IX deficiency is called *hemophilia B.* Both types are X-linked. Typical manifestations of hemophilia A include severe and protracted bleeding, after even minor trauma, and spontaneous bleeding into joints (hemarthroses), the central nervous system, and the abdominal cavity.

Treatment of hemophilia A involves infusion of factor VIII. With the availability of recombinant factor VIII, the risk of transmission of hepatitis B and C and HIV has now been mostly eliminated. However, about 5%–10% of patients with hemophilia A develop inhibiting antibodies, presumably due to sensitization following administration of factor VIII. These inhibitors bind to the infused factor VIII and render it ineffective; subsequently, the patient will need bypassing agents such as recombinant factor VIIa or an anti-inhibitor coagulant complex. Antibodies inhibiting coagulation can also develop in healthy older patients, in nonhemophilic patients after drug reactions, and in those with inherited vascular disorders. Clinical manifestations range from mild bleeding to full-blown hemophilia that correlates with level of factor deficiency. The aPTT is prolonged, while the PT is normal. Treatment involves various regimens of coagulation factor replacement and immunosuppression in an attempt to eliminate the inhibitor. However, during episodes of bleeding or as prophylaxis before surgery, patients with high titers of inhibitor should receive recombinant factor VIIa or an anti-inhibitor coagulant complex as first-line therapy. *Emicizumab,* a monoclonal antibody that binds factor IXa and supplants the need for factor VIIIa as a cofactor for factor X activation, was recently approved by the FDA. An investigational monoclonal antibody, *concizumab,* which inhibits the tissue factor pathway, is now in clinical trials. Gene therapy is currently in the developmental phase but could further transform the outlook for these patients.

Von Willebrand disease (vWD) is the most common inherited bleeding disorder: low levels of von Willebrand factor (vWF) are found in 1% of the population. The 2 main functions of vWF are stabilizing factor VIII to prevent degradation and promoting platelet adhesion. There are 3 major types of vWD. *Type 1* is autosomal dominant and accounts for 75% of cases. *Type 2* (15%–20% of cases) has 4 subtypes and is predominantly autosomal dominant, and *type 3* (5%) is autosomal recessive. Type 1 manifests with mild mucocutaneous bleeding, and most forms of type 2 are associated with mild to moderate bleeding. In contrast, the recessively inherited forms are associated with very low levels of factor VIII and severe bleeding. A form of vWD also occurs in patients with aortic valve stenosis and in some patients with thrombocythemia. Desmopressin, a synthetic form of vasopressin (antidiuretic hormone), may be used for episodes of bleeding and administered preoperatively to reduce risk of surgical bleeding. Plasma-derived concentrates to replace vWF are available for patients who cannot tolerate desmopressin or need prolonged treatment.

Bhat R, Cabey W. Evaluation and management of congenital bleeding disorders. *Hematol Oncol Clin North Am.* 2017;31(6):1105–1122.

Oldenberg J, Mahlangu JN, Kim B, et al. Emicizumab prophylaxis in hemophilia A with inhibitors. *N Engl J Med.* 2017;377(9):809–818.

Acquired coagulation disorders

Vitamin K deficiency Vitamin K is required for the production of factors II (prothrombin), VII, IX, and X in the liver. Normal diets contain large amounts of vitamin K, which is also synthesized by intestinal flora. Causes of vitamin K deficiency include biliary obstruction and various malabsorption syndromes (including sprue, cystic fibrosis, and celiac disease), in which intestinal absorption of vitamin K is reduced. Suppression of endogenous gastrointestinal flora, seen commonly in hospitalized patients on prolonged broad-spectrum antibiotic therapy, decreases intestinal production of vitamin K. However, clinical deficiency occurs only if dietary intake is also diminished. Nutritional deficiency is unusual but may occur with prolonged parenteral nutrition. Laboratory evaluation reveals prolongation of both PT and, later in the course of the disease, aPTT. Most forms of vitamin K deficiency respond to subcutaneous or intramuscular administration of 20 mg of vitamin K_1; coagulation defects normalize within 24 hours. Vitamin K_1 should not be given intravenously because of the risk of sudden death from an anaphylactoid reaction.

One special form of vitamin K deficiency is *hemorrhagic disease of the newborn,* which is the result of a normal mild deficiency of vitamin K–dependent factors during the first 5 days of life and the absence of the vitamin in maternal milk. This condition is now rare in developed countries because of the routine administration of vitamin K to newborns. (See also the section Antiphospholipid Syndrome in Chapter 9.)

Liver disease Hemostatic abnormalities of all types may be associated with disease of the liver, the site of production of all the coagulation factors except factor VIII and factor XIII A-subunit. As liver dysfunction develops, levels of the vitamin K–dependent factors decrease first, followed by those of factors V, XI, and XII; both PT and aPTT are prolonged. Thrombocytopenia, primarily the result of hypersplenism, and a prolonged bleeding time due to platelet dysfunction are common. In addition, intravascular coagulation and fibrinolysis are often present, further complicating the clinical picture.

Mild hemorrhagic symptoms are common in patients with significant liver disease. Severe bleeding is usually gastrointestinal in origin, arising from peptic ulcers, gastritis, or esophageal varices. Treatment is difficult at best and consists of blood and coagulation factor replacement. Local measures, such as vasopressin infusion or balloon tamponade of bleeding varices, can sometimes control potentially catastrophic bleeding.

Disseminated intravascular coagulation *Disseminated intravascular coagulation (DIC)* is a complex syndrome involving widespread activation of the coagulation and fibrinolytic systems within the general circulation. The syndrome is a secondary process, triggered by exposure of procoagulants to the bloodstream, which activates the coagulation cascade, resulting in formation of fibrin and fibrin degradation products (fibrin split products), resulting in occlusion of the microcirculation as well as various forms of organ failure and, occasionally, thrombosis of larger vessels. Subsequently, utilization and consumption of the coagulation factors and platelets produce bleeding. Laboratory findings may vary but usually include thrombocytopenia, hypofibrinogenemia, and elevated levels of fibrin split products. PT and aPTT are usually, but not invariably, prolonged.

Clinically, 2 forms of DIC are recognized. *Acute DIC* is characterized by the abrupt onset of severe, generalized bleeding. The most common causes are obstetric complications (most notably abruptio placentae and amniotic fluid embolism), septicemia, shock, massive trauma, malignancy (especially acute promyelocytic leukemia), ABO incompatibility, and major surgical procedures. Bleeding, thrombocytopenia, prolonged PT/aPTT, reduced procoagulant factors, low plasma fibrinogen, and reduced levels of coagulation inhibitors are characteristics of acute DIC. Treatment, other than specific measures aimed at the underlying disease, is controversial. Among the modalities used are heparinization and replacement of blood, platelets, and fibrinogen.

Chronic DIC is associated with disseminated solid-tumor neoplasms (pancreatic, ovarian, gastric, or brain) and autoimmune diseases. Laboratory values range from normal to moderately abnormal; levels of coagulation factors may even be elevated (high plasma fibrinogen). Bleeding and thrombosis (especially lower extremity deep venous thrombosis and pulmonary embolism) may occur, but the syndrome remains undiagnosed in most patients unless renal failure results from intravascular coagulation in the kidney. Many patients with chronic DIC do not require specific therapy for the coagulopathy because it is not severe enough to present a major risk of bleeding or thrombosis. On occasion, chronic DIC may convert to the acute form.

Thrombotic disorders

The hypercoagulable states encompass a group of inherited and acquired thrombotic disorders that increase the risk of thrombosis *(thrombophilia)*. The *primary hypercoagulable states* are caused by abnormalities of specific coagulation proteins resulting from inherited mutations in one of the antithrombotic factors. The trigger for a thrombotic event is often the development of one of the acquired secondary hypercoagulable states superimposed on an inherited state of hypercoagulability. The *secondary hypercoagulable states* lead to a thrombotic tendency by means of complex and often multifactorial mechanisms.

Primary Hypercoagulable States

Activated protein C resistance (factor V Leiden mutation)

Factor V is a procoagulant factor that amplifies thrombin production. Most patients with APC resistance harbor a single specific point mutation in the factor V gene, termed *factor V Leiden,* which renders both forms of factor V (active and inactive) insensitive to APC proteolysis. This mutation occurs with remarkable frequency (3%–7%) in healthy White populations but appears to be far less prevalent or even absent in certain Black and Asian populations. The major clinical manifestation of the heterozygous form is deep venous thrombosis or pulmonary embolism, for which there is a lifetime risk of 5% in the general population but up to 20% in families with history of thrombophilia. Asymptomatic heterozygotes with no history of thromboembolic events do not need to be routinely screened for other thrombophilias or treated with anticoagulants except in high-risk situations such as surgery or pregnancy.

Kujovich JL. Factor V Leiden thrombophilia. *Genet Med.* 2011;13(1):1–16.

Prothrombin G20210A gene mutation

The G20210A mutation in the prothrombin gene has been associated with elevated plasma levels of prothrombin. It is second only to factor V Leiden as a genetic risk factor for venous thrombosis and is also a risk factor for premature cardiovascular disease. It is much more common among White populations than in other populations. The risk of venous thromboembolism (VTE) increases 20-fold when both prothrombin G20210A and factor V Leiden mutation are present in the same individual.

Antithrombin deficiency

Antithrombin deficiency is rare. It leads to increased thrombin generation and, hence, fibrin accumulation with a lifelong propensity for thrombosis. A meta-analysis of case control and cohort studies showed a 16-fold increased risk of developing VTE in patients with antithrombin deficiency. This mutation may be acquired or hereditary.

Protein C deficiency

Protein C deficiency is also rare, affecting between 0.2% and 0.5% of the general population. This disorder leads to unregulated fibrin generation due to impaired inactivation of factors VIIIa and Va. The risk of VTE in patients who have protein C deficiency is increased 7-fold compared to that of persons without this deficiency.

Protein S deficiency

Protein S is the principal cofactor of APC; therefore, its deficiency mimics that of protein C. The prevalence of this condition in patients presenting with VTE is about 1%, and patients with protein S deficiency have 5 times the risk of developing VTE than those without this deficiency.

Screening for inherited thrombophilia

Screening for these conditions in the unselected general population is not recommended because of the low prevalence, low and variable penetrance among carriers, and lack of safe and cost-effective prophylaxis. Screening would be appropriate in the following groups:

- pedigrees that include multiple first-degree relatives with inherited thrombophilia and VTE onset before age 50
- family members of probands with symptomatic thrombophilia, particularly those who have protein C, protein S, or antithrombin deficiency
- women who plan to use oral contraceptives or hormone replacement therapy and have a family history of VTE with thrombophilia

Screening for methylenetetrahydrofolate reductase (*MTHFR*) gene variants, assaying homocysteine levels, or seeking plasminogen activator/promoter variants is not recommended, as there is no evidence that risk for blood clots is significantly higher or that prophylactic anticoagulation reduces risk.

De Stefano V, Rossi E. Testing for inherited thrombophilia and consequences for antithrombotic prophylaxis in patients with venous thromboembolism and their relatives. A review of the guidelines from scientific societies and working groups. *Thromb Haemost.* 2013;110(4):697–705.

Hyperhomocysteinemia

Hyperhomocysteinemia, which is caused by elevated blood levels of homocysteine, leads to severe neurologic developmental abnormalities in the homozygous state. Adults with the heterozygous state may have only thrombotic tendencies. Acquired causes of hyperhomocysteinemia in adults commonly involve nutritional deficiencies of pyridoxine, vitamin B_{12}, and folate, all of which are cofactors in homocysteine metabolism. High blood concentration of homocysteine constitutes an independent risk factor for both venous and arterial thrombosis; in contrast, all of the other primary hypercoagulable states are associated only with venous thromboembolic complications, usually involving the lower extremities. The initial treatment of acute venous thrombosis in these patients does not differ from that in patients without genetic defects.

Ophthalmic considerations Primary hypercoagulable states, particularly factor V Leiden mutation and subsequent APC resistance, are risk factors for central and branch retinal vein occlusion, especially in young patients.

Secondary Hypercoagulable States

Malignancy may stimulate thrombosis directly by elaborating procoagulant substances that initiate chronic DIC. This appears to be most prominent in patients with pancreatic cancer, adenocarcinoma of the gastrointestinal tract or lung, or ovarian cancer. *Myeloproliferative disorders* (see the earlier section "Thrombocytosis and essential thrombocythemia") are major causes of thrombosis and paradoxical bleeding, as is *paroxysmal nocturnal hemoglobinuria,* a related stem cell disorder.

Antiphospholipid syndrome is characterized by both venous and arterial thrombosis, including recurrent spontaneous abortions, deep venous thrombosis, and thrombotic events involving the cerebrovascular arteries. Evaluation of patients with this syndrome includes tests for anticardiolipin antibodies and lupus anticoagulants. See the section Antiphospholipid Syndrome in Chapter 9 for additional discussion.

Hypercoagulability associated with *pregnancy* involves a progressive state of DIC throughout the course of pregnancy, activated in the uteroplacental circulation. *Oral contraceptives* induce similar changes. The *postoperative state* and *trauma* are significant causes of venous thrombosis.

Ophthalmic considerations Ophthalmic complications of antiphospholipid syndrome include retinal vein and artery occlusion, retinal vasculitis, choroidal infarction, and nonarteritic anterior ischemic optic neuropathy, particularly in young patients without other traditional risk factors for thromboembolic disease.

Therapeutic anticoagulation

Many clinical situations require intentional disruption of the hemostatic process. The effect of aspirin on platelet function has already been discussed.

Unfractionated heparin (UFH) is a mucopolysaccharide that binds antithrombin III, potentiating its effects and inhibiting the formation of thrombin. It is given intravenously or subcutaneously, and therapy is assessed by measuring the aPTT. Aspirin should not be given to patients receiving heparin because the resultant platelet dysfunction may provoke bleeding. Low-molecular-weight (LMW) heparins are another type of parenteral anticoagulant. LMW heparins have a number of advantages over UFH, including greater bioavailability when given by subcutaneous injection and greater duration of anticoagulant effect, permitting once- or twice-daily administration. The dose is highly correlated with body weight, allowing administration of a fixed dose, and laboratory monitoring is not necessary. In addition, the risk of heparin-induced thrombocytopenia is lower. *Direct parenteral thrombin inhibitors*, such as lepirudin, argatroban, and bivalirudin, are utilized during percutaneous coronary intervention and for the treatment of heparin-induced thrombocytopenia.

There are 2 groups of *direct oral anticoagulants*: factor Xa inhibitors (eg, rivaroxaban, apixaban, and edoxaban) and direct thrombin inhibitors (eg, dabigatran). These are fixed-dose oral agents that, unlike vitamin K antagonists, do not require routine laboratory monitoring or dose adjustments. Another advantage is that they reach their peak efficacy in 1–4 hours after ingestion; therefore, a period of bridging therapy is not required when switching from the initial treatment (eg, heparin) to these agents. Furthermore, unlike heparin and vitamin K antagonists, these drugs bind to circulating as well as clot-bound thrombin or factor Xa. Until recently, the major disadvantage of these drugs was that no antidotes were readily available in case of bleeding events. However, idarucizumab, a dabigatran-specific Fab fragment, is now available and has been shown in vitro to reverse the effect of dabigatran within 15 minutes. More recently andexanet alfa, a recombinant factor Xa decoy molecule, has been approved for reversal of rivaroxaban and apixaban. Ciraparantag, which can potentially inhibit the anticoagulant effect of factor Xa inhibitors, is under investigation but is not yet FDA-approved. Fondaparinux, which binds to antithrombin, is a synthetic anticoagulant that is very similar to UFH and LMW heparin. It exclusively catalyzes antithrombin inhibition of factor Xa. Because it is eliminated in the kidney, it should be used cautiously in patients with renal disease. See Chapter 5, Table 5-1, in this volume for a list of direct oral antithrombotic agents.

The orally administered warfarin derivatives, of which warfarin sodium is the most widely used, inhibit the production of normal vitamin K–dependent coagulation factors (II, VII, IX, and X). Therapeutic effect is assessed by measuring the patient's INR. One critical issue is the long list of commonly used drugs that interact with warfarin. These interactions may cause an unintended increase or decrease in the INR, depending on the drug.

Heparin and the warfarin derivatives are used to prevent the formation of new thrombi and the propagation of existing thrombi, but neither affects the original clot. Thrombolytic agents such as streptokinase, urokinase, and tissue plasminogen activator (tPA) are sometimes indicated to lyse existing thrombi, as in the very early stages of myocardial infarction and in the early treatment of thrombotic stroke. See Chapter 5, Table 5-2, in this volume for a list of intravenous and subcutaneous antithrombotic agents.

Goldman L, Schafer AI. eds. *Goldman-Cecil Medicine.* 25th ed. Philadelphia: Elsevier/Saunders; 2015. Section XIV, Hematologic Diseases.

Milling TJ Jr, Kaatz S. Preclinical and clinical data for factor Xa and "universal" reversal agents. *Am J Med.* 2016;129(11 Suppl):S80–88.

Pollack CV Jr, Reilly PA, van Ryn J, et al. Idarucizumab for dabigatran reversal—full cohort analysis. *N Engl J Med.* 2017;377(5):431–441.

CHAPTER 9

Rheumatic Disorders

Highlights

- Effective biologic agents are continually being developed for the treatment of rheumatologic diseases. These agents target cytokines through various mechanisms: inhibiting tumor necrosis factor (TNF), blocking interleukin receptors, modifying T-cell or B-cell activity, or inhibiting the Janus kinase enzyme involved in mediating inflammation.
- Anti–TNF-α agents can be associated with significant adverse effects in rare instances, such as lymphoma or opportunistic infections, and may be linked to demyelinating disease, including optic neuritis.
- Actual body weight is more predictive than ideal body weight in assessing risk of maculopathy from the use of hydroxychloroquine.
- Undiagnosed spondyloarthritis may present with anterior uveitis.
- Children with the common forms of juvenile idiopathic arthritis should be periodically screened for uveitis, which is often asymptomatic.
- Clinicians should consider antiphospholipid syndrome when atypical ocular vaso-occlusive disease occurs in a patient younger than age 50.

Introduction

The rheumatic disorders are a heterogeneous collection of autoimmune and inflammatory diseases that include rheumatoid arthritis, spondyloarthritis, connective tissue diseases, and the vasculitides. Ocular involvement is common in autoimmune diseases, but its prevalence and manifestations vary among the different disorders. Ophthalmologists should be familiar with these conditions, their potential for ocular involvement, and the pharmacotherapy used. If a patient has been diagnosed with a rheumatic disorder, it is important for the ophthalmologist and the rheumatologist to communicate and to coordinate management. Treatment of rheumatic diseases commonly involves systemic anti-inflammatory and immunosuppressive therapy, some of which have ocular effects. Drug therapy is discussed at the end of this chapter.

Rheumatoid Arthritis

Rheumatoid arthritis (RA) is the most common rheumatic disorder, affecting approximately 1% of adults worldwide, and is 3 times more likely to occur in women than in men. RA is classically a progressive, symmetric, and deforming peripheral polyarthritis characterized by synovial inflammation and hypertrophy as well as autoantibody production. Although it can involve any joint, RA primarily affects the small joints of the hands and feet. Typically, affected joints are swollen and tender, with decreased range of motion and deformity from bone and cartilage destruction. Hand deformities (Fig 9-1) include nodules, ulnar deviation, Boutonnière deformity (abnormally flexed proximal interphalangeal [PIP] joint and extended distal interphalangeal [DIP] joint), and swan-neck deformity (abnormally hyperextended PIP and flexed DIP). Early diagnosis and treatment are critical in controlling the joint damage and associated disability.

Extra-articular Manifestations

Extra-articular involvement, which is an indicator of disease severity, occurs in about 40% of RA patients over the course of the illness. Risk factors for systemic involvement include the presence of rheumatoid factor (RF), anti–cyclic citrullinated peptide (CCP) antibodies, and smoking. RA can affect almost all systems; manifestations include

- subcutaneous rheumatoid nodules (in approximately 25% of patients)
- anemia of chronic disease (common in RA patients)
- increased risk of lymphoma
- Felty syndrome (seropositive RA, neutropenia, and splenomegaly)
- osteopenia and a higher risk of fractures
- pleural effusions, pulmonary nodules, and interstitial fibrosis
- cardiac disease (coronary artery disease, pericarditis and effusions, valvular disease from rheumatoid nodules, and cardiomyopathy from secondary amyloid deposition)
- peripheral vascular disease and vasculitis (small- to medium-sized vessels)
- carpal tunnel syndrome (from synovitis, compressive myelopathy, or radiculopathy)
- muscle weakness (primary or drug-induced myopathy)

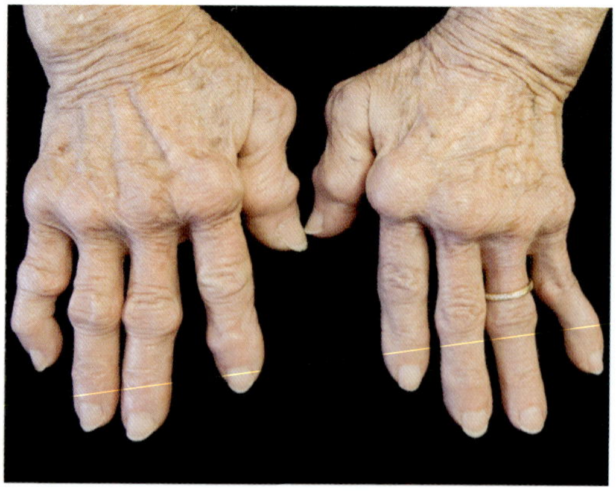

Figure 9-1 Rheumatoid arthritis showing characteristic ulnar deviation, swollen joints, and swan-neck deformities. *(Courtesy of Darin K. Bowers, MD.)*

Ocular involvement may include dry eye disease, scleritis, episcleritis, and corneal inflammation, melting, and infection. The ocular manifestations of RA are discussed in BCSC Section 8, *External Disease and Cornea*, and Section 9, *Uveitis and Ocular Inflammation*.

Laboratory Testing

Serologic testing is important in the workup and diagnosis of RA. *Rheumatoid factor (RF)* is present in 70%–80% of patients. However, it has limited specificity for the disease, as it can be positive in up to 10% of unaffected individuals and in about one-third of patients with systemic lupus erythematosus (SLE). *Anti-CCP antibody* is as sensitive as RF but has a higher specificity for RA (98%). Nevertheless, both of these tests may be negative in up to 50% of RA patients. Similarly, *anti–mutated citrullinated vimentin (anti-MCV) antibody* testing shows high specificity for the disease. *Erythrocyte sedimentation rate (ESR)* and *C-reactive protein (CRP)* levels are usually elevated. *Antinuclear antibody (ANA)* testing is nonspecific, because only 30% of RA patients have positive results, but it can help exclude other diseases such as SLE. Although genetic testing is not performed routinely, the *HLA-DRB1* gene appears to be the strongest known genetic risk factor for the development of RA.

Treatment

Treatment of RA involves an integrated approach, incorporating medications and nondrug therapies. Nonpharmacologic interventions include dietary counseling, exercise, physical therapy, smoking cessation, lipid control (to reduce the associated cardiovascular risks), and immunizations (to reduce the risk of infection linked with the use of immunosuppressive agents).

The ultimate goal of pharmacologic treatment (discussed in detail at the end of this chapter) is disease remission. Early diagnosis and treatment are imperative in preventing or delaying the long-term effects of disease progression. Mild symptoms of joint stiffness and pain can be treated with analgesics and *nonsteroidal anti-inflammatory drugs (NSAIDs)*, although these agents do not alter the long-term prognosis. *Glucocorticoids* are sometimes helpful in controlling the acute stages of inflammation; severe cases may require sustained low-dose therapy (<10 mg/day).

Disease-modifying antirheumatic drugs (DMARDs), which are divided into nonbiologic and biologic agents, have been shown to slow disease progression, reduce potential joint destruction, and maintain joint function while also limiting the need for long-term steroid use. In addition to their anti-inflammatory effect, these drugs reduce the body's heightened autoimmune reaction. Thus, the clinician should consider screening for preexisting infectious conditions such as hepatitis B and C and tuberculosis. Among *nonbiologic agents*, methotrexate is generally the first-line treatment, but other options are available. *Biologic agents*, developed through genetic engineering, are modified proteins that can target cytokines. The largest group of currently available agents consists of anti–tumor necrosis factor (TNF)-α inhibitors. Other biologics act by blocking interleukin (IL)-1 or IL-6 receptors or in modifying T-cell or B-cell activity. One emerging group of DMARDs, which are technically small-molecule drugs as opposed to true biologic agents, targets the inhibition of the Janus kinase (JAK) enzyme involved in mediating inflammation.

Angelotti F, Parma A, Cafaro G, Capecchi R, Alunno A, Puxeddu I. One year in review 2017: pathogenesis of rheumatoid arthritis. *Clin Exp Rheumatol.* 2017;35(3):368–378.

Singh JA, Saag KG, Bridges SL Jr, et al; American College of Rheumatology. 2015 American College of Rheumatology guideline for the treatment of rheumatoid arthritis. *Arthritis Care Res (Hoboken).* 2016;68(1):1–25.

Spondyloarthritis

Spondyloarthritis (SpA) represents a spectrum of HLA-B27–related rheumatic diseases that have a predilection for axial (spinal and sacroiliac joint) inflammation. The predominant symptom is low back pain, but a small subset of patients lacks axial symptoms and has primary peripheral disease characterized by pain and swelling in the arms and legs. Males are affected 2–3 times more often than females. Among these diseases are ankylosing spondylitis (AS), reactive arthritis, psoriatic arthritis, and the enteropathic arthropathies linked to inflammatory bowel disease (ulcerative colitis and Crohn disease). Syndromes that do not clearly fall into one of these categories and show no x-ray evidence of sacroiliitis are sometimes referred to as *nonradiographic axial spondyloarthritis.* What distinguishes SpA, in general, from other forms of arthritis is its tendency to cause inflammation in the ligaments and tendons that insert onto bone (*enthesitis*); the heel or Achilles tendon are common targets. Other features include asymmetric oligoarthritis and inflammation of fingers or toes (*dactylitis*), giving the appearance of "sausage digits." Axial radiographs or magnetic resonance imaging (MRI) of the sacroiliac joints can be helpful, although abnormalities are not always present in the early course of the disease.

Spondyloarthritis may occur in childhood, although it is rare before the second decade of life. The *juvenile-onset spondyloarthropathies* are generally classified as a type of juvenile idiopathic arthritis known as *enthesitis-related arthritis.* Because the radiographic findings are similar, SpA is sometimes misdiagnosed as the result of trauma. As in adults, most young patients are HLA-B27–positive, and more males than females seem to be affected. These patients may develop acute uveitis characteristic of HLA-B27–positive uveitis.

Ophthalmologists should be familiar with these diseases, as acute recurrent HLA-B27–associated anterior uveitis may be the presenting feature of SpA (see "Ophthalmic considerations"). With appropriate referral of suspected patients, early disease can be recognized and treated to limit future morbidity. See BCSC Section 9, *Uveitis and Ocular Inflammation,* for further discussion of the ophthalmic manifestations.

Ankylosing Spondylitis

Ankylosing spondylitis (AS) is the most common type of axial SpA. The cause is unknown, but the strong association with HLA-B27 (positive in 90% of patients with AS) suggests a genetic predisposition. The disease occurs most commonly in young men. Low back pain with limitation in spinal mobility is typical; complete spinal fusion may develop in later stages. Peripheral arthritis may also be present, most frequently affecting the ankles, hips, and knees. Extra-articular features of AS include a higher risk of cardiovascular disease, venous thromboembolism, stroke, and restrictive pulmonary disease.

NSAIDs are often the first-line treatment and are very effective, with 70%–80% of patients reporting significant improvement in symptoms. TNF-α inhibitors appear to be effective as a second-line treatment; most clinicians consider their use after failure of 2 separate NSAID trials. Nonbiologic DMARDs (eg, sulfasalazine or methotrexate) tend to work better for peripheral arthritis than for primary axial disease. Local glucocorticoid injection is helpful in some patients.

Reactive Arthritis

Reactive arthritis is an unusual form of SpA that occurs following an infection, usually originating in the gastrointestinal or genitourinary systems, and most commonly affects young adults, both men and women. The infectious agents associated with this disease include *Chlamydia trachomatis* in the genitourinary tract and *Salmonella, Shigella, Yersinia,* or *Campylobacter* in the gastrointestinal tract. Other microbes, including *Escherichia coli, Clostridium difficile,* and *Chlamydia pneumoniae* have recently been added to the list of causative agents. HLA-B27 and genetics appear to be involved in susceptibility to developing reactive arthritis after an infection.

The arthritic symptoms typically have their onset from days to weeks after the antecedent infection. The arthritis is aseptic, as no microbes have been identified in the joints. Joint involvement is typically asymmetric and episodic, primarily affecting the knees and ankles. In addition to a preceding urethritis or diarrhea, extra-articular findings may include enthesitis (often of the knees and ankles), dactylitis of the fingers and toes ("sausage digits"), and sacroiliitis. Oral ulceration, nail pitting, and the skin eruptions of keratoderma blennorrhagicum (Fig 9-2) and erythema nodosum (Fig 9-3) can also occur. Ocular findings may be present in up to 40% of patients (see "Ophthalmic considerations"). Historically, the term *Reiter syndrome* was used to describe the clinical triad of arthritis, urethritis, and conjunctivitis. However, individuals with all 3 findings represent only a small subset of patients.

The disease is often episodic, and most patients go into remission within 2 years. Any underlying infection should be treated with appropriate antibiotics. In most patients, NSAIDs are effective in managing inflammation. For refractory symptoms, glucocorticoid injection into inflamed joints or, more rarely, the use of biologic agents is sometimes necessary.

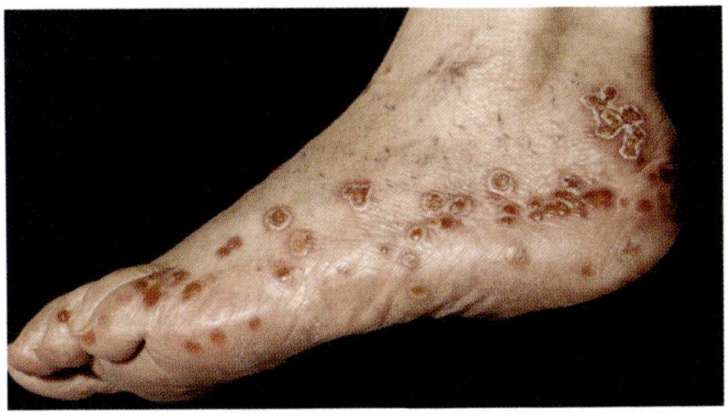

Figure 9-2 Keratoderma blennorrhagicum demonstrating hyperkeratotic lesions of the foot; it can also affect the palms of the hands, scalp, and trunk. The rash can resemble psoriasis. *(Used with permission from Wolff K, Johnson RA, Saavedra AP.* Fitzpatrick's Color Atlas and Synopsis of Clinical Dermatology. *7th ed. https://accessmedicine.mhmedical.com.)*

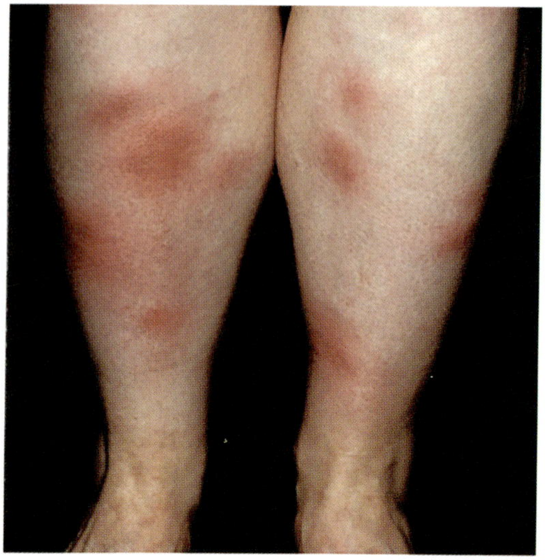

Figure 9-3 Erythema nodosum characterized by tender nodular eruptions, often involving the extensor surface of the legs below the knees. *(Used with permission from Wolff K, Johnson RA, Saavedra AP.* Fitzpatrick's Color Atlas and Synopsis of Clinical Dermatology. 7th ed. *https://accessmedicine.mhmedical.com.)*

Enteropathic Arthritis

Spondyloarthritis may occur in association with *inflammatory bowel disease (IBD),* of which ulcerative colitis and Crohn disease represent the majority of cases. Males and females are equally affected, although spondylitis is more common in men, and onset can be from childhood to adulthood. *Ulcerative colitis* is characterized by inflammation of the gastrointestinal mucosa with diffuse involvement of the colon. *Crohn disease,* also known as *regional enteritis, granulomatous ileocolitis,* or *granulomatous colitis,* is a focal granulomatous disease that can affect both the large and small intestines. Symptoms of both ulcerative colitis and Crohn disease include diarrhea (with or without bleeding) and cramping abdominal pain. Arthritis tends to occur more frequently in patients with large-bowel involvement or with extraenteric findings such as erythema nodosum (see Fig 9-3), stomatitis, or uveitis. HLA-B27 prevalence is as high as 75% in patients with axial involvement and is somewhat lower in those with primarily peripheral disease.

Radiographic findings of axial involvement are similar to those of AS but are of limited value in diagnosing early disease. MRI may also be helpful in demonstrating abnormal axial and sacroiliac findings in symptomatic patients. Elevated acute phase reactants, including ESR and CRP, often indicate heightened gastrointestinal (GI) inflammation but have limited benefit in assessing peripheral arthritis or spondylitis activity.

Psoriatic Arthritis

The skin disease psoriasis can be associated with SpA. Psoriatic arthritis has various presentations, including oligoarthritis (up to 4 joints), distal polyarthritis (more than 4 joints), and a more destructive type of arthritis known as *arthritis mutilans.* The prevalence of HLA-B27 is higher in these patients than in the general population (30% versus 6%), although not as high as in AS (90%). The course of the disease varies, but it is often similar to the progression seen with RA. Over half of individuals who have the disease for more than 10 years develop deforming arthritis in 5 or more joints. Although methotrexate is sometimes initially used for treatment, biologics and JAK inhibitors appear to be more effective in controlling disease progression.

Ophthalmic considerations Of all the known immune disorders in North America and Europe, SpA, including the subtypes reviewed here, has the strongest association with uveitis. A small percentage of patients presenting with idiopathic acute anterior uveitis have undiagnosed SpA. Up to 40% of patients with either AS or reactive arthritis develop the typical manifestations of acute nongranulomatous iridocyclitis, which can be recurrent and bilateral. Ocular involvement tends not to correlate with the activity of the joint disease.

Culture-negative bilateral conjunctivitis, which is typically self-limited, is also a common manifestation of reactive arthritis. IBD is more frequently associated with episcleritis. Uveitis presents in up to 3% of IBD patients, is significantly more common in females, and is not linked to the activity of the underlying disease. Ocular involvement with psoriatic arthritis is similar to that of other types of SpA, although the uveitis can be more insidious, posterior, and bilateral. See BCSC Section 9, *Uveitis and Ocular Inflammation.*

Parma A, Cometi L, Leone MC, Lepri G, Talarico R, Guiducci S. One year in review 2016: spondyloarthritis. *Clin Exp Rheumatol.* 2017;35(1):3–17.

Juvenile Idiopathic Arthritis

The term *juvenile idiopathic arthritis (JIA)* has replaced the older name, juvenile rheumatoid arthritis, because the disease has no direct relationship with adult-onset RA. Girls are affected more often than boys by a 3:1 ratio. Age of onset tends to be younger for girls (1–4 years) than for boys (8–10 years), and JIA is somewhat less common in African American and Asian populations than in White populations. As with many other autoimmune disorders, the pathogenesis of JIA is unclear.

Although classification of JIA has always been challenging, the International League of Associations for Rheumatology divides JIA into the 5 categories shown in Table 9-1. Ocular involvement is most common in the oligoarticular group, less common in the polyarticular group, and least common in the systemic group. Patients with oligoarticular or polyarticular (especially RF-negative subtype) disease should be periodically screened for ocular involvement because it is often asymptomatic. Furthermore, a positive ANA in either of these 2 groups is associated with an increased risk of developing uveitis.

Systemic JIA may present with variable onset of intermittent fever, arthritis, macular skin rash, lymphadenopathy, hepatosplenomegaly, pericarditis, and pulmonary effusions. Although laboratory findings of elevated ESR, CRP, and thrombocytosis are usual, ANA and RF are rarely present. The arthritis can involve any number of joints. Ocular involvement is not typical for this form of JIA.

Table 9-1 International League of Associations for Rheumatology Classification of Juvenile Idiopathic Arthritis (JIA)

Subtype	% of JIA Cases	Sex	% of Patients With Uveitis
Oligoarticular	40–50	F>M	30
Polyarticular			
RF-negative subtype	20–25	F>M	15
RF-positive subtype	5	F>M	<1
Systemic	5–10	F=M	<1
Psoriatic	5–10	F>M	10
Enthesitis-related	5–10	M>F	7

The last 2 subtypes, *psoriatic arthritis* and *enthesitis-related arthritis*, were added to help in categorizing patients who did not fit into more common entities. Uveitis can occur in both of these subtypes.

Systemic Lupus Erythematosus

Systemic lupus erythematosus (SLE) is a heterogeneous autoimmune disease of undetermined cause that presents with a wide range of clinical manifestations and can involve any organ. It is characterized by remissions and relapses, from mild to severe. The disease is estimated to affect 1.5 million people in the United States. Women are affected far more frequently than men, and the median age of onset is between 35 and 50 years. Individuals of African, Asian, and Native American heritage are more likely than White individuals to develop SLE. It is associated with B-cell hyperactivity, hypergammaglobulinemia, and a plethora of autoantibodies. These include antinuclear antibodies (ANAs) as well as antibodies to DNA and cytoplasmic components. SLE has classically been considered an immune complex disease that leads to an inflammatory response and tissue damage.

Signs and Symptoms

Patients may present with single-organ involvement, such as nephritis, or with a multisystem disease. The characteristic cutaneous manifestation of SLE is the *butterfly rash* (or *malar rash*) across the nose and cheeks, which appears in 70%–80% of patients (Fig 9-4). Other cutaneous manifestations include discoid lesions, which often lead to scarring, and alopecia. Mucosal lesions, usually painless oral or nasal ulcers, are present in up to 40% of patients. Acute or chronic photosensitivity occurs in many patients.

Approximately 90% of SLE patients experience articular disease, as either a polyarthralgia or a nondeforming migratory polyarthritis. Constitutional symptoms, such as fatigue, fever, myalgia, and weight loss, are common. Renal disease affects approximately 50% of patients; it can present with a range of manifestations from hematuria, proteinuria, and nephrotic syndrome to fulminant glomerulonephritis and renal failure.

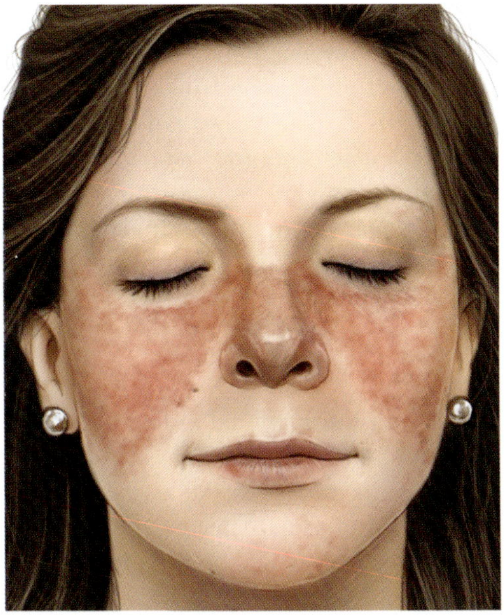

Figure 9-4 Malar "butterfly" rash in a patient with systemic lupus erythematosus. *(Used with permission from Mayo Foundation for Medical Education and Research. All rights reserved.)*

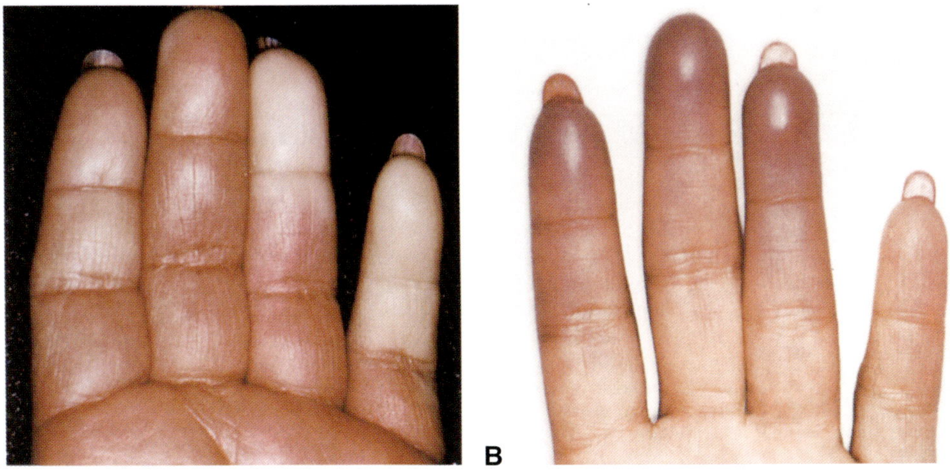

A B

Figure 9-5 Raynaud phenomenon. **A,** Sharply demarcated pallor resulting from the closure of digital arteries. **B,** Digital cyanosis of the fingertips in a patient with primary Raynaud phenomenon. *(Reproduced with permission from Wigley FM. Clinical practice. Raynaud's phenomenon.* N Engl J Med. *2002;347(13):1001. Copyright ©2002 Massachusetts Medical Society.)*

Raynaud phenomenon occurs in up to 50% of patients with SLE (Fig 9-5). Anemia of chronic disease is common, along with reduction in leukocytes and platelets. The rate of coronary artery disease is significantly greater in SLE patients than in unaffected individuals. Other, less common cardiac manifestations include pericarditis, myocarditis, and Libman-Sacks endocarditis. Valvular disease has been reported in more than 50%

of patients. Thromboembolism is more common in SLE, especially in the presence of antiphospholipid antibodies and lupus anticoagulant. Pulmonary involvement includes pleuritis, interstitial lung disease, and pulmonary hypertension. Gastrointestinal manifestations are varied and include dysphagia, esophagitis, hepatitis, and pancreatitis (GI symptoms are sometimes related to medications). Central nervous system (CNS) involvement occurs in more than one-third of patients, and symptoms are typically transient. The most common presentations of neurologic lupus are headache, cognitive impairment, seizures, psychosis, and peripheral neuropathy. See "Ophthalmic considerations" for ocular manifestations.

Diagnosis

Table 9-2 lists the classification criteria developed by an international SLE study group. Although this schema is intended primarily for research purposes, clinicians have found it useful in diagnosing and documenting the disease. Patients must satisfy at least 4 of the 17 criteria, including at least 1 clinical and 1 immunologic criterion. Alternatively, SLE can be diagnosed in patients with biopsy-proven nephritis with positive ANA or anti–double-stranded DNA (anti-dsDNA) antibodies. More recently, the British Society for Rheumatology released new UK-based guidelines for the diagnosis, assessment, and treatment of nonrenal manifestations of SLE (referenced in the Treatment section).

ANA testing should be ordered for suspected cases of SLE, as virtually all patients with SLE have positive titers of 1:160 or higher. Lower ANA titers limit the test specificity,

Table 9-2 SLICC Criteria for Diagnosis of Systemic Lupus Erythematosus

Clinical criteria
Acute cutaneous lupus
Chronic cutaneous lupus
Hematologic findings: hemolytic anemia, leukopenia, thrombocytopenia
Neurologic involvement[a]
Nonscarring alopecia[a]
Oral ulcers[a]
Renal involvement
Serositis[a]
Synovitis
Immunologic criteria
ANA
Anti-dsDNA antibody
Antiphospholipid antibody
Anti-Sm antibody
Direct Coombs test
Low levels of complement

ANA = antinuclear antibody; dsDNA = double-stranded DNA; SLICC = Systemic Lupus International Collaborating Clinics; Sm = Smith.
[a]In the absence of an alternative cause.

Modified with permission from Petri M, Orbai AM, Alarcón GS, et al. Derivation and validation of the Systemic Lupus International Collaborating Clinics Classification criteria for systemic lupus erythematosus. *Arthritis Rheum.* 2012;64(8):2682. Copyright ©2012 by the American College of Rheumatology.

as up to a third of unaffected individuals have a titer of 1:40. Thus, testing should be reserved for cases of high clinical suspicion. Three other immunologic tests that are highly specific for SLE are anti-dsDNA, anti-Smith (anti-Sm), and antiphospholipid antibodies. The presence of any 1 of these is considered an acceptable immunologic criterion. Additionally, antiribosomal P protein antibodies have a high specificity and can be helpful when the diagnosis is uncertain. Several other autoantibodies (anti-Ro/SS-A, anti-La/SS-B, anti-RNP, and anti-RA33) may indicate a predisposition to SLE or other autoimmune disease, but they are not included within the classification system.

Treatment

The treatment of SLE depends on disease severity. It can have a varied clinical course, ranging from a relatively benign illness to fulminant organ failure and death. Most patients have a relapsing and remitting course that requires frequent titration of medications.

Nonpharmacologic measures include sun protection to address photosensitivity, smoking cessation to reduce cardiovascular risks, and immunizations to decrease infection risk (if immunosuppressive agents are used). The most commonly prescribed medication is hydroxychloroquine. Alternatively, treatment may include NSAIDs, glucocorticoids (preferably low dose and short term), and immunosuppressive drugs. If antiphospholipid antibodies are present, low-dose aspirin appears to reduce the risk of thrombosis. Refractory cases of SLE and severe disease with CNS involvement may require high-dose pulse therapy with glucocorticoids and belimumab or rituximab, which have been shown to modulate B-cell activity.

Gordon C, Amissah-Arthur MB, Gayed M, et al. The British Society for Rheumatology guideline for the management of systemic lupus erythematosus in adults. *Rheumatology (Oxford)*. 2018;57(1):e1–e45.

La Paglia GMC, Leone MC, Lepri G, et al. One year in review 2017: systemic lupus erythematosus. *Clin Exp Rheumatol*. 2017;35(4):551–561.

Ophthalmic considerations Ocular involvement of SLE may correlate with systemic disease activity and can precede other systemic symptoms. The most common ocular manifestation of SLE is keratoconjunctivitis sicca from secondary Sjögren syndrome. Other manifestations include discoid cutaneous lesions of the eyelids as well as retinal or choroidal microvascular lesions. Cotton-wool spots, hemorrhages, vascular occlusions, and neovascularization may be present. The prevalence of ocular manifestations varies from 3% of outpatients to 29% of hospitalized patients. The inflammatory vasculopathy of SLE should be distinguished from vascular damage caused by secondary problems such as hypertension from renal disease or occlusions due to embolic disease or antiphospholipid antibodies. Typical anterior or intermediate uveitis is not a common feature of SLE. Neuro-ophthalmic involvement in SLE includes cranial nerve palsies, lupus optic neuropathy, and central retrochiasmal disorders of vision. Cerebral disorders of vision include hallucinations, visual field defects, and cortical blindness. (See also BCSC Section 9, *Uveitis and Ocular Inflammation,* and Section 12, *Retina and Vitreous.*)

Silpa-archa S, Lee JJ, Foster CS. Ocular manifestations in systemic lupus erythematosus. *Br J Ophthalmol.* 2016;100(1):135–141.

Sarcoidosis

Sarcoidosis is a multisystem disease of unknown cause in which noncaseating granulomas are present in affected tissues. The disease occurs primarily in young adults. Although any organ can be affected, there is a tendency for hilar adenopathy and pulmonary infiltrates, as well as joint and skin involvement. Common symptoms include cough, fever, weight loss, dyspnea, arthralgias, and erythema nodosum (see Fig 9-3).

Signs and Symptoms

Although pulmonary findings are the most typical (present in about 30% of patients), extrapulmonary manifestations vary widely by ethnicity and sex. African American individuals have a greater tendency for skin, liver, and eye involvement than White individuals. Females have more frequent skin and ocular manifestations, while males have a higher incidence of cardiac involvement. Cutaneous findings are variable and include various papules, plaques, and nodules, such as the painful nodules of erythema nodosum. Arthropathy occurs in 10%–15% of affected individuals. It tends to be acute rather than chronic and can be mistakenly diagnosed as reactive arthritis.

Ophthalmic considerations Ocular manifestations of sarcoidosis occur in approximately 25% of patients and can be the presenting symptom in 5% of cases. Eye involvement can include any periocular structure (skin, orbit, lacrimal gland, and muscles) as well as anterior and posterior segments. Uveitis and retinitis associated with sarcoidosis are discussed in greater detail in BCSC Section 9, *Uveitis and Ocular Inflammation,* and Section 12, *Retina and Vitreous,* respectively.

Diagnosis

Histopathology is valuable in confirming the diagnosis whenever possible, and common sites include lung, lymph node, skin, liver, and bone marrow. Pathology reveals granulomatous inflammation (usually noncaseating). In 3 situations, however, a diagnosis can be reasonably established without biopsy: Löfgren syndrome (erythema nodosum, hilar adenopathy, migratory polyarthralgia, and fever), Heerfordt-Waldenström syndrome (parotid gland swelling, facial nerve palsy, uveitis, and fever), and asymptomatic bilateral hilar adenopathy. Biopsy of erythema nodosum skin lesions is not helpful, as granulomas are not associated with the eruption.

No serologic test is pathognomonic for sarcoidosis. Although serum angiotensin-converting enzyme (ACE) is elevated in 75% of patients, poor sensitivity and reduced specificity limit its usefulness. Pulmonary imaging is helpful and may include radiography, computed tomography, or positron-emission tomography scans. An ophthalmologic exam is important as part of the workup of any patient suspected of having sarcoidosis.

Treatment

Patients with asymptomatic disease often do not require treatment. Spontaneous remission is common for mild disease. For patients with more extensive manifestations, treatment is tailored to the affected systems. Glucocorticoids are typically the first line of treatment, and maintenance doses are sometimes required for years. For refractory cases, DMARDs are sometimes employed. See also BCSC Section 9, *Uveitis and Ocular Inflammation.*

Antiphospholipid Syndrome

Antiphospholipid syndrome (APS) is an autoimmune disorder that predisposes patients to arterial or venous thrombosis. It occurs as a primary condition or in association with other autoimmune diseases, especially SLE.

Signs and Symptoms

Deep venous thrombosis is the most common type of thrombosis, occurring in approximately one-third of patients with APS. Episodes of thrombosis can recur, particularly in patients with high antiphospholipid antibody titers. Patients may also have pulmonary embolism and superficial thrombophlebitis. CNS disease can include strokes, transient ischemic attacks, dementia, and even psychosis. APS should be considered when thrombosis or cerebrovascular disease occurs in a young patient without other risk factors for stroke.

This syndrome can cause complications during pregnancy. Patients may have multiple first-trimester spontaneous abortions and premature births due to preeclampsia or placental insufficiency; late-term fetal death may also occur.

Other manifestations of APS include thrombocytopenia, hemolytic anemia, nephropathy, and livedo reticularis. Cardiac manifestations include valvular thickening and nodules (*Libman-Sacks endocarditis*). In rare instances, a severe form of APS can occur with multiple vessel occlusions and multiorgan failure. This form of the disease is called *catastrophic antiphospholipid syndrome* and has a mortality rate of 48%.

Diagnosis

In patients suspected of having APS, immunoassays are performed to detect the presence of anticardiolipin antibodies, anti-β_2 glycoprotein antibodies, and lupus anticoagulants. Additional testing for underlying autoimmune disease in newly diagnosed APS patients should be considered because SLE, in particular, is present in up to 36% of cases.

Ophthalmic considerations Ocular manifestations of APS include transient monocular blindness, ischemic optic neuropathy, and retinal vascular occlusion. Visual field loss, diplopia, and even proliferative retinopathy have also been reported. Clinicians should consider APS when atypical ocular vaso-occlusive disease occurs in patients who are younger than 50 years or who have bilateral findings. Coordination with the patient's primary care physician or rheumatologist is important in the workup.

Treatment

Therapy for thrombosis usually consists of heparin, followed by warfarin. The optimal duration of treatment is not known: some experts believe that anticoagulation can be discontinued if the antiphospholipid antibody titers decrease, but lifelong treatment is recommended for patients with recurrent disease. Associated autoimmune disorders are often treated with such drugs as hydroxychloroquine to help reduce risk of APS complications. Treatment of pregnant patients remains controversial; it may include some combination of heparin or low-molecular-weight heparin and aspirin, as warfarin is teratogenic. Patients with antiphospholipid antibodies without a history of thrombosis may benefit from prophylactic aspirin. The use of autologous stem cell transplantation or rituximab has been investigated, but the benefits remain questionable.

Meroni PL, Chighizola CB, Rovelli F, Gerosa M. Antiphospholipid syndrome in 2014: more clinical manifestations, novel pathogenic players and emerging biomarkers. *Arthritis Res Ther.* 2014;16(2):209.

Systemic Sclerosis

Systemic sclerosis (SSc), formerly known as scleroderma, is a relatively uncommon connective tissue disorder characterized by fibrous and degenerative changes in the skin and other organ systems. The term *scleroderma* is often used for sclerosis affecting only the skin. SSc is further classified into *limited* and *diffuse* subtypes, depending mainly on the extent of skin involvement. The etiology of this disease is poorly understood but involves activation of fibroblasts that produce excessive collagen deposition, inflammation, and fibrosis. SSc is 4 times more common in women than in men, with age of onset typically in the third or fourth decade of life. African American individuals seem to be more prone to the diffuse form of the disease, although it can affect other groups as well. The limited form of SSc rarely involves internal organs and has a better prognosis, often with a normal life span. It is frequently associated with the *CREST syndrome* (*c*alcinosis, *R*aynaud phenomenon, *e*sophageal involvement, *s*clerodactyly, and *t*elangiectasia).

Signs and Symptoms

The hallmark of SSc is changes to the skin, namely thickening, tightening, and induration, with subsequent loss of mobility and contracture (Fig 9-6). The disease usually begins

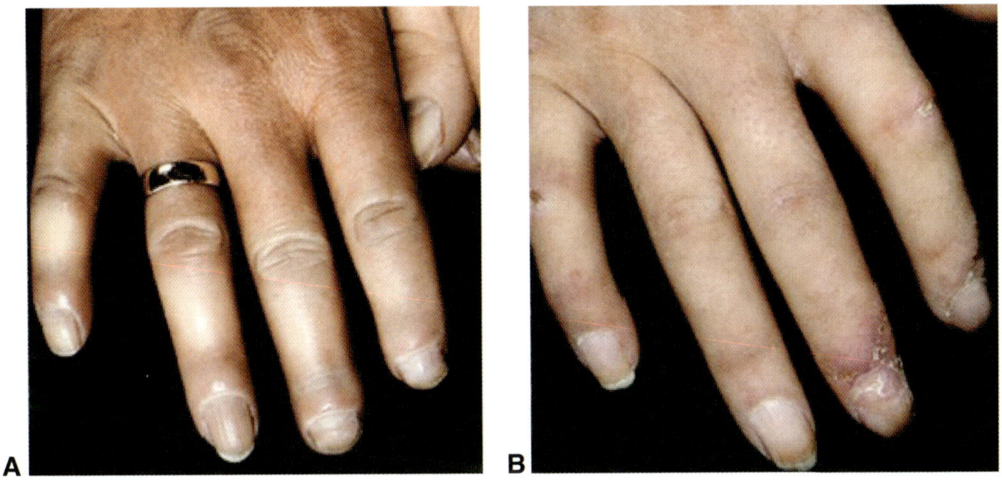

Figure 9-6 Typical skin changes in systemic sclerosis. **A,** Thickening and tightening of the fingers. **B,** Associated ischemic changes in the peripheral digits. *(Used with permission from Wolff K, Johnson RA, Saavedra AP.* Fitzpatrick's Color Atlas and Synopsis of Clinical Dermatology. *7th ed. https://accessmedicine.mhmedical.com.)*

peripherally, in the fingers and hands, and subsequently spreads centripetally up the arms to involve the face and body. Telangiectasia and calcinosis are common. Vascular effects also occur; more than 95% of SSc patients experience Raynaud phenomenon (see Fig 9-5). Less frequently, permanent damage to blood vessels can result in digital ulcers and ischemia.

Organ involvement is present in more than 90% of patients; the most common is esophageal dysmotility with gastroesophageal reflux secondary to stricture formation and submucosal fibrosis. The small and large intestines may also be affected, with decreased motility, malabsorption, and diverticulosis. Cardiopulmonary disease is manifested primarily by pulmonary vascular fibrosis leading to restrictive lung disease and decreased diffusing capacity, pulmonary hypertension, and right-sided heart failure. These complications, along with arrhythmias arising from cardiac fibrosis, account for a cumulative 5-year survival rate around 75% from the time of diagnosis. Musculoskeletal characteristics include polyarthralgias, tendon friction rubs, and occasionally myositis. Renal disease is seen in approximately 50% of patients.

Diagnosis

The great majority of patients with SSc test positive for ANA. Other useful serological tests include anti-DNA topoisomerase I and anti-RNA polymerase III, which are highly specific for the disease. Anticentromere antibody is often present in the limited subtype of SSc. These specific serologies help classify the disease and various syndromes that overlap with SSc.

Treatment

Treatment is aimed at controlling problems in the specific organ systems involved. Several agents in the antihypertensive class of endothelin-1 receptor antagonists are sometimes beneficial in patients with pulmonary hypertension. ACE inhibitors are recommended for the treatment of hypertension due to renal disease. Patients with Raynaud phenomenon are treated with calcium channel blockers. Immunosuppressive agents, including methotrexate and cyclophosphamide, have proved effective in the treatment of diffuse SSc cutaneous manifestations and may slow the progression of disease. Management of inflammatory joint disease is similar to that of rheumatoid arthritis.

Kowal-Bielecka O, Fransen J, Avouac J, et al; EUSTAR Coauthors. Update of EULAR recommendations for the treatment of systemic sclerosis. *Ann Rheum Dis.* 2017;76(8):1327–1339.

Ophthalmic considerations Ocular involvement occurs in about 50% of SSc patients; the most common manifestations are periocular skin fibrosis and tightening, along with keratoconjunctivitis sicca. The skin changes may lead to blepharophimosis or lagophthalmos. Patchy choroidal nonperfusion related to diffuse microvascular damage may appear on fluorescein angiography. Occasionally, as a result of renal involvement, a patient can develop retinopathy from malignant hypertension, with cotton-wool spots, intraretinal hemorrhages, and optic nerve head edema.

Sjögren Syndrome

Sjögren syndrome is a chronic autoimmune disorder characterized by lymphocytic infiltration of exocrine glands. It can occur as a primary disease alone or as a secondary form linked with other autoimmune disorders, especially RA, SLE, or SSc. The syndrome can present at any age and in either sex, although women in the fifth and sixth decades of life are the most commonly affected. Typical symptoms include dry eyes, dry mouth, and dry skin (xerosis). The ophthalmologist may be the first physician to see these patients because of their ocular symptoms. Parotid and lacrimal gland enlargement (*Mikulicz syndrome*) can occur in more severely affected individuals.

Patients with primary Sjögren syndrome may have a number of systemic manifestations, including upper-airway dryness, mucous plug development, purpuric vasculitis, and hyperglobulinemia. Although about 50% of patients report symptoms of arthralgia, arthritis is less common; and some patients may have subclinical inflammatory myopathy. Mild anemia across all cell lines is found in approximately 20% of patients, and the overall risk of non-Hodgkin lymphoma is increased. Central and peripheral neurologic involvement may be present and mimic multiple sclerosis or psychiatric disorders.

The American College of Rheumatology and European League Against Rheumatism recently updated their classification criteria for primary Sjögren syndrome based on 5 objective measures. These include specific findings on labial salivary gland biopsy, presence of anti-Ro antibodies, ocular staining, abnormal Schirmer testing, and reduced unstimulated salivary flow. The benefit of minor salivary gland biopsy is to confirm the disease, to rule out other disease processes (eg, sarcoidosis, amyloidosis), and to serve as a prognostic indicator for the development of future lymphoma. Serum level of *Fms-like tyrosine kinase 3 ligand (Flt-3L)* also shows promise as a potential predictor for the development of this malignancy. Ongoing research is directed at finding key biomarkers for Sjögren syndrome to provide more sensitive and specific testing. Among those being studied are *profilin* and *carbonic anhydrase I (CA-I)* in saliva and *cathepsin S* in tears.

Treatment is aimed at relief of symptoms and substitution or supplementation for reduced or absent secretions. Immunosuppression may be necessary in patients with systemic manifestations. (See also BCSC Section 8, *External Disease and Cornea.*)

Chen W, Cao H, Lin J, et al. Biomarkers for primary Sjögren's syndrome. *Genomics Proteomics Bioinformatics.* 2015;13(4):219–223.

Shiboski CH, Shiboski SC, Seror R, et al; International Sjögren's Syndrome Criteria Working Group. American College of Rheumatology/European League Against Rheumatism classification criteria for primary Sjögren's syndrome: a consensus and data-driven methodology involving three international patient cohorts. *Ann Rheum Dis.* 2017;76(1):9–16.

Polymyositis and Dermatomyositis

Polymyositis and *dermatomyositis* are idiopathic inflammatory diseases of skeletal muscle characterized by progressive weakness affecting proximal muscle groups, particularly those of the shoulders and hips. Women are more commonly affected than men (2:1), with a peak age incidence between 40 and 50 years. Both disorders are associated with polyarthritis, dysphagia, and interstitial pulmonary disease. Ocular involvement is relatively uncommon, apart from the heliotrope rash of dermatomyositis, which is very specific but not often present (Fig 9-7). In rare cases, the extraocular muscles may be involved, resulting in ophthalmoplegia.

Dermatomyositis is distinguished from polymyositis by the presence of cutaneous lesions. These skin lesions appear as an erythematous to violaceous rash variably affecting the eyelids (*heliotrope rash*; see Fig 9-7), cheeks, nose, chest (*V-neck sign*), and extensor surfaces (*Gottron sign*). Pathogenically, dermatomyositis is associated with immune complex deposition in the vessels, whereas polymyositis appears to reflect T-cell–mediated muscle injury.

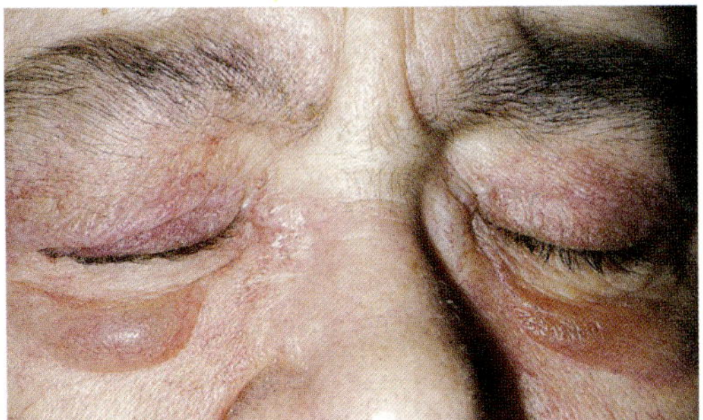

Figure 9-7 Heliotrope rash in dermatomyositis, with typical reddish-purple appearance and associated eyelid swelling. *(Used with permission from Wolff K, Johnson RA, Saavedra AP.* Fitzpatrick's Color Atlas and Synopsis of Clinical Dermatology. *https://accessmedicine.mhmedical.com.)*

Laboratory findings in both disorders include elevated serum muscle enzymes, serum and urine myoglobin, and abnormal electromyography results. A wide range of autoantibodies is found in most patients, including several that are specific to myositis. Muscle biopsy may confirm the muscle damage from inflammation.

Glucocorticoids are typically initiated at the time of diagnosis and are usually tapered over a period of 9–12 months. Immunosuppressive agents, such as azathioprine or methotrexate, are sometimes used in patients unresponsive to steroid treatment or in those who develop adverse effects.

Polymyalgia Rheumatica

Polymyalgia rheumatica (PMR) is a relatively common chronic inflammatory condition affecting older adults that is characterized by proximal myalgia and morning stiffness of the neck, shoulders, and hip girdle. Among rheumatic conditions in adults, the lifetime risk of this disease is second only to rheumatoid arthritis. PMR is significant for its association with giant cell arteritis (GCA), which approximately 10% of PMR patients will develop. Similarly, up to 50% of patients diagnosed with GCA have manifestations of PMR. Although the etiology of both is unclear, many believe that the 2 entities share a common pathophysiology. People of European descent are at greatest risk, while those of Asian, Latino, and African American heritage are the least susceptible.

The onset of symptoms can be abrupt. They are most noticeable upon arising from bed in the morning; in fact, the absence of morning stiffness helps to exclude the diagnosis. Associated synovitis can limit range of motion in affected joints: the classic finding in a patient with PMR is the inability to raise the arms above 90°. ESR and CRP are often elevated. Patients with PMR should be asked about symptoms typical of GCA. Temporal artery biopsy is not indicated in patients without signs and symptoms of GCA, as it rarely yields positive results.

Prednisone typically brings dramatic relief in 2–3 days, with complete recovery often occurring within 3 weeks. Patients without relapses can usually be tapered off by 1 year. If patients need longer-term treatment, methotrexate may be helpful in reducing the steroid requirement. Other biologics have not shown consistent results.

Relapsing Polychondritis

Relapsing polychondritis is a rare, episodic autoimmune disorder characterized by widespread, potentially destructive inflammation of cartilage throughout the body, including ears (most commonly involved), nose, cardiac and respiratory structures, joints, and eye. Males and females of all ages and races can be affected, although White individuals seem more susceptible. The disease is variable in duration and severity. Nasal bridge involvement can progress to cause saddle nose deformity from cartilage collapse. Laryngotracheobronchial disease may be insidious but can lead to the fatal complication of laryngeal collapse. Involvement of the inner ear, cardiovascular system, and skin is less common. Cardiovascular problems include aortic insufficiency (due to progressive dilation of the aortic root) and vasculitis. Skin lesions are most often caused by cutaneous vasculitis.

In up to one-third of patients, relapsing polychondritis can be associated with other connective tissue diseases (eg, SLE or RA), systemic vasculitis, or malignancy. Ocular manifestations, which occur in up to 60% of patients, include episcleritis, scleritis, uveitis, and, rarely, retinal vasculitis.

Treatment focuses on reducing symptoms and preserving the integrity of cartilaginous structures. Pharmacotherapy includes systemic corticosteroids, dapsone, methotrexate, and cyclophosphamide. Patients may require surgical interventions such as tracheostomy, aortic aneurysm repair, and cardiac valve replacement.

Vasculitis

The systemic vasculitides are a group of diseases whose principal pathology involves autoimmune damage to blood vessels, which can result in ischemia and necrosis of supplied tissues. These diseases are grouped according to size and location of affected vessels. Vasculitis can occur as a primary disease state or as a secondary condition associated with other immune disorders or with exogenous factors such as infection, neoplasia, or medication. Table 9-3 outlines the most recent classification created by the Chapel Hill

Table 9-3 Names of Vasculitides Adopted by the Chapel Hill Consensus Conference on the Nomenclature of Systemic Vasculitides[a]

Large-vessel vasculitis
Giant cell (temporal) arteritis
Takayasu arteritis
Medium-sized–vessel vasculitis
Polyarteritis nodosa[b]
Kawasaki disease
Small-vessel vasculitis
ANCA-associated small-vessel vasculitis
Granulomatosis with polyangiitis (Wegener granulomatosis)
Eosinophilic granulomatosis with polyangiitis (Churg-Strauss syndrome)
Microscopic polyangiitis
Immune complex vasculitis
IgA vasculitis (Henoch-Schönlein purpura)
Cryoglobulinemic vasculitis
Anti-GBM disease
Variable-vessel vasculitis
Behçet disease
Cogan syndrome

ANCA = antineutrophil cytoplasmic autoantibody; GBM = glomerular basement membrane; IgA = immunoglobulin A.

[a]*Large vessel* refers to the aorta and the largest branches directed toward major body regions (eg, to the extremities and the head and neck); *medium-sized vessel* refers to the main visceral arteries (eg, renal, hepatic, coronary, and mesenteric arteries); and *small vessel* refers to venules, capillaries, arterioles, and the intraparenchymal distal arterial radicals that connect the arterioles.

[b]Strongly associated with ANCA.

Modified with permission from Jeanette JC, Falk RJ, Bacon PA, et al. 2012 Revised International Chapel Hill Consensus Conference Nomenclature of Vasculitides. *Arthritis Rheum.* 2013;65(1):1–11. Copyright ©2013 by the American College of Rheumatology.

Consensus Conference on these diseases. The following subsections emphasize the primary vasculitides that are more likely to have ophthalmic involvement.

Jennette JC, Falk RJ, Bacon PA, et al. 2012 revised international Chapel Hill consensus conference nomenclature of vasculitides. *Arthritis Rheum.* 2013;65(1):1–11.

Large-Vessel Vasculitis

Giant cell arteritis

Giant cell (temporal) arteritis, which affects older adults, is a potentially blinding granulomatous inflammatory disease involving the aorta and its branches. It is of particular concern to ophthalmologists and is discussed at length in BCSC Section 5, *Neuro-Ophthalmology.*

Takayasu arteritis

Like giant cell arteritis, *Takayasu arteritis* affects large arteries, particularly branches of the aorta; but, in contrast, it occurs primarily in children and young women. The disease is rare in Western countries but is more common in Asia, particularly Japan. Other names include *aortic arch arteritis, aortitis syndrome,* and *pulseless disease.*

This disease may involve the entire aorta or be localized to any segment of the aorta or its primary branches. The inflammatory process is characterized by panarteritis with granulomatous inflammation. The involved vessels may ultimately become narrowed or obliterated, resulting in ischemia of the supplied tissues. Areas of weakened vascular walls may develop dissections or aneurysms.

Systemic features such as fatigue, headache, weight loss, and low-grade fever are common. Evidence of vascular insufficiency due to large-artery narrowing leads to the characteristic pulseless phase. Angiography, including magnetic resonance angiography, is essential in confirming the diagnosis. Treatment is generally with systemic corticosteroids, which may successfully suppress the disease. Cyclophosphamide or methotrexate is added in resistant cases. Surgical reconstruction of stenotic vessels may be necessary.

Ophthalmic considerations Patients with Takayasu arteritis may report transient visual disturbances and blindness due to decreased perfusion. The most characteristic ocular findings are retinal arteriovenous anastomoses, best demonstrated by fluorescein angiography. Milder changes found earlier in the course of the disease include small-vessel dilation and microaneurysm formation. More severe ischemia may result in peripheral retinal nonperfusion, iris and retinal neovascularization, and vitreous hemorrhage.

Medium-Sized–Vessel Vasculitis

Polyarteritis nodosa

Classic *polyarteritis nodosa (PAN)* is characterized by necrotizing vasculitis of medium and small muscular arteries. The lesions are segmental, and aneurysms may develop, which are detectable by angiography. *Mononeuritis multiplex,* a painful vasculitic neuropathy involving peripheral motor or sensory nerves, may be a presenting feature. CNS lesions can also occur. Renal involvement is common and is often associated with hypertension due to glomerular ischemia. Gastrointestinal disease with infarction of the viscera is also common. PAN may be limited to a single organ, such as the appendix, uterus, or testes. Although most cases of PAN are idiopathic, hepatitis B and C viral infections as well as hairy cell leukemia have been linked to its onset. Biopsy of involved tissues or organs is helpful in confirming the diagnosis.

The mean age of onset of PAN is in the fifth and six decades of life, with men affected more often than women. Survival in patients with untreated PAN is poor. However, most patients can be treated with a combination of corticosteroids and an immunosuppressive drug such as cyclophosphamide. Therapy appears to improve disease control and long-term outcomes. Systemic antivirals may be helpful in treating PAN related to hepatitis B or C. See BCSC Section 9, *Uveitis and Ocular Inflammation.*

Ophthalmic considerations Ocular manifestations, which occur in up to 20% of patients with PAN, may include hypertensive retinopathy, retinal vasculitis, and visual field loss from CNS lesions. Cranial nerve palsies can occur, as well as scleritis and marginal corneal ulceration. Choroidal vasculitis is often overlooked in PAN and may cause transient visual symptoms, exudative retinal detachments, and pigmentary changes. Fluorescein angiography may be necessary to identify choroidal involvement.

Kawasaki disease

Kawasaki disease, also known as *mucocutaneous lymph node syndrome,* is a condition associated with inflammation in the walls of medium-sized vessels throughout the body. The disease typically affects infants and young children. Patients often develop a persistent high fever, swollen lymph nodes, bilateral conjunctivitis, and truncal rash. A characteristic feature of Kawasaki disease is *strawberry tongue*—an extremely red, swollen tongue.

Although the disease is typically self-limited, it can lead to associated cardiovascular complications including coronary artery aneurysms, myocarditis, and dysrhythmias. Prompt treatment, which includes intravenous immunoglobulin and aspirin, reduces the potential for long-term complications.

Small-Vessel Vasculitis

Inflammation in small-vessel disease predominantly affects the arterioles, venules, and capillaries. This group of vasculitic disorders is further categorized based on the presence or relative absence of vessel-wall deposition of immunoglobulin and/or complement components. Subtypes include antineutrophil cytoplasmic autoantibody (ANCA)–associated small-vessel vasculitis and immune complex small-vessel vasculitis.

ANCA-associated vasculitis

Granulomatosis with polyangiitis Formerly known as Wegener granulomatosis, *granulomatosis with polyangiitis (GPA)* is an immune-mediated necrotizing granulomatous vasculitis affecting small vessels. The disease strikes older adults and both sexes equally, with White individuals more commonly affected. The clinical features of GPA include granulomatous inflammation of the paranasal sinuses or nasopharyngeal tissues in a majority of cases. Glomerulonephritis occurs in up to 85% of patients and can be asymptomatic until later stages. Other findings include cutaneous vasculitis and, less commonly, neurovasculitis. Limited forms of the disease may occur without significant systemic involvement, making diagnosis difficult. Ocular disease, found in up to 50% of patients, may be the presenting feature. Ocular findings include scleritis with or without peripheral keratitis, idiopathic orbital inflammatory disease, and vasculitis-mediated retinal vascular or neuro-ophthalmic lesions. Over 85% of patients with GPA are seropositive for ANCA. Histopathology remains the definitive way to confirm the diagnosis. (See also BCSC Section 7, *Oculofacial Plastic and Orbital Surgery,* and BCSC Section 9, *Uveitis and Ocular Inflammation.*)

Early and aggressive treatment of systemic GPA is critical, as the mortality rate of untreated severe disease approaches 90% within 2 years of onset. Glucocorticoids in combination with either cyclophosphamide or rituximab are highly effective in inducing and maintaining remission of disease. Trimethoprim-sulfamethoxazole prophylaxis is sometimes used to help prevent opportunistic infections during treatment. Plasma exchange may be beneficial in severe cases with rapidly deteriorating renal or pulmonary function.

Eosinophilic granulomatosis with polyangiitis Formerly known as Churg-Strauss syndrome, *eosinophilic granulomatosis with polyangiitis (EGPA)* is a vasculitis of small- to medium-sized arteries characterized by chronic rhinosinusitis, asthma, and eosinophilia. The cause is unknown. Average age of onset is between 50 and 60 years, with no sex predominance.

Any organ can be affected, but the lungs and skin (tender subcutaneous nodules) are most commonly involved. Cardiovascular involvement is responsible for half of the deaths among affected patients. Peripheral mononeuropathy or polyneuropathy is common. Renal and gastrointestinal involvement is sometimes evident. Ophthalmic manifestations include conjunctival granulomas, retinal vasculitis and occlusion, uveitis, and cranial nerve palsies.

Diagnosis of EGPA depends on the presence of several criteria, including asthma, eosinophilia, eosinophilic vasculitis, transient pulmonary infiltrates, and neuropathy. Biopsy of tissue from the lung or a skin nodule is helpful in establishing the diagnosis; pathologic examination often shows granulomas with eosinophilic tissue infiltration of smaller vessels. ANCA titers are positive in about 50% of patients. Many patients achieve remission with glucocorticoids alone, although additional immunosuppressive therapy may be necessary in more severe cases.

Microscopic polyangiitis *Microscopic polyangiitis (MPA)* is a systemic necrotizing vasculitis that is similar to GPA in targeting small vessels, and it is sometimes difficult to differentiate between the 2 entities. On histologic examination, however, MPA lacks the necrotizing granulomatous formation seen in GPA. Patients with MPA are also less likely to relapse. In both conditions, the majority of patients are ANCA-positive; but patients with GPA tend to have high proteinase 3 (PR3)-ANCA levels, whereas patients with MPA tend to have higher myeloperoxidase (MPO)-ANCA levels. Treatment of MPA is similar to that of GPA.

Variable-Vessel Vasculitis

As the name suggests, *variable-vessel vasculitis* has no predilection for a specific type of vessel. Two examples are Behçet disease and Cogan syndrome vasculitis.

Behçet disease

Behçet disease was initially described as a triad of oral ulcers, genital ulcers, and uveitis with hypopyon. It is now recognized as a multisystem vasculitis of unknown etiology that can affect arterial and venous vessels of any size. The disease is most common in the Middle East and Asia, affects males more often than females, and usually has its onset during the third or fourth decade of life.

Signs and symptoms Oral ulcers are the most common clinical feature, affecting over 95% of patients. Genital ulcers and skin involvement each occur in about 75% of cases. Skin disease can include erythema nodosum (see Fig 9-3), superficial thrombophlebitis, pyoderma, and pathergy (pustular response to skin injury). Approximately half of patients have asymmetric, nondeforming arthritis that commonly affects the knees, wrists, and ankles.

Vascular disease can present as migratory superficial thrombophlebitis, major-vessel thrombosis, arterial aneurysms, or even peripheral gangrene. CNS disease is found in 20% of patients and includes brainstem syndrome, meningoencephalitis, and confusional states. The major causes of mortality are from CNS involvement and large-vessel disease, including arterial aneurysm.

Diagnosis Behçet disease may be associated with a number of nonspecific laboratory abnormalities, including elevated ESR, CRP, and circulating immune complexes. Patients may also have serologic evidence of a hypercoagulable state, and the prevalence of HLA-B51 is higher than among unaffected individuals. However, no specific laboratory tests are pathognomonic for this disease. The diagnosis is based on clinical criteria that include oral ulcers and any 2 of the following: uveitis, genital ulcers, skin involvement, and pathergy. Other criteria may be used, depending on regional differences in disease presentation.

Treatment Management varies according to disease severity and organ systems involved. Patients with mild disease may benefit from colchicine for treatment of arthritis and ulcers. Oral and genital lesions may respond to topical steroid solutions or require systemic therapy if severe. The use of corticosteroids alone may control acute exacerbations but does not seem to alter disease outcome. As a result, 1 or more immunosuppressive agents are usually added as therapy. Interferon-alfa has also been effective, especially for mucocutaneous manifestations. Treatment of posterior uveitis typically begins with azathioprine and steroids. Alkylating agents such as cyclophosphamide may be used in refractory cases, although these drugs may have significant toxicity. Tumor necrosis factor (TNF)-α inhibitors may also be helpful.

Zeidan MJ, Saadoun D, Garrido M, Klatzmann D, Six A, Cacoub P. Behçet's disease physiopathology: a contemporary review. *Auto Immun Highlights.* 2016;7(1):4.

Ophthalmic considerations Ocular disease is a significant cause of morbidity in Behçet disease, affecting up to 70% of patients, often bilaterally. The most common ocular manifestations are iridocyclitis, with or without hypopyon, and retinal vasculitis. Posterior uveitis and retinal vasculitis are often associated with ischemia, macular edema, and exudates, leading to significant vision loss. See also BCSC Section 9, *Uveitis and Ocular Inflammation.*

Cogan syndrome

Cogan syndrome is an immune-mediated disorder that affects young adults and is characterized by inflammatory lesions of the eye and inner ear. Patients may present with nonspecific symptoms such as fatigue, fever, and weight loss. Medium- or large-vessel vasculitis, including aortitis, occurs in 10% of cases. Ophthalmic findings may include uveitis, interstitial keratitis, and scleritis. Dizziness and hearing problems may reflect inner ear disease such as vestibular dysfunction and sensorineural hearing loss, respectively. Recurrent untreated inflammation may lead to blindness and deafness. Patients are commonly treated with oral corticosteroids and other immunosuppressive medications, including methotrexate and azathioprine. See BCSC Section 8, *External Disease and Cornea,* for further discussion.

Medical Therapy for Rheumatic Disorders

Medications are used in rheumatology for several purposes, including analgesia, control of inflammation, and immunosuppression. The use of these drugs in treating ocular inflammatory diseases is discussed in BCSC Section 9, *Uveitis and Ocular Inflammation.*

Corticosteroids

Glucocorticoids decrease inflammation by inhibiting the breakdown of phospholipid to arachidonic acid and blocking the production of inflammatory mediators, including prostaglandins and leukotrienes. Glucocorticoids have a variety of other systemic effects apart from their anti-inflammatory activity. They promote gluconeogenesis, with a concomitant negative nitrogen balance and reduction in protein production. Fat oxidation, synthesis, storage, and mobilization are also affected. After glucocorticoid administration, the number of circulating neutrophils increases because mature neutrophils are released from bone marrow, and their movement from the blood into other tissues is reduced, while the number of other circulating leukocytes decreases. Associated mineralocorticoid activity increases sodium retention and potassium excretion.

Table 9-4 lists the relative potency of commonly used glucocorticoid preparations. The molecular structure of the corticosteroid nucleus can be modified to dissociate glucocorticoid from mineralocorticoid activity. Unfortunately, isolating the beneficial anti-inflammatory effects from the less desirable glucocorticoid effects has not been fully achieved. The ophthalmologist must be aware of the ocular and systemic toxicities associated with systemic corticosteroids.

Table 9-4 Potency of Commonly Used Glucocorticoids

Glucocorticoid	Approximate Equivalent Dose, mg	Relative Anti-inflammatory Potency
Hydrocortisone	20	1.0
Cortisone	25	0.8
Prednisone	5	4.0
Prednisolone	5	4.0
Methylprednisolone	4	5.0
Triamcinolone	4	5.0
Dexamethasone	0.75	25.0

Adverse effects

Ocular adverse effects of systemic corticosteroids include posterior subcapsular cataracts, glaucoma, mydriasis, ptosis, papilledema associated with idiopathic intracranial hypertension, worsening of ocular infection, and delay in wound healing. Systemic complications may include peptic ulceration, osteoporosis, and aseptic necrosis of the femoral head, as well as muscle and skin atrophy. Steroids can also cause hyperglycemia, hypertension, edema, weight gain, and changes in body fat distribution, resulting in a cushingoid habitus. Other adverse effects include hyperosmolar nonketotic states, hypokalemia, and growth delay in children. Mental changes are a common problem, ranging from mild mood alterations to severe psychological reactions, including psychological dependence.

Osteoporosis is a significant problem that can increase the risk of fractures as early as a few months after beginning corticosteroid therapy. Bone mineral density testing is used to assess the degree of osteoporosis. In addition to calcium and vitamin D supplementation, hormone replacement therapy and bisphosphonates are sometimes initiated.

Cessation of therapy

Rapid withdrawal of systemic corticosteroid therapy can cause complications. The rate of corticosteroid withdrawal is determined by 2 criteria: (1) the degree of hypothalamic-pituitary-adrenal (HPA) suppression, which in turn is related to steroid potency, dose, and duration of therapy, and (2) the response of the underlying disease to the corticosteroid withdrawal. HPA suppression is likely present in patients who have a cushingoid appearance or who have received a glucocorticoid equivalent daily dose greater than or equal to 10 mg of prednisone (alternatively, a continuous evening or bedtime dose of ≥5 mg) for more than 3 weeks. HPA suppression is reduced below these parameters. When tapering becomes necessary, a practical approach is to reduce steroid requirement by 5% to 10% every 2 to 4 weeks while monitoring response carefully. Otherwise, sudden cessation of corticosteroid therapy could result in adrenal insufficiency, with symptoms such as fatigue, weakness, arthralgias, nausea, orthostatic hypotension, and hypoglycemia. In severe cases, adrenal suppression may be fatal.

After corticosteroid therapy has been discontinued, adrenal function may not return to normal for a year or more, and coverage with supplementary corticosteroids may be required if the patient has a serious illness or undergoes surgery during this recovery period.

Other considerations

Ophthalmologists who initiate systemic corticosteroid therapy for ophthalmic diseases should consider requesting assistance from the patient's primary care provider to monitor for adverse effects. For patients who require high-dose or extended corticosteroid treatment, clinicians should strongly consider early use of other immunosuppressive medications, which can decrease patient dependency on, and long-term complications of, corticosteroid use.

Nonsteroidal Anti-inflammatory Drugs

Clinicians use a wide variety of NSAIDs to treat RA and other rheumatic diseases. These agents decrease synthesis of inflammatory mediators such as prostaglandins by inhibiting the enzyme *cyclooxygenase (COX),* and all are analgesic, antipyretic, and anti-inflammatory. The COX enzyme has 2 isoforms. *COX-1* is present in most cells and appears to be involved in various aspects of cellular metabolism, such as gastric cytoprotection, platelet aggregation, and renal function. *COX-2* is present in some tissues, including brain and bone, but is also expressed at other sites in response to inflammation.

Complications from the use of oral NSAIDs account for approximately 12% of hospital admissions and more than 16,000 deaths each year in the United States. Their most significant adverse effects include gastrointestinal bleeding, renal failure, hypertension, and heart failure, as well as induction of asthma in aspirin-sensitive individuals. Oral NSAIDs can also interfere with platelet function and can cause bone marrow suppression, hepatic toxicity, and CNS symptoms including headache, dizziness, and confusion. In rare cases, NSAIDs have been associated with ocular adverse effects such as nonspecific blurred vision and diplopia. There have also been reports of possible optic neuropathy and macular edema, especially with use of ibuprofen.

The *traditional NSAIDs* inhibit both isoforms of COX. *Selective COX-2 inhibitors* have a lower risk of gastrointestinal damage and have less effect on platelet function. Two of these drugs (rofecoxib and valdecoxib) have been removed from the market worldwide because of adverse cardiovascular events. However, parecoxib, a prodrug of valdecoxib, remains available in many European countries. Similar concerns have been raised about celecoxib; although it is still available, this drug carries significant warnings. It has been proposed that the selective blocking of COX-2 decreases the production of prostacyclins, which cause vasodilation and inhibit platelet aggregation, leading to increased prothrombotic activity. Etoricoxib, another COX-2–selective NSAID, is available outside the United States. Ophthalmologists should be aware that conjunctivitis, temporary blindness, and blurred vision have been reported with use of COX-2 inhibitors.

Systemic NSAIDs may be useful in helping to control uveitis or scleritis in some patients, but they are not as effective as corticosteroids. Several topical NSAIDs have been approved for ocular use; they are discussed in BCSC Section 8, *External Disease and Cornea,* and Section 9, *Uveitis and Ocular Inflammation.*

Disease-Modifying Antirheumatic Drugs

There are 2 major categories of DMARDs: nonbiologic and biologic agents. See Table 9-5 for the classification, mechanism, and toxicities of these drugs.

Table 9-5 Disease-Modifying Antirheumatic Drugs

Drugs	Mechanism of Action	Toxicities
Nonbiologic agents		
Methotrexate	Inhibits folate metabolism/DNA synthesis	GI, liver, pneumonitis, cytopenia, sterility, teratogenicity
Leflunomide	Inhibits DNA/RNA synthesis	GI, liver, pneumonitis (rare)
Hydroxychloroquine	Inhibits lysosomal enzymes	GI, retina, hemolytic anemia in G6PD deficiency
Sulfasalazine	Exact mechanism unknown	GI, allergic, hemolytic anemia in G6PD deficiency
Azathioprine	Inhibits purine synthesis/DNA replication	GI, infection, cytopenia, lymphoma
Cyclophosphamide, chlorambucil	Cytotoxic effect/DNA crosslinking	Cytopenia, infection, infertility, malignancy
Cyclosporine, tacrolimus	Inhibits T-cell activation	Hypertension, renal toxicity
Mycophenolate mofetil	Inhibits T-cell/B-cell proliferation	GI, cytopenia, infection
Biologic agents		
Anti-TNF agents	Cytokine inhibition	Allergy, rash, infection, lymphoma
Adalimumab		
Certolizumab pegol		
Etanercept		
Golimumab		
Infliximab		
IL inhibitors	IL cytokine inhibition	
Anakinra	IL-1 cytokine inhibition	Neutropenia, infection
Canakinumab	IL-1 cytokine inhibition	Neutropenia, infection
Rilonacept	IL-1 cytokine inhibition	Neutropenia, infection
Sarilumab	IL-6 cytokine inhibition	Neutropenia, thrombocytopenia, elevated cholesterol and triglycerides, infection
Tocilizumab	IL-6 cytokine inhibition	Neutropenia, thrombocytopenia, elevated cholesterol and triglycerides, infection
Secukinumab	IL-17 cytokine inhibition	Allergy, infection
Ixekizumab	IL-17 cytokine inhibition	Allergy, infection
Ustekinumab	IL-12/23 cytokine inhibition	GI, infection, nasopharyngitis
Other biologic agents		
Abatacept	Inhibition of T-cell activation	Infusion reaction, infection
Alemtuzumab	Lymphocyte depletion	GI, infection, cytopenia
Belimumab	Inhibits B-cell activation	GI, allergy, leukopenia
Rituximab	B-cell lysis/suppression	Infusion reaction (may be severe), PML
Kinase inhibitors		
Tofacitinib	Janus kinase/cytokine inhibition	GI, infection, anemia
Baricitnib	Janus kinase/cytokine inhibition	GI, infection, anemia

DMARDs = disease-modifying antirheumatic drugs; G6PD = glucose-6-phosphate dehydrogenase; GI = gastrointestinal; IL = interleukin; PML = progressive multifocal leukoencephalopathy; TNF = tumor necrosis factor.

Nonbiologic drugs

Methotrexate A structural analogue of folic acid, *methotrexate* interferes both with folate-dependent metabolic pathways, such as purine, and with pyrimidine metabolism. Its disease-modifying effect may be mediated partly through increased extracellular adenosine, which has intrinsic anti-inflammatory activity. Methotrexate is given weekly, usually beginning at a dose of 7.5–10 mg, gradually increasing to a maximum dose of 25 mg, depending on disease response. All patients are supplemented with folic acid to decrease adverse effects associated with methotrexate use. Major adverse effects include hepatic fibrosis, interstitial lung disease, bone marrow toxicity, teratogenicity, sterility, and, in higher dosages, renal toxicity. Baseline and periodic monitoring should include blood counts, liver enzymes, and albumin and creatinine levels.

Leflunomide The immunosuppressive agent *leflunomide* targets rapidly dividing cell populations such as activated lymphocytes. It is most commonly used to treat RA, although it has also been effective in managing other conditions including psoriatic arthritis, juvenile polyarthritis, refractory dermatomyositis, and SLE. This drug is similar in efficacy to methotrexate, and the 2 are sometimes combined if methotrexate alone is ineffective. Adverse reactions include GI side effects, hepatotoxicity, and hypertension (especially if taken with NSAIDs). Close monitoring of patients is advised.

Hydroxychloroquine An antimalarial compound, *hydroxychloroquine* is also commonly used to treat rheumatologic diseases. In addition to its anti-inflammatory activity, the drug raises the pH of various cellular compartments, which decreases both cytokine production and lymphocyte proliferation. Response to treatment may take weeks to months, in part because of the drug's long half-life (1–2 months) and the time required to achieve steady-state levels.

Hydroxychloroquine is one of the safest immunosuppressive drugs used in managing rheumatologic disease. Retinopathy (bull's-eye maculopathy) due to hydroxychloroquine use is a relatively unusual complication, but it can cause irreversible vision loss if not detected early.

Ophthalmic considerations Recently updated recommendations suggest that *actual* body weight is more predictive than *ideal* body weight in assessing risk of retinopathy from hydroxychloroquine (at a maximum daily dose of 5 mg/kg). A baseline eye examination is advised within the first year of therapy. Annual follow-up exams can be delayed until 5 years after initiation, although this recommendation remains somewhat controversial in the ophthalmic community. More frequent exams are indicated for higher-risk patients. Duration of treatment is one of the risk factors, as 20% of patients develop toxicity with 20 years of medication usage. Other risk factors include preexisting retinal disease, presence of renal disease, and concurrent tamoxifen use. In addition to comprehensive dilated examinations, spectral domain optical coherence tomography and 10-2 visual field (VF) testing should be performed regularly. Asian patients appear to have a different clinical presentation, with more peripheral retinal findings, so a 24-2 or 30-2 VF assessment should be considered instead. The American Academy of Ophthalmology's recommendations and guidelines are available at www.aao.org/clinical-statement/revised-recommendations-on-screening-chloroquine-h. Retinopathy is discussed more fully in BCSC Section 12, *Retina and Vitreous.*

Marmor MF, Kellner U, Lai TY, Melles RB, Mieler WF; American Academy of Ophthalmology. Recommendations on screening for chloroquine and hydroxychloroquine retinopathy (2016 revision). *Ophthalmology.* 2016;123(6):1386–1394.

Sulfasalazine Although its exact mechanism of action is unclear, *sulfasalazine* is effective in treating RA. It is often used in combination with other drugs, such as hydroxychloroquine and methotrexate.

Azathioprine An antimetabolite, *azathioprine* interferes with purine metabolism. Its use, especially in inflammatory bowel disease, is limited due to its toxicity. The most common adverse effects are gastrointestinal symptoms, risk of infection, and bone marrow suppression. Patients treated with this drug have up to a 4-fold increase in the risk of lymphoma.

Alkylating agents *Cyclophosphamide* and *chlorambucil* are alkylating agents that are very potent immunosuppressive drugs. Their primary mechanism of action involves cross-linking DNA molecules, which blocks DNA replication. They also have potentially severe adverse effects, including infertility, bone marrow suppression, increased risk of infection, and late malignancy. Consequently, these drugs are reserved for very resistant or life-threatening diseases such as granulomatosis with polyangiitis, for which the benefits outweigh the risks. Cyclophosphamide is available as an oral or intravenous agent. The oral form is associated with increased rates of bladder cancer.

Calcineurin inhibitors *Cyclosporine* and *tacrolimus* block calcineurin, thereby inhibiting the transcription of IL-2 and other cytokines, primarily in helper T cells. These drugs are used chiefly to prevent rejection in patients who have undergone transplants, but clinicians are increasingly recognizing their benefit in treating autoimmune diseases. The main adverse effects of both drugs are nephrotoxicity and hypertension. Other potential problems include infections and nonmelanoma skin cancers. Because of such risks, these agents are reserved for recalcitrant cases that do not respond to standard therapies.

Mycophenolate Initially used as an antirejection drug in the United States, *mycophenolate mofetil* is increasingly being employed in patients with immunologic diseases. It inhibits the production of guanosine in lymphocytes, thereby decreasing cellular proliferation and antibody production. Primary adverse effects include gastrointestinal symptoms, bone marrow suppression, and increased risk of infection. An enteric-coated formulation of *mycophenolate sodium* typically reduces the incidence of gastrointestinal adverse effects. Overall, the drug seems to be well tolerated by patients and may serve as an adjunct to other medications.

Biologic and other anticytokine agents

TNF-α inhibitors Research that facilitated improved understanding of the immune response has led to the development of drugs targeting specific mediators. Cytokines, which are cell-signaling proteins generated by activated immune cells, can enhance or inhibit the immune response. *Tumor necrosis factor (TNF)-α* is a major proinflammatory cytokine involved in the pathogenesis of inflammatory diseases. The US Food and Drug Administration (FDA) has approved 5 TNF-α antagonists: *adalimumab, certolizumab pegol, etanercept, golimumab,* and *infliximab.* Certolizumab pegol is unique in this group as being an FDA category B drug and, therefore, is a treatment option for patients who are pregnant or nursing.

The drugs are usually well tolerated, but there is potential for severe adverse effects (see Table 9-5). Although not established, there may be a link between TNF-α inhibition and demyelinating disease, including optic neuritis, as well as potential risk of various malignancies. All patients on immunosuppressive therapy require close monitoring for the development of serious adverse effects. The cost of these drugs can also become a barrier for patients.

Interleukin inhibitors Biologic agents have been developed to block several types of interleukin (IL). Although these agents are not as potent as the TNF-α inhibitors, IL-1 drugs, including *anakinra, canakinumab,* and *rilonacept,* are used in many autoimmune disorders. The IL-6 inhibitor *tocilizumab* is used primarily for RA and JIA but may also be effective in treating giant cell arteritis and polymyalgia rheumatica. The drugs *secukinumab* and *ixekizumab* block the IL-17 pathway and are mainly used in psoriatic arthritis, as is the IL-12/23 inhibitor, *ustekinumab.*

Other biologic agents *Abatacept* is used in the treatment of RA and JIA. This drug blocks the CD28 receptor, which is involved in T-cell activation. It can be very effective in treating refractory disease.

Rituximab is a B-cell–depleting monoclonal antibody used primarily in chemotherapy but also in cases of RA that are unresponsive to other agents.

Belimumab is a human monoclonal antibody that inhibits B-cell activation. It was approved by the FDA for the treatment of SLE, but it may also be helpful for other immune disorders.

Alemtuzumab is a monoclonal antibody that binds to CD52, a protein on mature lymphocytes. The drug is used to treat chronic lymphocytic leukemia and has shown promise in the treatment of autoimmune diseases.

JAK inhibitors Kinase inhibitors are another group of immunosuppressive agents showing promise in treating rheumatologic disease. Janus kinase is one such enzyme these drugs target. *Tofacitinib* is a small-molecule oral agent that inhibits JAK-1 and JAK-3. *Baricitinib* inhibits JAK-1 and JAK-2. Both are approved by the FDA for rheumatoid arthritis. Their role may be in cases that are refractory to other classes of agents, including nonbiologic agents and TNF-α inhibitors.

Biosimilar agents The expiration of patent protection on some biologic agents has led to the development of *biosimilar agents.* A biosimilar has amino acid sequencing that is analogous (not identical) to the original compound (*reference product*) on which it is based. The FDA requires a biosimilar to be "highly similar to" and to have "no clinically meaningful differences" from the reference product for approval. The use of *infliximab-dyyb,* the biosimilar for infliximab, has grown worldwide and is particularly effective in treating inflammatory bowel disease. This agent, along with the biosimilars for etanercept and adalimumab, was approved in 2016 by the FDA for the treatment of RA, psoriatic arthritis, and ankylosing spondylitis. Other biosimilar agents continue to be developed.

Diehl R, Ferrara F, Müller C, et al. Immunosuppression for in vivo research: state-of-the-art protocols and experimental approaches. *Cell Mol Immunol.* 2017;14(2):146–179.

Wiseman AC. Immunosuppressive medications. *Clin J Am Soc Nephrol.* 2016;11(2):332–343.

CHAPTER 10

Geriatrics

Highlights

- Cataract, age-related macular degeneration (AMD), ischemic optic neuropathy, giant cell arteritis, diabetic retinopathy, and glaucoma are all diseases that disproportionately affect older persons.
- The subspecialty of geriatrics emphasizes a different medical paradigm of functional assessment and a more holistic approach to patient care compared with the traditional medical paradigm.
- The ophthalmologist is uniquely qualified to assess the visual limitations and visual needs of the elderly patient and communicate them to the geriatrician.
- Referral for vision rehabilitation is appropriate for patients with visual acuity less than 20/40, central scotomata, visual field loss, or contrast sensitivity loss.
- The median age of the world's population is increasing almost exponentially. This expanding older population presents a growing challenge to primary care physicians and medical subspecialists in the United States and Western Europe.

Introduction

The median age of the world's population is increasing almost exponentially. In the United States, the population aged 65 years and older is projected to more than double, from 46 million in 2016 to over 98 million by 2060, representing 14.9% and nearly 25% of the total population, respectively. In addition, the number of persons aged 85 years and older is expected to triple, from 6.2 million in 2014 to 19.7 million in 2060. Worldwide, over the same period, the population aged 65 years and older is projected to increase by approximately 617 million, up to 1.6 billion, from 8.5% to 16.7%. In the next 15 years, the number of older persons is expected to grow fastest in Latin America and the Caribbean with a projected 71% increase, followed by Asia at 66%, Africa at 64%, Oceania at 47%, and Europe at 23%.

This expanding older population presents a growing challenge to primary care physicians and medical subspecialists in the United States and Western Europe. The subspecialty of geriatrics emphasizes a different medical paradigm of functional assessment and a more holistic approach to patient care compared with the traditional medical paradigm.

Physiologic Aging and Pathologic Findings of the Aging Eye

Age-related changes in sensation and perception can isolate individuals from their surrounding environments and trigger complex psychological reactions. These changes may include diminished hearing and vision, slowed intellectual and physical response times, and increased difficulty with memory. However, many physical and intellectual abilities are retained throughout the life span, and their loss should not be assumed to be part of the normal aging process. These include the senses of taste and smell, intelligence, the ability to learn, and sexuality. Any change in physical, intellectual, or emotional capabilities may reflect underlying organic or psychological disease.

Age-related changes in the eye affect individuals differently. The periorbital and eyelid skin and soft tissues atrophy with age. Dermatochalasis and levator dehiscence may produce secondary ptosis. Eyelid laxity may cause entropion, ectropion, and trichiasis. Lacrimal gland dysfunction, decreased tear production, meibomian gland dysfunction, and goblet cell dysfunction may cause dry eye symptoms. As a result of the aging process, the conjunctiva undergoes atrophic changes and corneal sensitivity is reduced. The pupils become progressively miotic and less reactive to light. There is an increasing incidence of presbyopia, cataract, glaucoma, AMD, and diabetic retinopathy. Contrast sensitivity and visual field sensitivity are reduced. In addition, refractive error (of some type) is present in more than 90% of older patients and remains a significant cause of visual disability in the nursing home patient.

Worldwide, the 4 leading causes of vision loss in the older population are AMD, glaucoma, cataract, and diabetic retinopathy. It is estimated that by 2030, 3.7 million persons in the United States will have AMD. Glaucoma will affect 4.3 million individuals by 2030 and becomes more common with increasing age; thus, screening is recommended for patients older than 50 years. Cataract accounts for 50% of visual impairment in adults over the age of 40; it affects 1 in every 6 people in this age group. It is projected that by 2030, 38.7 million Americans will have cataracts. Diabetic retinopathy is a leading cause of new cases of legal blindness among working-aged Americans. The prevalence of retinopathy in individuals with diabetes mellitus aged 40 years and older in the United States is 28.5% (4.2 million persons), and the prevalence of vision-threatening retinopathy is 4.4% (0.7 million persons). Assuming a similar prevalence for diabetes mellitus, the projected numbers in 2050 would be 16.0 million persons with diabetic retinopathy and 3.4 million persons with vision-threatening diabetic retinopathy.

National Eye Institute website; www.nei.nih.gov. Accessed September 10, 2021.

Saaddine JB, Honeycutt AA, Narayan KM, Zhang X, Klein R, Boyle JP. Projection of diabetic retinopathy and other major eye diseases among people with diabetes mellitus: United States, 2005–2050. *Arch Ophthalmol.* 2008;126(12):1740–1741.

Ophthalmic considerations Ophthalmology is largely an outpatient specialty. For older patients, access to the ophthalmologist's office can be a major physical barrier to eye care. The ideal outpatient office should be designed to accommodate older patients with various disabilities; such an office environment should include the following:

- a safe, well-lit office that is close to drop-off areas and parking
- automatic or assisted doors (doorways with pull levers or handles, not doorknobs)
- large-print, legible, well-placed signs
- wheelchair-accessible entryways and waiting rooms
- obstacle-free and well-lit, high-contrast walkways, hallways, and waiting areas (free of rugs, electrical cords, and tripping hazards, such as toys)
- accessible bathrooms with elevated toilet seats, grab bars, and a wheelchair-accessible sink
- staff trained to assist patients with disabilities to and from the examination room
- a private area where patients with decreased hearing and vision can receive assistance from office staff to complete forms

The American Academy of Ophthalmology's Initiative in Vision Rehabilitation page on the ONE Network (www.aao.org/low-vision-and-vision-rehab) provides resources for low vision management, including patient handouts and information about additional vision rehabilitation opportunities beyond those provided by the ophthalmologist.

American Academy of Ophthalmology Vision Rehabilitation Committee, Hoskins Center for Quality Eye Care. Preferred Practice Pattern® Guidelines. *Vision Rehabilitation*. San Francisco: American Academy of Ophthalmology; 2017. Available at www.aao.org/ppp.

Elder Abuse

Elder abuse is an important public health problem. It is a violation of human rights and is a significant cause of illness, injury, loss of productivity, isolation, and despair, according to the World Health Organization. The National Elder Abuse Incidence Study (1998) found that in 1996, nearly half a million persons aged 60 years or older had been physically abused, neglected, or in some way mistreated. This study, which was based on Adult Protective Service records and sentinel reports (eg, reports from community professionals), very likely greatly underestimated the true scope of the problem of abuse of older Americans, because the majority of elder abuse cases are unreported and are undetected by monitoring agents. A 2017 study that summarized 52 studies in 28 countries from diverse regions estimated that over the past year, 15.7% of people aged 60 and over were subjected to some form of abuse. In the United States, the prevalence of elder maltreatment was reported as 7.6%–10% of study participants and is estimated to affect 11.4% of adults aged 60 years and older. Worldwide, it is estimated that only 1 in 24 cases of elder abuse is reported, in part because elderly individuals are often afraid to report the abuse to family, friends, or the authorities. The EU Charter of Fundamental Rights, Article 25, states that "The Union recognizes and respects the rights of the elderly to lead a life of dignity and independence and to participate in social and cultural life," yet 47% of European people believe that poor treatment, neglect, and abuse of older people are common in their countries.

Major risk factors for elder abuse include external stresses due to marital, financial, and legal difficulties; dependent relationships (eg, the abuser may be dependent on the older patient for finances or housing, or vice versa); mental illness and substance abuse; social isolation; and misinformation about normal aging or about the patient's medical or nutritional needs. Maltreatment can occur at home, in assisted living facilities, or in nursing homes. It can take the form of physical or psychological abuse, material misappropriation, neglect and abandonment, or sexual abuse.

Physical abuse means inflicting physical pain or injury upon an older adult. Psychological abuse includes verbal assaults, threats of abuse, harassment, and intimidation. Material misappropriation or financial abuse of the elderly includes taking money or property or using/misusing money or property without the owner's knowledge or permission; forging or forcing an elderly person's signature; misusing ATM cards or credit cards; and persuading an elderly individual to change a will or an insurance policy. Passive neglect is a caregiver's failure to provide an older adult with life's necessities such as food, water, hygiene, clothing, shelter, medical care, or medication. Neglect may be intentional or unintentional and may be related to financial constraints or lack of other resources (eg, transportation, supervision). Elder abuse also includes deprivation of basic rights (eg, decision-making for care, privacy) and abandonment.

The ophthalmologist may be the first physician to see an older patient who is being abused or neglected. The signs may be subtle, and early recognition is key. The ophthalmologist should suspect elder abuse in the following circumstances:

- broken eyeglasses, with a report by the patient of being slapped or abused
- evidence of physical abuse (eg, bruises, black eyes, fractures, lacerations, wounds in various stages of healing, burns, welts, patches of hair loss, or unexplained subconjunctival, retinal, or vitreous hemorrhage)
- repeated visits to the emergency department or office
- conflicting or noncredible history from caregiver or patient
- unexplained delay in seeking treatment
- unexplained, inconsistent, vague, or poorly explained injuries
- history of being "accident prone"
- expressions of ambivalence, anger, hostility, or fear by the patient toward the caregiver
- poor adherence to follow-up or care instructions

Sometimes it is necessary to obtain the patient history with the caregiver out of the room. Directed questions for the patient include "Has anyone at home tried to harm you?"; "Has anyone tried to make you do things that you don't wish to do?"; and "Has anyone taken anything from you without your consent?"

Any suspected case of elder neglect or abuse should prompt a complete written report. Documentation of any suspicious injuries is mandatory, including type, size, location, and characteristics of injury and stage of healing. Requirements for reporting elder abuse vary from state to state, and many areas have abuse hotlines for reporting maltreatment. The physician should be aware of local services for adult protection, community social services, and law enforcement agencies.

Acierno R, Hernandez MA, Amstadter AB, et al. Prevalence and correlates of emotional, physical, sexual, and financial abuse and potential neglect in the United States: the National Elder Mistreatment Study. *Am J Public Health.* 2010;100(2):292–297.

National Council on Aging website: Elder Abuse Facts. www.ncoa.org/advocates/public-policy/issues/aging-services/elder-justice. Accessed September 10, 2021.

Perioperative Considerations in the Management of Elderly Patients

There are several considerations that the ophthalmologist should take into account in the preoperative evaluation and perioperative management of elderly patients; loss of vision alone may not be an appropriate sole indication for surgical intervention (eg, cataract surgery). Functional assessment includes determining how vision loss affects instrumental activities of daily living (IADLs) such as reading, driving, taking medications properly, and using the telephone independently; IADLs should be documented preoperatively. All prescription medications should also be documented to ensure that they do not interact with perioperative medications. An elderly patient may have multiple medical conditions that require use of numerous prescription medications. Some of these medications can even have ocular side effects. Please see Chapter 16 for further discussion. The management of informed consent should be considered; this process may be different in patients with mild dementia and in those who have legal guardians or caregivers who will need to participate in the process.

Elderly patients undergoing surgery may be prone to confusion or delirium perioperatively. Delirium is estimated to occur in approximately 4%–5% of patients after cataract surgery. Many causes for confusion are preventable. Minimization of preoperative sedation or psychotropic medications, appropriate patient and family orientation by nursing or ancillary staff, and careful supervision and reassurance in the postoperative period can diminish confusion. Often, a confused older patient simply needs a familiar face or reassurance to regain calm. The use of restraints should be minimized.

Confusion may be exacerbated in patients with vision loss or in those who require vision rehabilitation. In a monocular older patient, patching of the eye after surgery may aggravate confusion and disorientation. Having a family member in the recovery room can be very helpful. The patch should be removed as soon as possible, and the patient should be provided with appropriate eye protection. Topical anesthetic may not be indicated because of comorbidities such as cognitive impairment and inability to cooperate during surgery. In addition, patients with decreased vision following intraocular surgery may experience limited mobility or be at increased risk for falls. Bed rest and immobilization can lead to disuse of extremities, development of pressure ulcers, and other problems. For these patients, active rehabilitation should be encouraged as soon as possible.

Though rare in outpatient ophthalmic surgery, surgical or anesthesia complications may result in life-threatening conditions. The surgeon must pay careful attention to any preexisting directives (eg, do-not-resuscitate order or living will) prior to any surgical intervention (including laser treatments and periocular injections or anesthetics). By discussing possible treatment decisions with the patient and family members early—preferably before any serious illness arises or, if a serious illness is present, early in its course—the surgeon can avoid emergency decisions.

Some potential issues for discussion include limits of treatment, antibiotics, and changes in the patient's living situation. Candidly and openly discussing these important issues with the patient and the family (especially in cases of dementia) in the preoperative period allows them to consider these matters in the context of their belief systems and without the disorientation and confusion created by an emergency. The content, context, time, and date of such discussions should be well documented in the medical record and communicated to the patient, the family, and the primary care physician or geriatrician.

Psychology of Aging

The psychology of aging is influenced by a wide range of factors, including physical changes, adaptive mechanisms, and psychopathology. Each older patient has a unique psychological profile and social life history. Deleterious changes are not universal; in fact, in the absence of disease, growth of character and the ability to learn continue throughout life.

With age, the issue of loss becomes more prevalent. Losses—of status, physical abilities, loved ones, and income—become more frequent. A fear of loss of social and individual power, and the attendant loss of independence, is common. In addition, the reality of death has increasing influence on a person's psychological status. All of these losses increase the incidence of depression.

Depression

Depression is the most frequent psychiatric problem in the older population. Approximately one-quarter of older patients seen in primary care settings are clinically depressed. The prevalence of depression in patients with macular degeneration is even higher, at 30%–40%. The suicide rate in White American men older than 65 years is 5 times greater than that of the general population; loneliness is the main reason cited, along with financial problems and poor health. Successful suicide is much less common in older American women, but older women attempt suicide more often than do men.

The criteria set forth in the *Diagnostic and Statistical Manual of Mental Disorders,* Fifth Edition (DSM-5), make a clear separation between depressive symptoms that result from a general medical condition and the medication used to treat it from late-life depression. An alternative diagnosis of mood disorder is preferred for the former.

Major depressive disorder is characterized by episodes of at least 2 weeks of depressed mood or loss of interest or pleasure in activities with 4 or more of the following symptoms:

- changes in appetite with associated weight loss or gain
- significant weight loss or gain
- sleep disturbance
- agitation
- diminished libido
- retardation (slowing down)
- loss of energy
- feelings of worthlessness or guilt
- difficulties in concentration and decision-making
- recurrent thoughts of suicide or death

Although the signs and symptoms of depression in older individuals are similar to those seen in younger age groups, older depressed patients are *more likely* than younger patients to have somatic or hypochondriacal complaints, minimize depression symptoms (masked depression), and have psychotic delusional disease. However, they are *less likely* to report symptoms of guilt. The most frequent presentations of subclinical depression include new medical complaints, fatigue, poor concentration, exacerbation of existing symptoms and medical problems, preoccupation with health, and diminished interest in pleasurable activities.

The ophthalmologist's role is to recognize and refer the patient with depression or to be aware of precipitating factors. For instance, loss of function, such as moderate or severe vision loss, can precipitate depression, as can recent death of a spouse. Ophthalmic medications such as β-blockers and α-agonists can cause fatigue, depression, and diminished cognition. Red flags may include frequent visits to the ophthalmology office and unexplained vision loss. Though not prevalent in the ophthalmology setting, testing patients for depression might be enormously helpful in attaining care for those patients who have this disorder; an appropriate referral for such testing may be necessary.

Many targeted screening tests, also called case-finding instruments, ask about depressed mood and *anhedonia*, a psychological condition characterized by inability to experience pleasure in acts that normally produce it. Most of these instruments require more time than is available during a typical office visit. A briefer case-finding instrument, the Patient Health Questionnaire-2 (PHQ-2), is a suggested screening device. It is sensitive, but not specific; it does not suggest or establish a final diagnosis or monitor depression severity, but screens for depression in a "first step" approach. The self-report questionnaire consists of the following 2 questions:

1. During the past month, have you been bothered by feeling down, depressed, or hopeless?
2. During the past month, have you often been bothered by little interest or pleasure in doing things?

If the first question is answered in the affirmative, it is highly likely that the patient has depression. The added sensitivity and greater specificity provided by the second question, if answered in the affirmative, makes it worthwhile to ask the questions. A score of 2 or 3 on either question is considered a positive response to this 2-question test and is in line with DSM criteria for depression. Further information on the PHQ-2 is available on the website of the American Psychological Association (www.apa.org/pi/about/publications/caregivers/practice-settings/assessment/tools/patient-health). After using the PHQ-2 to evaluate a patient, the ophthalmologist may conclude that further evaluation by the patient's primary care physician is necessary.

Kroenke K, Spitzer RL, Williams JB. The Patient Health Questionnaire-2: validity of a two-item depression screener. *Med Care.* 2003;41(11):1284–1292.

Miguel A, Henriques F, Azevedo LF, Pereira AC. Ophthalmic adverse drug reactions to systemic drugs: a systematic review. *Pharmacoepidemiol Drug Saf.* 2014;23(3):221–233.

Alzheimer Disease and Dementia

Alzheimer disease and dementia are discussed in Chapter 11 of this volume.

Osteoporosis

Osteoporosis is defined by the World Health Organization as a disease "characterized by low bone mass and micro-architectural deterioration of bone tissue, leading to bone fragility and a consequent increase in risk of fracture." Osteoporosis is a significant, worldwide public health problem that is becoming increasingly common. It is estimated that globally, 1 of every 2 women and 1 of every 4 men older than 50 years will have an osteoporosis-related fracture. In the United States, 1.5 million fractures related to osteoporosis occur annually, with the estimated cost of caring for these patients approaching $18 billion. This number is expected to triple by the year 2040. In older patients, a broken hip can increase mortality fourfold. Those with hip fractures have a 20% risk of entering a nursing home within a year of their fracture, and it is estimated that almost 50% of women with hip fractures do not fully regain previous function. Many patients with hip fractures experience a decline in function, along with increased feelings of isolation, depression, and fear of falling. In an individual with osteoporosis, the potential for falling becomes even more important.

Ophthalmic considerations It is important to note what medications are being taken by a patient with osteoporosis. The class of drugs known as bisphosphonates, which are often prescribed for postmenopausal women to inhibit bone resorption, can affect eye health. These drugs are associated with inflammatory disease of the eye, including conjunctivitis, uveitis, and episcleritis. Scleritis, which can be vision threatening, has also been reported. On the other hand, a study of veterans determined that the rates of uveitis and/or scleritis following dispensing of a bisphosphonate drug were low and did not differ significantly from those of the control group.

French DD, Margo CE. Postmarketing surveillance rates of uveitis and scleritis with bisphosphonates among a national veteran cohort. *Retina.* 2008;28(6):889–893.

Falls

Falls are a leading cause of injury and death in older Americans. The incidence and severity of falls rises with increasing age. Approximately one-third of US adults older than 65 years fall each year, yet less than half talk to their physicians about it. In 2010, about 21,700 older adults in the United States died as a result of unintentional fall injuries. In 2014 alone, older Americans experienced 29 million falls, resulting in 7 million injuries and incurring about $31 billion in annual Medicare costs. Falls are responsible for more than 60% of all traumatic brain injuries (TBIs) in people over 65 years old. In the United States, fall-related TBIs are responsible for 14,347 deaths per year. Men are more likely to die from a fall. Older White individuals are 2.4 times more likely to die from falls than are older Black individuals. Also, there are differences in fatal fall rates among ethnic groups; older non-Hispanic persons have higher fatal fall rates than do older Hispanic persons. Fear of falling may cause elderly persons to limit activities, leading to reduced physical fitness, which, in turn, increases the actual risk of falling.

Prevention of falls is key. Older adults may reduce their chances of falling by

- exercising regularly
- increasing leg strength and balance
- asking their physician or pharmacist to review any of their medications that might cause dizziness or drowsiness
- having their eyes checked annually to update glasses or evaluate for eye diseases that limit vision
- getting assistance to make their living areas safer by
  - removing tripping hazards
  - installing grab bars in the bathroom and railings on the side of stairways (such as the entry to the home)
  - improving lighting

Visual disorders are a frequent cause of falls. Recent studies in the United States and the United Kingdom suggest that elderly individuals are almost twice as likely to fall if they are visually impaired. An ophthalmologist may help patients reduce the risk of falls by

- asking patients appropriate questions about the activities listed above that might reduce fall risk
- recognizing and treating visual disorders, including refractive errors, to identify and minimize ocular reasons for falls

Patients with reduced vision from eye disease, most often macular degeneration, are at the highest risk of falling. Once a history of falls is obtained, it is incumbent upon the ophthalmologist to notify the patient's primary care physician about this finding or refer the patient to a multidisciplinary medical facility with resources for managing falls in the elderly.

Centers for Disease Control and Prevention (CDC). Stopping elderly accidents, deaths & injuries (STEADI): Older adult fall prevention. www.cdc.gov/steadi. Updated July 9, 2020. Accessed September 10, 2021.

Stevens JA, Ballesteros MF, Mack KA, Rudd RA, DeCaro E, Adler G. Gender differences in seeking care for falls in the aged Medicare population. *Am J Prev Med.* 2012;43(1):59–62.

Ophthalmic considerations Many activities of daily living require adequate functioning of different visual components such as near, intermediate, and distance vision, as well as peripheral vision, binocular vision, depth perception, contrast sensitivity, and color vision. Cataract surgery improves functional visual status, resulting in overall improved health-related quality of life, mental health, and emotional well-being. Visual function plays an important role in physical performance, especially in terms of mobility. The rate of falls in the elderly is diminished after cataract removal, with a lower incidence of hip fracture 1 year after the procedure when compared with patients with cataract who did not have cataract surgery.

American Academy of Ophthalmology Cataract/Anterior Segment Panel, Hoskins Center for Quality Eye Care. Preferred Practice Pattern® Guidelines. *Cataract in the Adult Eye.* San Francisco: American Academy of Ophthalmology; 2016. www.aao.org/ppp.

American Academy of Ophthalmology Committee, Hoskins Center for Quality Eye Care. Preferred Practice Pattern® Guidelines. *Comprehensive Adult Medical Eye Evaluation.* San Francisco: American Academy of Ophthalmology; 2015. www.aao.org/ppp.

American Academy of Ophthalmology Retina/Vitreous Panel, Hoskins Center for Quality Eye Care. Preferred Practice Pattern® Guidelines. *Age-Related Macular Degeneration.* San Francisco: American Academy of Ophthalmology; 2015. www.aao.org/ppp.

American Academy of Ophthalmology Retina/Vitreous Panel, Hoskins Center for Quality Eye Care. Preferred Practice Pattern® Guidelines. *Diabetic Retinopathy.* San Francisco: American Academy of Ophthalmology; 2017. www.aao.org/ppp.

Tseng VL, Yu F, Lum F, Coleman AL. Risks of fractures following cataract surgery in Medicare beneficiaries. *JAMA.* 2012;308(5):493–501.

US Census Bureau website; www.census.gov.

United Nations Statistics Division Demographics and Social Statistics: Population Censuses' Datasets (1995–Present). New York, NY. https://unstats.un.org/unsd/demographic-social/products/dyb/dybcensusdata.cshtml. Accessed September 10, 2021.

CHAPTER 11

Behavioral and Neurologic Disorders

Highlights

- Each year, 1 in 5 adults is affected with a mental health disorder, of which only half are ever diagnosed by a physician.
- Newer therapeutic agents for psychiatric diseases allow for more effective treatment with generally fewer adverse effects compared with older agents.
- Visual impairment almost doubles the risk of acquired depression.
- Second-generation antipsychotics (SGAs) such as olanzapine, quetiapine, and clozapine may be associated with the onset or worsening of diabetes mellitus and its associated ocular findings.
- The use of the antiepileptic medication vigabatrin is associated with irreversible and often asymptomatic concentric visual field loss in up to 50% of patients.
- Some new treatments for Parkinson disease may be neuroprotective and are therefore considered potential disease-modifying agents.

Introduction

Since the 1980s, the World Health Organization (WHO) has focused its efforts on common behavioral and neurologic disorders that cause substantial disability and challenges to individuals, families, and societies. The WHO approach is based on epidemiologic evidence and the assessment of disease burden using disability-adjusted life-years (DALYs). In 2010, the Global Burden of Disease Study (GBD) demonstrated that mental, neurological, and substance abuse disorders accounted for 10.4% of global DALYs, an increase of 41% since 1990. It is estimated that this figure will increase another 5% by the year 2030. Some of the disorders that contribute to this overall burden include schizophrenia, epilepsy, dementias (in particular, Alzheimer disease), multiple sclerosis, Parkinson disease, stroke, and brain injury. The global economic consequences of these health issues are significant as well, with an estimated economic loss of $16.3 trillion between 2011 and 2030.

Patel V, Chisholm D, Parikh R, et al; DCP MNS Author Group. Addressing the burden of mental, neurological, and substance use disorders: key messages from Disease Control Priorities, 3rd edition. *Lancet.* 2016;387(10028):1672–1685.

Behavioral Disorders

Behavioral disorders encompass a wide range of conditions in which the common factor is disordered functioning of thinking, behavior, and/or interpersonal relationships. In the absence of screening, only approximately 50% of persons with depression and other mental health conditions are ever diagnosed. Recent reports indicate that less than 5% of adults in primary care settings are ever formally screened for depression. Because electronic health records are starting to include standardized screening tools, including questions targeting depression, this percentage may improve. The prevalence of these disorders is staggering: each year, 1 in 5 adults will experience a mental health condition, and 75% of these conditions develop by the age of 24. The goal of the WHO's Mental Health Gap Action Program is to raise awareness of the challenges related to mental health disorders and to facilitate solutions for the growing need for services, particularly in resource-poor regions.

Behavioral Disorders Associated With Medical Conditions

Behavioral disorders are sometimes associated with other conditions, which can present a challenge to clinicians in understanding their cause and determining the best course of treatment. Sometimes the disorder is caused by the medical condition itself, and sometimes the etiology is multifactorial. Potential causes include adverse effects from medication or stressors related to dealing with the medical condition such as the associated financial burden, limited access to appropriate care, or the lack of an adequate support network.

Because almost any disease can result in behavioral changes in an individual, it is imperative for clinicians to look for indicators of underlying causal factors. For example, mental disorders that develop in patients later in life are more likely to be related to an underlying medical condition that would explain the delayed onset. In addition, more acute changes may be the result of a physiological change, such as a neurovascular event, an infection, an environmental exposure, an electrolyte imbalance, or a hormonal change. Finally, behavioral abnormalities associated with disorders of the motor system, such as gait and balance problems, speech irregularities, or unusual tics, suggest a possible underlying neuropathology, warranting further investigation. Neurologic disease states that can cause behavioral changes include head trauma and post-concussion syndrome, stroke, multiple sclerosis, and brain tumors, especially tumors involving the frontal lobe.

Chronic disease states, such as disabling rheumatoid arthritis, chronic pulmonary illness, or cardiovascular disease, are associated with higher rates of depression in adults. Other illnesses associated with behavioral changes in patients include untreated thyroid disorders, Lyme disease, hemochromatosis, and Wilson disease. Some diseases may present with only minor mood changes, whereas others present with major depression, hallucinations, and delusions. As noted, behavioral changes may be induced by medications, for example, carbonic anhydrase inhibitors, steroids, and chemotherapeutic agents, among others.

Schizophrenia

WHO lists schizophrenia as one of the top 10 disorders contributing to the global burden of disease. Schizophrenia usually begins when patients are young and continues to a greater or lesser extent throughout their lives. The prevalence is estimated at 1% of the global population.

The hallmarks of schizophrenia include hallucinations, delusions, disorganized thinking, and "negative" symptoms such as emotional and cognitive blunting. Motor disturbances range from uncontrolled, aimless activity to catatonic stupor, in which the patient may be immobile, mute, and unresponsive, yet fully conscious. Also common are repetitive, purposeless mannerisms and an inability to complete goal-directed tasks. Patients with schizophrenia may have other mental health conditions, such as major depression and anxiety disorders. Alternatively, manifestations of schizophrenia can be confused with symptoms of depression or anxiety. The lifetime occurrence of substance abuse in individuals with this disorder is approximately 50%. Associated illnesses include *schizophreniform disorder,* in which schizophrenic manifestations occur for less than 6 months, and *brief psychotic disorder,* which lasts less than 1 month. Patients with *schizoaffective disorder* have a significant mood disorder, such as depression, in addition to the psychotic manifestations.

Mood Disorders

Mood disorders, also called affective disorders, represent a spectrum of mental health illnesses in which prolonged periods of sadness (depression) are on one end and signs of excessive elation (mania) are on the other end. Manifestations of both ends of the spectrum at different times in an individual is termed bipolar disorder.

Major depression manifests as significant depressive episodes without any manic symptoms, often referred to as unipolar depression; it is far more common than mania alone. The lifetime risk for a major depressive disorder is 9% for men and approximately 17% for women. In developed countries, the prevalence of this disorder is around 18%, whereas in underdeveloped nations, it is around 9%. Major depression may occur at any age, but it most commonly affects middle-aged persons. Elderly individuals who live in health care facilities and individuals affected with a wide range of acute and chronic disease also appear to be at higher risk.

Major depression is a disabling condition that causes impairment of basic physical functions, as manifested by sleep disturbances, changes in appetite with associated weight loss or gain, diminished libido, and an inability to experience pleasure *(anhedonia).* Affective changes include pervasive and persistent low mood, slowed thought processes, low self-esteem, and loss of interest or pleasure in normal activities. Social withdrawal and psychomotor retardation are observed, although agitation can also occur. Patients commonly report somatic symptoms such as fatigue and headache, as well as other nonspecific symptoms. The risk of suicide in the depressed patient is over 25 times that of the general population; factors associated with suicide risk include the degree or longevity of the disorder, male sex, the family history of psychiatric disorder, and the presence of comorbidity. Patients with *dysthymic disorder* have chronic, less severe depressive symptoms that do not meet the criteria for major depression.

Mania is a period of abnormally and persistently elevated or irritable mood that is sufficiently severe to impair social or occupational functioning. Typical symptoms include euphoria or irritability, grandiosity, decreased need for sleep, increased speed of thought and speech (flight of ideas), and increased goal-directed activity. Formerly called manic depression, *bipolar disorder* is found in approximately 3% of people. It manifests in 2 forms. Bipolar I disorder describes any illness in which mania is present, whether or not depression occurs. Bipolar II disorder refers to patients with major depressive episodes and at least one mild manic episode (hypomania). *Cyclothymic disorder* describes cyclical episodes of mania and mild depression.

For the nonpsychiatric clinician, depression creates several problems. In some patients, mood change may not be apparent, and the illness may manifest in somatic symptoms, leading to time-consuming, expensive workups. Conversely, in patients known to be depressed, an organic disease may be overlooked as psychosomatic. Recommendations for psychotherapeutic intervention may be met with resistance, anger, or denial, disrupting the patient–physician relationship. Patients may have difficulty adhering to diagnostic and treatment regimens for medical disorders and surgical procedures. A screening study of older patients attending an ophthalmology clinic showed that 1 in 5 patients suffered from depression. Visual impairment almost doubles the risk of depression. In a recent study, the prevalence of depression in patients with macular degeneration was as high as 39%. The American Academy of Ophthalmology's Preferred Practice Pattern Guidelines recommend screening all macular degeneration patients and providing appropriate referrals for those suspected of having depression.

American Academy of Ophthalmology Retina/Vitreous PPP Panel, Hoskins Center for Quality Eye Care. Preferred Practice Pattern® Guidelines. *Age-Related Macular Degeneration.* San Francisco: American Academy of Ophthalmology; 2015. Available at www.aao.org/ppp.

Cimarolli V, Casten RJ, Rovner BW, Heyl V, Sörensen S, Horowitz A. Anxiety and depression in patients with advanced macular degeneration: current perspectives. *Clin Ophthalmol.* 2015;10:55–63.

Somatization, Anxiety, and Stress-Related Disorders

Somatic symptom and related disorders

The *Diagnostic and Statistical Manual of Mental Disorders,* Fifth Edition (DSM-5), has recategorized "somatoform disorders" as *somatic symptom and related disorders.* The term somatoform disorder is still recognized, however, by the WHO *International Classification of Diseases,* 10th Revision (ICD-10). (In ICD-11, which is now in development and is scheduled for approval by January 2022, this designation may be replaced with the term *bodily distress disorder.*) The term "somatization" is a more general description of the syndrome of symptoms that suggest physical illness or injury in the absence of objective findings or a known physiological mechanism. These symptoms may be result from anxiety, depression, or interpersonal conflicts.

The syndrome is not uncommon; the prevalence in the general population is approximately 6%. Risk factors associated with somatization include female sex, lower socioeconomic or educational level, and ethnic minority status. Somatization is a known problem among outpatient clinics, emergency department visits, and admittances to hospitals because each case requires investigation to rule out underlying disease. However, the disorder has significant ramifications for the individual affected because it can cause impaired functioning and disability. The most common presentation includes pain (eg, headache, back pain), gastrointestinal complaints, cardiopulmonary symptoms, and various neurological symptoms. The manifestation can involve any system; ophthalmologists should be aware of this syndrome because patients may present with ophthalmic-related symptoms such as blurred or double vision.

Entities under the DSM-5 designation of somatic symptom and related disorders include conversion disorder, illness anxiety disorder, and factitious disorder.

Conversion disorder *Conversion disorder* is characterized by temporary and involuntary loss or alteration of physical functioning caused by psychosocial stress. Symptoms are typically neurologic and may include functional vision loss. Psychotherapy is the primary treatment. Diagnosis may be difficult because of the subjective nature of the symptoms.

Illness anxiety disorder Formerly called hypochondriasis, *illness anxiety disorder* is a preoccupation with the fear of having or developing a serious disease. Physical examination fails to support the patient's belief, and reassurance by the examining physician often fails to allay the fear. A subcategory of this entity relevant to ophthalmologists is *body dysmorphic disorder,* in which the patient believes that his or her body is deformed, even though there is no physical defect, or the patient has an exaggerated concern about a mild physical anomaly. Ophthalmologists performing reconstructive and cosmetic surgery should be aware of this disorder because surgical repair of the "defect" is rarely successful in the patient's mind.

Factitious disorder and malingering *Factitious disorder* (previously known as Munchausen syndrome) is characterized by the willful production, feigning, or exaggeration of physical or psychological signs or symptoms in the absence of external causes. Treatment requires discovery of the true nature of the physical illness, a carefully planned confrontation, and psychotherapy. Prognosis for recovery is guarded. Self-inflicted chronic conjunctivitis, keratitis, and even scleritis are the usual ophthalmic presentations of factitious disease. Although related, *malingering* is not classified as a mental illness because it involves the fabrication of symptoms for secondary personal gain (eg, money, drugs); malingering should be considered when symptoms and findings do not make sense. Ophthalmologists should be familiar with techniques for detecting malingerers because patients are occasionally encountered in practice settings. See BCSC Section 5, *Neuro-Ophthalmology,* for a description of some of these techniques.

Generalized anxiety disorder

Anxiety disorders represent another group of diseases that can significantly interfere with normal functioning. *Generalized anxiety disorder (GAD)* is common, with a lifetime prevalence of 5%. GAD affects women twice as frequently as men. The disorder is characterized by unrealistic or excessive anxiety and worry that is not focused on one particular life event. GAD is associated with depression in a majority of cases and carries an increased risk of substance abuse. Pharmacologic therapy and psychotherapy may be successful in treating patients with this disease.

Panic disorder

Patients with *panic disorder* report discrete periods of intense terror and impending doom with associated physical symptoms (eg, trembling, difficulty breathing) that are almost intolerable. These episodes can occur abruptly, either in certain predictable situations or without any situational trigger. Mild cases may be treated with psychotherapy, but more significant disease may require treatment with antidepressant medication such as selective serotonin reuptake inhibitors (SSRIs).

Post-traumatic stress disorder

Post-traumatic stress disorder (PTSD) occurs after an individual has been exposed to a traumatic event associated with intense fear. When exposed to reminders of the event, the patient then persistently re-experiences the event through intrusive recollections, nightmares, flashbacks, or distress. The lifetime prevalence of PTSD is variable but has been reported at rates as high as 12% in the general population of North America and significantly lower rates (approximately 1%) in other countries. This difference is poorly understood. Combat soldiers and victims of assault are at particular risk. Treatment usually includes cognitive behavioral therapy, psychotherapy, and antidepressants.

Personality disorders

Personality disorders, which affect approximately 6% of the global population, merit discussion here because they may be associated with substance abuse and poor adherence to treatment. These disorders are diagnosed when personality traits become so inflexible and maladaptive that they create significant occupational and/or interpersonal dysfunction. Patients usually have little or no insight into their disorder. DSM-5 categorizes these disorders into 3 types:

- *Cluster A personality disorders* include paranoid, schizotypal, and schizoid disorders.
- *Cluster B personality disorders* include antisocial, borderline, histrionic, and narcissistic personality disorders. Patients with these disorders may display dramatic or irrational behavior and may have a tendency for disruptive behavior in clinical settings.
- *Cluster C personality disorders* include avoidant, dependent, and obsessive-compulsive personality disorders.

Psychotherapy is generally the treatment of choice for all of these entities. There are no medications indicated specifically for personality disorders, although psychotropic agents may be helpful in treating coexisting mental health disorders (eg, depression or substance abuse).

Miller NR. Functional neuro-ophthalmology. *Handb Clin Neurol.* 2011;102:493–513.

Substance Abuse Disorders

Drug dependence is the abuse of a drug to the point that one's physical health, psychological functioning, or ability to exist within the demands of society is threatened. Drug abuse and addiction are often considered strictly social problems. However, there is overwhelming evidence that in addition to the detrimental short-term effects, drug abuse has long-term effects on brain metabolism and activity. With habitual use, changes occur in the brain, turning drug abuse into an illness of addiction. Individuals who are addicted to drugs have compulsive drug cravings and are typically unable to quit by themselves; treatment is necessary to end the compulsive behavior.

Ophthalmic considerations Pupil changes can occur as a result of drug use. Pupillary constriction commonly occurs with the use of opiates, while dilation occurs with the use of cocaine, amphetamines, or lysergic acid diethylamide (LSD). Pupillary dilation may also be observed in individuals undergoing opiate withdrawal.

Sustained horizontal gaze-evoked nystagmus can be a sign of sedative or ethanol use. Toxic optic neuropathy is observed in patients with alcohol dependence as either a direct effect of the disease or in association with the malnutrition that often accompanies alcoholism. Wernicke disease, which is most often associated with chronic alcoholism, is caused by thiamine deficiency; individuals with Wernicke disease present with ocular palsies, nystagmus, memory disturbance, and peripheral neuropathy. Children born to mothers with alcoholism may have fetal alcohol syndrome (FAS). Ocular manifestations of FAS include epicanthal folds, ptosis, strabismus, optic nerve hypoplasia, microphthalmia, and retinal vascular anomalies. See BCSC Section 6, *Pediatric Ophthalmology and Strabismus,* for further discussion of FAS.

Patients who abuse intravenous drugs are at risk of retinovascular occlusion and endophthalmitis and are more likely to have an HIV infection, which has associated ocular findings. Cocaine use can lead to optic neuropathy, intracranial microinfarcts causing internuclear ophthalmoplegia, and visual field defects. Its use during pregnancy can cause intrauterine growth retardation, microcephaly, developmental delay, and learning disabilities. Affected infants also have an increased risk of strabismus and neonatal retinal hemorrhages. Crack cocaine use in particular should be considered in young patients who present with corneal ulcers or epithelial defects without an obvious cause.

Pharmacologic Treatment of Psychiatric Disorders

Antipsychotic Drugs

Antipsychotic drugs have been used for over 60 years and are broadly divided into 2 groups: first-generation ("typical") antipsychotics (FGAs) and second-generation ("atypical") antipsychotics (SGAs) (Table 11-1). The distinction between the 2 categories is based on differences in receptor activity, adverse effects, and overall efficacy, although there is

Table 11-1 Antipsychotic Medications

First-generation (typical) agents	
Chlorpromazine	Perphenazine
Droperidol	Pimozide
Fluphenazine	Prochlorperazine
Haloperidol	Thioridazine
Loxapine	Thiothixene
Mesoridazine	Trifluoperazine
Molindone	
Second-generation (atypical) agents	
Aripiprazole	Olanzapine
Asenapine	Paliperidone
Brexpiprazole	Pimavanserin
Cariprazine	Quetiapine
Clozapine	Risperidone
Iloperidone	Ziprasidone
Lurasidone	

overlap in both classes. Both are used in the treatment of schizophrenia as well as in the management of bipolar disorder and other psychiatric conditions. FGAs are primarily dopamine receptor blockers, whereas SGAs inhibit both serotonin and dopamine. FGAs are more likely to cause extrapyramidal "Parkinson-like" side effects (including rigidity and tremor) and tardive dyskinesia (involuntary movements of the face, tongue, trunk, and extremities).

Antipsychotic medications effectively reduce many symptoms of acute and chronic psychoses, allowing more patients to function outside psychiatric institutions. In addition to potential extrapyramidal reactions, other adverse effects include drowsiness, orthostatic hypotension, anticholinergic effects, and weight gain. Less common problems include cholestatic jaundice, blood dyscrasias, photosensitivity, and a rare idiosyncratic reaction known as *neuroleptic malignant syndrome (NMS).* NMS is characterized by "lead-pipe" muscle rigidity and hyperthermia and can lead to rhabdomyolysis and possible death if not recognized and treated. The SGAs may be less likely to cause these adverse effects, although higher doses may still cause problems.

Ophthalmic considerations Second-generation antipsychotics (SGAs) such as olanzapine, quetiapine, and clozapine may be associated with a number of ocular manifestations, including the onset or worsening of diabetes mellitus and its associated ocular findings. This may be in part due to weight gain, which is an adverse effect associated with these medications. Anticholinergic effects may lead to secondary dry eye syndrome, accommodative symptoms, and the precipitation of angle-closure glaucoma. A few studies have suggested an increase in cataract formation in patients taking antipsychotic drugs, particularly first-generation antipsychotics (FGAs). Eye examinations are recommended by the drug manufacturers every 2 years for patients up to age 40, and annually thereafter.

Other potential ocular findings, more commonly associated with FGAs, include periorbital and conjunctival pigmentation, corneal deposition, and vision loss from retinal pigmentary degeneration typically associated with the use of thioridazine. Blepharospasm and other ocular motility problems can occur in association with extrapyramidal side effects.

Packer S. Ocular side effects of psychotropics: special considerations. *Psychiatr Times.* 2014;31(6). www.psychiatrictimes.com/view/ocular-side-effects-psychotropics-special-considerations. Published June 12, 2014. Accessed September 10, 2021.

Antianxiety and Hypnotic Drugs

Benzodiazepines

The benzodiazepine class of medications is often the first-line therapy for patients with GAD. They are also beneficial as an adjunct to anesthesia or for management of alcohol withdrawal, treatment of seizures, alleviation of muscle spasm, treatment of insomnia, and treatment of nocturnal myoclonus. Table 11-2 lists the common antianxiety and hypnotic medications as well as the older class of barbiturates. The use of barbiturate drugs has declined due to their high potential for addiction and abuse. Although effective in treating these disorders, benzodiazepine use has also diminished over concerns related to dependency. Benzodiazepines are often prescribed to patients to manage the acute stage of chronic anxiety to allow time for prescribed serotonin–norepinephrine reuptake

Table 11-2 Antianxiety and Hypnotic Medications

Benzodiazepines	
Alprazolam	Halazepam
Chlordiazepoxide	Lorazepam
Clobazam	Midazolam
Clonazepam	Oxazepam
Clorazepate	Quazepam
Diazepam	Temazepam
Estazolam	Triazolam
Flurazepam	
Barbiturates	
Amobarbital	Phenobarbital
Pentobarbital	Secobarbital
Nonbenzodiazepine Nonbarbiturates	
Antianxiety agents	Hypnotic agents
Buspirone	Eszopiclone
Hydroxyzine	Ramelteon[a]
Meprobamate	Suvorexant[b]
	Zaleplon
	Zolpidem

[a]Melatonin receptor agonist.
[b]Orexin receptor antagonist.

inhibitors (SNRIs) or selective serotonin reuptake inhibitors (SSRIs), which may be safer for prolonged use, to take effect.

The mechanism of action for benzodiazepines is centered around their effect on gamma-aminobutyric acid (GABA) receptors in the central nervous system. Although these agents are similar in their effects, there is variation in the time of onset, half-life, and how they are metabolized. Withdrawal symptoms, including anxiety, tremors, psychosis, and even seizures, are more likely if intake is abruptly stopped after long-term use. All of the benzodiazepine drugs have the potential to cause retrograde amnesia, and respiratory depression is possible, especially if combined with alcohol. Benzodiazepines are involved in overdose suicide attempts in about 5% of cases.

Ophthalmic considerations The abuse potential of benzodiazepines is mild compared with other drugs such as hydromorphone and cocaine. Nevertheless, long-term administration of these agents can cause physical dependence. Ocular adverse effects can occur, although they tend to be dose-related and transient. Decreased accommodation, induced phorias, and nystagmus are sometimes associated with benzodiazepine use.

Antidepressants

A growing number of patients with major depression are being managed with medication alone, despite reports that demonstrate the benefits of combining pharmacologic treatment with psychotherapy. Nevertheless, this group of drugs is effective in managing the symptoms associated with depression, improving the rate of recovery, reducing the risk of suicide, and aiding in social and occupational rehabilitation.

In general, antidepressants can take up to 6 weeks to show significant effect; treatment is generally continued for up to 12 weeks, although long-term management may be needed in select cases. Antidepressants are associated with a 50%–60% response rate among patients with major depression in the primary care setting. These drugs can result in mood elevation, improved appetite, better sleep, and increased mental and physical activity.

Table 11-3 lists the various classes of antidepressants. The first-generation tricyclic antidepressants and monoamine oxidase inhibitors (MAOIs) are generally no longer prescribed as first-line treatment due to safety concerns (in particular, overdose) and adverse effects. Second-generation options include SSRIs, SNRIs, atypical antidepressants, and serotonin modulators. Of these, SSRIs are the most widely prescribed; they are very effective and tend to be better tolerated. Occasional adverse effects associated with SSRIs include sexual dysfunction, drowsiness, insomnia, weight gain, dizziness, headache, and blurred vision (likely related to dry eye and, to a lesser extent, mydriasis). Rare cases of angle-closure glaucoma have been reported. SSRIs may also cause inhibition of platelet function, and some studies suggest a possible increase in risk of bleeding, especially involving the upper gastrointestinal system.

Because major depression is now thought to affect 5% of children and adolescents, the use of SSRIs has steadily increased in this population as well. There have been some

Table 11-3 Antidepressant Medications

Tricyclic and tetracyclic antidepressants	
Amitriptyline	Imipramine
Amoxapine	Maprotiline
Clomipramine	Nortriptyline
Desipramine	Protriptyline
Doxepin	Trimipramine
Selective serotonin reuptake inhibitors	
Citalopram	Fluvoxamine
Escitalopram	Paroxetine
Fluoxetine	Sertraline
Dopamine–norepinephrine reuptake inhibitor	
Bupropion	
Serotonin–norepinephrine reuptake inhibitors	
Desvenlafaxine	Venlafaxine
Duloxetine	
Serotonin modulators	
Nefazodone	Trazodone
Noradrenergic and specific serotonergic antidepressant	
Mirtazapine	
Monoamine oxidase inhibitors	
Isocarboxazid	Selegiline (skin patch)
Phenelzine	Tranylcypromine

reports of antidepressants leading to increased suicidal ideation in a small percentage of children and adolescents. Close monitoring for abnormal behavior, agitation, and suicidal thoughts is advised, especially within the first 4 weeks after the individual begins antidepressant therapy.

Mood stabilizers

Mood stabilizers are a heterogeneous group of medications that do not clearly share a common mechanism of action. They are the drugs of choice for the treatment of bipolar disorder. *Lithium carbonate* was the first drug to be developed in this class and has been the most widely studied. Other mood stabilizers include the antiepileptic agents *valproic acid, carbamazepine,* and *lamotrigine.* Potential ocular adverse effects of lithium use include blurred vision, nystagmus (usually downbeat), and exophthalmos associated with lithium-induced changes in thyroid function.

Ophthalmic considerations Although behavioral disorders do not directly affect the eye, several related issues are important for ophthalmologists to be aware of. Patient education and reassurance may be required because the underlying mental disorder may mean that anticholinergic side effects, such as dry eye and accommodative changes, are more concerning to patients. Poor adherence to treatment is another common problem among patients with mental health issues. Malingering and functional vision loss require a high index of suspicion and special diagnostic skills on the part of the clinician. Some medications used to treat eye disease, including carbonic anhydrase inhibitors, brimonidine, and oral corticosteroids, may induce or exacerbate depression. Although β-blockers were thought to increase the risk of depression, recent studies suggest this correlation is not as strong as was previously believed.

Richa S, Yazbek JC. Ocular adverse effects of common psychotropic agents: a review. *CNS Drugs.* 2010;24(6):501–526.

Neurologic Disorders

Parkinson Disease

Parkinson disease (PD), also known as paralysis agitans, is a neurodegenerative condition that is characterized by tremor, bradykinesia, and rigidity. Parkinson disease usually affects persons older than 50 years, and its incidence rises dramatically after age 60. Early-onset PD (prior to age 50) is seen in less than 10% of cases; risk factors for early onset are still unclear. Worldwide, approximately 7.5 million people are affected with the disease; this number is estimated to rise to over 9 million by 2030. Many studies indicate a male predominance. The differential diagnosis for Parkinson disease includes other neurodegenerative disorders such as dementia with Lewy bodies, corticobasal degeneration, multiple system atrophy, and progressive supranuclear palsy.

Etiology

The basal ganglia are a complex of deep gray-matter nuclei that includes the corpus striatum, globus pallidus, and substantia nigra. These structures regulate the initiation and control of movement. Patients with Parkinson disease have typically lost 80% or more of the dopamine-producing neurons in the substantia nigra. Depletion of dopamine in the complex nigrostriatal pathway produces an imbalance in inhibitory and excitatory neuronal signals, leading to the cardinal signs of Parkinson disease.

Although most cases are sporadic, genetic factors are implicated in the pathogenesis, especially in early-onset cases. At least 5 possible causative genes have been identified, and the number of Parkinson-like disorders associated with specific genetic defects is increasing. Many of these defects appear to be involved in cellular protein metabolism. Overall, Parkinson disease seems to have a multifactorial etiology that includes genetic predisposition, environmental factors, and age-related changes in neuron metabolism.

Symptoms

The first symptom of Parkinson disease is usually tremor of a limb at rest. Other common symptoms include bradykinesia, rigidity, a shuffling gait, postural instability, and stooped posture. Persons with Parkinson disease often have reduced facial expressions and speak in a soft voice. The disease is associated with nonmotor features such as depression (in up to 50% of cases), dementia, personality changes, sexual difficulties, sleep disorders, and hallucinations.

Treatment

There is currently no cure for Parkinson disease. Dopamine replacement, with medications such as *levodopa*, is the main treatment. Dopamine itself cannot be given because it does not cross the blood–brain barrier. Although levodopa helps at least three-fourths of patients with Parkinson disease, not all symptoms respond equally to the drug. Bradykinesia and rigidity respond best, whereas tremor may only be marginally reduced. Problems with balance and other symptoms may not be alleviated at all. Patients are often given levodopa combined with *carbidopa*. The combination of the 2 together delays the conversion of levodopa into dopamine until it reaches the brain, diminishing some of the adverse effects that often accompany levodopa therapy alone.

After years of therapy, patients may experience a "wearing-off" effect that occurs about 4 hours after a dose of levodopa, when symptoms may return. Catechol *O*-methyltransferase inhibitors such as *entacapone* extend the duration of the levodopa effect and reduce the "off" time by inhibiting the methylation of levodopa and dopamine.

Several additional therapies for Parkinson disease exist, and research is dedicated to finding more effective modalities. Dopamine agonists *(bromocriptine, pramipexole, ropinirole, rotigotine,* and *apomorphine)* stimulate dopamine receptors in the brain and may delay the need for levodopa. The monoamine oxidase (MAO) type B inhibitors *selegiline, rasagiline,* and *safinamide* may modestly improve symptoms of Parkinson disease. Based on information obtained from animal studies, the first 2 may also have neuroprotective properties and are therefore considered to be potential disease-modifying agents. The glucagon-like peptide-1 (GLP-1) drug *exenatide*, which is used in the treatment of type 2 diabetes mellitus, has also demonstrated some potential neuroprotective effect and is currently being studied. Anticholinergic drugs such as *trihexyphenidyl* and *benztropine* have a short-lived effect controlling tremor and rigidity. However, only about half of patients respond to anticholinergics, and typical anticholinergic adverse effects can be problematic.

Amantadine, an antiviral drug, may be used during the early stages of the disease, either alone or in combination with anticholinergics or levodopa. After several months, the effectiveness of amantadine wears off in one-third to one-half of patients.

Modern surgical treatments consist primarily of deep-brain stimulation and pallidotomy or thalamotomy. The dopamine deficiency in patients with Parkinson disease results in excitation of the globus pallidus, which in turn inhibits thalamic activity. Both surgical techniques serve to suppress this excessive globus pallidus activity. Deep-brain stimulation is initially safer than pallidotomy but requires intensive adjustments and lifelong maintenance, given the risk of hardware complications and infection. Pallidotomy carries the risk of complications such as stroke and hemorrhage, as well as the risk of irreversible adverse effects, and is seldom performed.

Ferreira M, Massano J. An updated review of Parkinson's disease genetics and clinicopathological correlations. *Acta Neurol Scand.* 2017;135(3):273–284.

Kalia LV, Kalia, SK, Lang AE. Disease-modifying strategies for Parkinson's disease. *Mov Disord.* 2015;30(11):1442–1450.

Ophthalmic considerations Patients with Parkinson disease may present with numerous ophthalmologic findings. These findings can be divided into eyelid disorders and ocular motor abnormalities. Eyelid disorders include seborrheic dermatitis and blepharitis, apraxia of eyelid opening, eyelid retraction, decreased blinking (with secondary dry eye), and blepharospasm. Ocular motor abnormalities include convergence insufficiency, limitation of upgaze, saccadic abnormalities, square-wave jerks, and oculogyric crisis. Patients commonly report difficulty with reading and symptoms related to ocular surface abnormalities.

Drug-related adverse effects may also be superimposed, especially for patients on anticholinergic medications, which may exacerbate dry eyes and cause accommodative changes or precipitate angle-closure glaucoma. Over 30% of patients with coexisting ocular disease and reduced vision may experience formed recurrent hallucinations characteristic of Charles Bonnet syndrome. However, this syndrome is not specific to Parkinson disease because it can be seen with other neurodegenerative conditions. Likewise, visual hallucinations can also occur as a result of treatment. This adverse effect has been reported in particular with the use of levodopa and anticholinergic agents. The drug amantadine has been reported to cause corneal infiltrates and edema in rare cases.

Multiple Sclerosis

See BCSC Section 5, *Neuro-Ophthalmology.*

Epilepsy

Epilepsy is characterized by recurrent seizures due to a genetically inherited or acquired brain disorder. The prevalence of epilepsy increases with age, especially after 65, and occurs in 2%–5% of adults in general. Even patients with epilepsy under relative control can experience problems with depression, driving, employment, and insurance.

Etiology

Epilepsy has many possible causes. Seizures result from synchronized electrical activity of neuronal networks in the cerebral cortex. Any disturbance of normal neuronal activity, including injury, infection, and abnormal brain development, can lead to seizures. Cerebral vascular disease is the most common cause in older adults; however, about half of all seizures have no identifiable cause. Seizures may develop because of an abnormality in brain wiring, an imbalance of neurotransmitters, or some combination of these factors. Epilepsy can also be associated with a variety of developmental and metabolic disorders, including cerebral palsy, neurofibromatosis, tuberous sclerosis, and autism.

Typically, seizures are divided into 2 major categories: partial and generalized. *Partial seizures* occur in only 1 part of the brain and are further divided into *simple* (without impairment of consciousness) and *complex* (with impairment of consciousness). Symptoms of simple partial seizures (also called *auras*) depend on the part of the brain from which the seizures originate and include motor symptoms, sensory symptoms (which can resemble a migraine aura), and even autonomic symptoms. Complex partial seizures are the most common type of seizures in adults with epilepsy. During the seizure, patients may appear to be awake but do not interact with others around them and do not respond normally to instructions or questions. They often stare into space and either remain motionless or engage in repetitive behaviors, called *automatisms*, such as facial grimacing or gesturing.

Generalized seizures cause impaired consciousness and abnormal activity in both hemispheres at the onset of the seizure. These events may follow partial seizures. They can be nonconvulsive (absence, or "petit mal") or convulsive (tonic–clonic, or "grand mal"; or some variation of tonic–clonic). Absence seizures almost always begin in childhood or adolescence and are frequently familial, suggesting a genetic cause. During seizures, some patients make purposeless movements, such as jerking an arm or rapidly blinking their eyes. Others have no noticeable symptoms except for brief periods of "absence." Childhood absence epilepsy often stops when the child reaches puberty. A generalized tonic–clonic seizure is the most dramatic, in that it begins with an abrupt alteration in consciousness, sometimes in association with a scream or shriek. All of the muscles stiffen, and the patient may become cyanotic during the tonic phase. Within a short time, the muscles begin to jerk and twitch for 1–2 minutes, and then the patient goes into a deep sleep.

The end of a seizure is referred to as the *postictal period* and signifies the recovery period for the brain. This period may last from several seconds up to a few days, though typically no more than a few hours. Postictal paresis (Todd paralysis) is a transient focal motor deficit that lasts for hours or, in rare cases, days after an epileptic convulsion. It is thought to be related either to neuronal exhaustion (from electrical overactivity during the seizure) or to active inhibition.

Diagnosis

Electroencephalography (EEG) is the most common diagnostic test for epilepsy, although a normal EEG result does not rule out the disorder. Computed tomography (CT), magnetic resonance imaging (MRI), positron emission tomography (PET), and single-photon emission computed tomography (SPECT) are useful tools for revealing abnormalities in the brain that cause epilepsy. Patients with epilepsy have a higher overall mortality rate that is about twice that of the general global population. Occurrence of other associated mood disorders, particularly depression, is also higher in these patients.

Treatment

Currently available treatments help control seizure activity in 80% of patients with epilepsy. The medication used is determined by the type of epilepsy, comorbidities, age of the patient, and potential drug interactions. This latter concern specifically applies to the medication's effect on patients who are concurrently being treated with warfarin or certain antibiotics, or who are taking oral contraceptives. For generalized tonic–clonic seizures, the first-line therapy includes *valproic acid, lamotrigine,* and *topiramate*. For partial seizures, *carbamazepine, phenytoin, oxcarbazepine,* or *ethosuximide* are often used (especially in children). To minimize side effects, monotherapy is the goal; however, use of a second agent is sometimes necessary to control breakout seizures. Adverse effects vary; they may include nausea, rash, anorexia, somnolence, dizziness, and confusion. The neurologic effects often become the dose-limiting factor. Some of these drugs used for the treatment of epilepsy can also promote hyperlipidemia, which may increase the risk of cardiovascular disease. Rare, but serious, drug reactions include Stevens-Johnson syndrome and toxic epidermal necrolysis (TEN).

When medications inadequately control seizure activity, surgery is a potential option. The most commonly performed procedure for epilepsy is removal of a seizure focus via lobectomy or lesionectomy. Other, less common surgical procedures for epilepsy include multiple subpial transections, corpus callosotomy, and hemispherectomy. An implanted vagus nerve stimulation (VNS) device can be effective in helping to control seizures in children when medication alone is not sufficient.

Fountain NB, Van Ness PC, Swain-Eng R, Tonn S, Bever CT Jr; American Academy of Neurology Epilepsy Measure Development Panel and the American Medical Association-Convened Physician Consortium for Performance Improvement Independent Measure Development Process. Quality improvement in neurology: AAN epilepsy quality measures. Report of the Quality Measurement and Reporting Subcommittee of the American Academy of Neurology. *Neurology.* 2011;76(1):94–99.

Noe KH. Seizures: diagnosis and management in the outpatient setting. *Semin Neurol.* 2011;31(1):54–64.

Ophthalmic considerations Transient unilateral or bilateral mydriasis can occur as an expression of seizure activity, during or after the event; it is most common in children. Horizontal or vertical gaze deviations are commonly associated with seizure activity. The gaze tends to be directed away from the side of the cortical seizure activity during the event and then toward the side of the prior activity after the seizure. Some patients experience conjugate, convergent, or monocular nystagmus during the clonic stage of a seizure. Clonic eyelid retraction has also been described in patients with absence or myoclonic seizures. It is unusual for patients with true seizures to shut their eyes during the episode, whereas patients who are feigning a seizure often keep their eyes closed.

Certain antiepileptic drugs have potential ocular side effects. Phenytoin can cause dose-related nystagmus, and maternal use of this medication is associated with fetal hydantoin syndrome, which includes hypertelorism, epicanthal folds, glaucoma, optic nerve hypoplasia, and retinal colobomas. Carbamazepine can cause blurred vision, diplopia, and nystagmus. Topiramate has been associated with acute angle-closure glaucoma, anterior chamber shallowing, acute myopia, and choroidal effusions, usually within the first 2 weeks of therapy. These effects may be an idiopathic response related to the presence of sulfa in topiramate. Treatment of the glaucoma includes cessation of the drug and use of cycloplegics and topical hypotensives.

Vigabatrin, used in refractory seizure disorders, is associated with irreversible concentric visual field loss in up to 50% of patients that is often asymptomatic. Central vision can also be affected. A complete ophthalmic examination and visual field testing should be performed before starting therapy and repeated every 3 months. The onset and progression of vision loss from vigabatrin are unpredictable and irreversible.

Stroke

See Chapter 6, Cerebrovascular Disease, in this volume.

Alzheimer Disease and Dementia

Dementia is a disorder characterized by a decline in cognitive ability to a point of interfering with daily function. The diagnosis can be challenging due to its insidious onset; early symptoms may only be apparent to close family members. Globally, the prevalence of dementia in individuals aged 60 and over is between 5%–8%. Of the 50 million people affected worldwide, approximately 60% live in low- to middle-income regions. Several specific syndromes fall under the category of dementia, including Alzheimer disease, vascular (multi-infarct) dementia, and Lewy body dementia.

Alzheimer disease

Alzheimer disease (AD) is the most common cause of dementia in people older than 65 years. Memory impairment is its cardinal feature, with language and behavioral deficits occurring over time. In addition to age, family history appears to be a risk factor, suggesting a genetic link; the early-onset form of the disease seems to have the strongest genetic tie. The pathologic hallmarks of AD are extraneuronal amyloid plaques and neurofibrillary degeneration. These 2 findings are associated with neuronal death and decreased levels of the neurotransmitter acetylcholine. As the disease progresses, the basal forebrain and eventually the cerebral cortex become involved.

Diagnosis of AD is made clinically; serological testing and neuroimaging studies are used to rule out other causes. Epidemiological data from the European Community Concerted Action Epidemiology of Dementia Group (EURODEM) found that 70% of patients with dementia have AD. In 2015, the estimated global cost of the disease was $808 billion. Life expectancy in individuals with AD is shortened relative to the degree of impairment at the time of diagnosis. The disease presents significant challenges to family and caregivers in dealing with a variety of related issues, including emotional lability, risk of wandering, and potential for injury. Resources are available to assist patients and their families with these matters, such as the Alzheimer's Association (www.alz.org).

An atypical presentation of AD can result from neuropathological abnormalities concentrated in particular areas of the brain. For example, posterior cortical atrophy can lead to progressive cortical impairment and ocular manifestations from pathology that involves the visual pathways. As a result, many of these patients may present early in the progression of their disease to an optometrist or ophthalmologist with a variety of visual symptoms and findings, including homonymous visual field defects.

Cholinesterase inhibitors such as donepezil and the neuropeptide-modifying agent *memantine* are helpful, used either alone or in combination therapy, in treating AD. Recently, the FDA granted approval for the drug Aduhelm (aducanumab, Biogen/Eisai), which has shown limited clinical efficiency while targeting the underlying pathophysiology of AD.

Vascular dementia

Vascular dementia is the second most common form of dementia and accounts for 10%–20% of cases in North America and Europe. The disease is associated with findings on neurologic examination consistent with prior strokes; neuroimaging studies typically show evidence of multiple infarcts. As in other vascular diseases, patients with hypertension, diabetes mellitus, or abnormal lipid profiles are at increased risk. Although *donepezil* and *memantine* are sometimes used in treatment, their benefit appears to be limited. Management is usually directed at treating any comorbidities, including the behavioral symptoms that often accompany this disease.

Lewy body dementia

Lewy body dementia (LBD) is another common form of neurodegenerative dementia. The disease is characterized pathologically by the presence of eosinophilic intracytoplasmic inclusions (Lewy bodies) in the deep cortical regions of the brain. There may be considerable clinical and pathologic overlap between LBD, AD, and Parkinson disease. Ophthalmologists should be aware of LBD, however, because patients with this syndrome often present with complex (or formed) visual hallucinations. The Dementia with Lewy Body Consortium has recently revised the criteria used to diagnose the disorder, including interpretation of certain biomarkers and the significance of the presence of an REM sleep behavior disorder in the patient. There are no specific pharmacotherapy options for patients affected, although cholinesterase inhibiters have shown some benefit in select cases.

Ophthalmic considerations Patients with dementia may report a host of visual symptoms and manifest a variety of findings depending on the extent of the disease. Reduced contrast sensitivity, depth perception, and motion perception have been reported in cases of Alzheimer disease (AD). Because this disease is associated with an impaired cholinergic system, a reduced pupillary constriction response may be observed, which improves after treatment with the anticholinesterase agent donepezil.

Unfortunately, there is currently no reliable test specific to the diagnosis of AD. Ocular motility disorders, especially saccadic latency, have been observed. Because the retina is an extension of the nervous system, researchers are investigating ways to help detect neurodegenerative disease using optical coherence tomography (OCT); thinning of the retinal nerve fiber layer (RNFL) may be an associated finding.

James BD, Leurgans SE, Hebert LE, Scherr PA, Yaffe K, Bennett DA. Contribution of Alzheimer disease to mortality in the United States. *Neurology.* 2014;82(12):1045–1050.

Moretti, D, ed. *Update on Dementia.* London, United Kingdom: InTechOpen Limited; 2016.

Prion-Associated Neurologic Disorders

Prion diseases (also known as transmissible spongiform encephalopathies) are chronic and progressive neurodegenerative disorders that can affect both humans and animals. Prions are pathogenic agents that are transmissible and consist of abnormal proteins. Known human forms include kuru, Creutzfeldt-Jakob disease (CJD), Gerstmann-Sträussler-Scheinker (GSS) syndrome, and fatal familial insomnia (FFI). Kuru, which was the first prion disease to be identified, in a tribe in Papua New Guinea, is thought to be transmitted through cannibalism practices. Most prion diseases have overlapping clinical features, including tremor, ataxia, involuntary movements, and dementia.

CJD is the most commonly recognized form of prion disease. The worldwide incidence is about 1 case per million population. Males and females are equally affected, and the median age of onset is 60. An iatrogenic form can occur following various surgical procedures, including corneal transplantation. Rapidly progressive mental deterioration, behavioral abnormalities, and myoclonus are characteristic of the disease. Ophthalmic disturbances are not uncommon and may include diplopia, supranuclear palsies, hallucinations, and various visual field deficits. CJD is distinguished from more common causes of dementia by its rapid onset and progression as well as the presence of myoclonus and associated gait disturbances. Brain biopsy is the gold standard in diagnosing the disorder but is rarely necessary. MRI, EEG, and cerebral spinal fluid (CSF) analysis are generally sufficient to rule out other disease etiologies and help establish the diagnosis. The presence of the CSF protein 14-3-3 is highly specific for the disease itself, but the sensitivity of the test is lower, so the usefulness of the test is limited. There is no treatment for CJD, and death often occurs within a year of onset.

Informed Consent in Patients with Behavioral and Neurologic Disorders

Every physician-patient interaction involves some assessment to determine whether patients have adequate capacity to make an informed decision about their own care. Assessing decision-making capacity in patients with mental health disease or specific neurologic conditions can present challenges to the clinician caring for these patients. A patient's cognition is the main determinant affecting this capacity; patients with impairment from any underlying cause, including behavioral and neurodegenerative disorders, are therefore at risk of impaired cognitive ability. At highest risk of such impairment are patients affected by Alzheimer disease, Parkinson disease, schizophrenia, depression, substance abuse, and traumatic brain injury.

When cognitive impairment is suspected, the clinician should consider initiating a formal assessment of capacity by a trained professional. This assessment consists of open-ended questions that relate to the medical decision being investigated. The questions are designed to formally evaluate the 4 decision-making attributes: understanding, appreciation, reasoning, and expression of a choice. Several assessment tools are available to help in testing for decision-making capacity, such as the MacArthur Competence Assessment Tool for Treatment (MacCAT-T), the Assessment of Capacity for Everyday Decision-Making (ACED), and the Capacity to Consent to Treatment Instrument (CCTI). It is imperative for clinicians to understand the potential challenges; if patients refuse to be tested, it may be an issue of trust, particularly if the patients feel that their abilities to understand are being questioned. It may be effective to assist such patients in their understanding that this assessment is required, and that all information obtained during this assessment will result in the best medical care.

When it is determined that a patient has significant impairment and lacks the capacity to make an informed decision, there is an ethical obligation to find an individual who is capable of making decisions for that patient. It is helpful when patient preferences are established prior to the patient's incapacity. Without this, local laws can determine who may serve as the patient's proxy; generally, the order prioritizes the spouse first, followed by any adult children, then parents, siblings, or other relatives. If the treatment dilemma is urgent and no surrogate is found, formal guardianship can be assigned by a judge based upon a legal determination of incompetence.

Fields LM, Calvert JD. Informed consent procedures with cognitively impaired patients: A review of ethics and best practices. *Psychiatry Clin Neurosci.* 2015; 69(8):462–471.

CHAPTER 12

Preventive Medicine

Highlights

- Multiple studies support the life-saving value of mammography in breast cancer screening. The frequency of mammography and other tests should be based on an assessment of the individual patient's risk of breast cancer.
- Screening for colorectal cancer can be accomplished via a number of procedures or through stool testing. Fecal immunochemical testing is more sensitive than guaiac-based fecal occult blood testing.
- More than 99% of all cervical cancers are positive for human papillomavirus (HPV). A vaccine against HPV is now available.
- Tdap (tetanus toxoid, diphtheria, and acellular pertussis vaccine) is recommended for all unvaccinated health care professionals as a means of preventing nosocomial outbreaks of pertussis.
- In 2017, the US Food and Drug Administration (FDA) approved an inactivated recombinant varicella zoster vaccine that is far more effective than the previous zoster vaccine for prevention of clinical zoster in patients over age 50.
- The US Centers for Disease Control and Prevention (CDC) recommends one-time testing for hepatitis C for all persons born in the United States between 1945 and 1965. Many individuals are unaware that they have a chronic, asymptomatic infection with the hepatitis C virus.

Screening Procedures

The goal of preventive medicine is not only to reduce premature morbidity and mortality but also to preserve function and quality of life.

Screening techniques can be used for research and for practical disease prevention or treatment. Screening for nonresearch purposes is useful if the disease in question is

- detectable with some measurable degree of reliability
- treatable or preventable
- significant because of its impact (prevalence or severity)
- progressive
- generally asymptomatic (or has symptoms a patient might deny or might not recognize)

Screening techniques should not be applied to a certain population until the following concerns have been addressed:

- sensitivity and specificity of the test
- convenience and comfort of the test
- cost of finding a problem
- cost of not finding a problem

The term *sensitivity* describes how often a test result is positive among persons with a target disease. *Specificity* measures the test's ability to exclude truly negative results. *Relative risk* is the probability of a disease based on a specific finding divided by the probability of that disease in the absence of that specific finding. (See Chapter 1 in this volume for additional discussion of these terms.)

Cost can and should be measured in both economic and human terms, including the cost of discomfort, losing function, or dying.

Screening can be done as a one-time venture or by the sequential application of screening tests. Initially, a more sensitive test is administered; when appropriate, it is followed by a more specific test (which is often more costly or difficult to use). When judging the predictive value of the screens for an individual patient, the physician should account for the patient's clinical history, current medications, and results from a physical examination.

Cardiovascular Diseases

Hypertension

The American College of Cardiology (ACC) and the American Heart Association (AHA) guidelines published in November 2017 define hypertension as systolic blood pressure that is greater than or equal to 130 mm Hg and/or diastolic blood pressure greater than or equal to 80 mm Hg. Hypertension currently afflicts approximately 1.4 billion people worldwide. In the United States, it affects an estimated 103 million persons aged 20 years and older; only about half of these cases are under control with treatment. In adults in the United States, the prevalence of hypertension is approximately 46% under the 2017 ACC/AHA guidelines. Hypertension in children is also becoming a more widely recognized problem.

The consequences of uncontrolled hypertension include significantly increased risk of thrombotic and hemorrhagic stroke, atherosclerotic heart disease, atrial fibrillation, congestive heart failure, left ventricular hypertrophy, aortic aneurysm and dissection, peripheral arterial disease, and renal failure. Approximately 30% of end-stage renal disease is related to hypertension.

Hypertension meets all 5 of the screening criteria mentioned previously: it is detectable, treatable, highly prevalent, progressively damaging, and characteristically asymptomatic until late in its course. See Chapter 3 in this volume for discussion of the classification, evaluation, and pharmacologic treatment of hypertension.

Whelton PK, Carey RM, Aronow WS, et al. 2017 ACC/AHA/AAPA/ABC/ACPM/AGS/APhA/ASH/ASPC/NMA/PCNA Guideline for the prevention, detection, evaluation and management of high blood pressure in adults: a report of the American College of Cardiology/American Heart Association Task Force on Clinical Practice Guidelines. *Hypertension.* 2018;71(6):e13–e115.

Atherosclerotic cardiovascular disease

In the United States, atherosclerosis is responsible for approximately one-half of deaths in individuals of all ages and for one-third of deaths in individuals between 35 and 65 years of age. Three-fourths of deaths related to atherosclerosis result from *coronary heart disease (CHD).* Atherosclerosis is the leading cause of permanent disability and accounts for more hospital days than any other illness.

The rationale for early screening emerged after it was demonstrated that a reduction in risk factors correlated to a reduction in the incidence of coronary disease events. For further discussion on identifying and modifying cardiovascular risk factors, see Chapter 4 in this volume.

Screening for significant coronary artery atherosclerosis is more expensive and time-consuming than screening for associated reversible risk factors. In general, it is reasonable to screen for a history of cardiovascular symptoms and events (eg, chest pain, dyspnea, syncope, arrhythmias, claudication, stroke) and reserve more specific testing (eg, exercise stress testing, cardiac computed tomography [CT], or magnetic resonance imaging [MRI]) for individuals in higher-risk categories.

Cancer

In women, the most common cancers are breast, lung, and colorectal. In men, they are prostate, lung, and colorectal. The types of cancer that best meet the criteria for screening are breast cancer, cervical cancer, colorectal cancer, lung cancer, melanoma, and urologic cancer. Table 12-1 presents the American Cancer Society's 2017 recommendations for early cancer detection. See also Chapter 13 in this volume.

Siegel RL, Miller KD, Jemal A. Cancer statistics, 2017. *CA Cancer J Clin.* 2017;67(1):7–30.

Smith RA, Brooks D, Cokkinides V, Saslow D, Brawley OW. Cancer screening in the United States, 2013: a review of current American Cancer Society guidelines, current issues in cancer screening, and new guidance on cervical cancer screening and lung cancer screening. *CA Cancer J Clin.* 2013;63(2):88–105.

Breast cancer

Though now surpassed by lung cancer as the most common cause of death in women older than 40 years, breast cancer remains the most common malignancy in women. The overall prevalence of breast cancer in the United States is 10%–12%. The age-adjusted incidence of breast cancer declined by 6.7% in 2003 (12% decline in women older than 50 years). This decrease was mostly due to a 50% reduction in the use of hormone replacement therapy (HRT). In the Women's Health Initiative, a US National Institutes of Health randomized trial, HRT with estrogen and progesterone was associated with an increased risk of invasive breast cancer and abnormal mammograms. From 1989 to 2015, the breast cancer death rate in the United States decreased by 39%, although Black women had a significantly higher death rate than White women. More than 75% of all breast cancers are cured with current therapy. Nevertheless, approximately 266,000 new cases of breast cancer and more than 41,000 related deaths were projected for the United States alone for 2018.

The importance of specific screening is increased by the presence of known risk factors, all of which are identifiable by patient history: (1) first-degree relative with breast,

Table 12-1 American Cancer Society Recommendations for Early Cancer Detection in Asymptomatic Adult Patients, 2017

Test or Procedure, by Cancer Type	Population Sex	Population Age, Years	Frequency
Colorectal			
Stool DNA testing	M, F	>50	Every 3 years
Fecal immunochemical or gFOBT test	M, F	>50	Annually
Colonoscopy	M, F	>50	Every 10 years if patient not high risk
CT colonography	M, F	>50	Every 5 years
Double-contrast barium enema	M, F	>50	Every 5 years
Sigmoidoscopy	M, F	>50	Every 5 years
Cervical			
Papanicolaou test ("pap smear")	F	21–29; <20, if high risk	Every 3 years
		30–65	With HPV testing every 5 years
Endometrial			
Endometrial tissue sample	F	Women at high risk[a]	When indicated
Breast			
Mammography	F	40–44	Optional
		45–54	Baseline, then annually
		55+	Every 2 years
Prostate			
Serum PSA, with or without rectal examination	M	>50	Discuss risks/benefits of testing
		Men at high risk[b]	Annually for high-risk patients
Lung			
Low-dose helical CT	M, F	55–74, smoker	Annually if patient identified as high risk
General			
Health counseling and cancer checkup[c]	M, F	>20	At time of general checkup

CT = computed tomography; gFOBT = guaiac-based fecal occult blood test; HPV = human papillomavirus; PSA = prostate specific antigen.

[a]History of infertility, obesity, failure to ovulate, abnormal uterine bleeding, or use of estrogen therapy.

[b]Positive family history of prostate cancer, African American race.

[c]To include examination for cancers of the thyroid, testis, prostate, ovary, lymph nodes, oral region, and skin.

ovarian, or tubal cancer, (2) prior breast, ovarian, or tubal cancer, (3) nulliparity, (4) first pregnancy after age 30, (5) early menarche or late menopause, (6) radiotherapy to the chest between the ages 10 and 30, and (7) *BRCA* mutation status. Additional risk factors are high breast density, elevated serum estrogen or testosterone levels, a high-fat diet, obesity, and a sedentary lifestyle.

Approximately 42% of breast cancers detectable by mammography are not detectable by physical examination alone, and one-third of those found during mammographic screening are noninvasive or, if invasive, less than 1 cm in size. Because mammograms can yield false-negative results, the best detection strategy involves a physical examination plus mammography, followed by fine-needle aspiration or biopsy if either reveals an abnormality. Mammography has been shown to be safe as well as effective; the current low-dose radiation associated with it does not significantly increase the risk of radiation-induced cancer. False-positive results may lead to overtreatment; in the Canadian National Breast Screening study, the incidence of over-diagnosis was 22%.

Counseling alone is generally recommended for women with an average risk of breast cancer until 40 years of age. According to the recommendation by the US Preventive Services Task Force, mammographic screening should be performed every 2 years for average-risk women aged 50–75 years, and screening should be discussed with women from age 40. The American Cancer Society continues to recommend yearly mammography after age 45. In addition to general screening recommendations, assessment tools can help estimate an individual patient's risk of breast cancer, for example, the Gail model (www.mdcalc.com/gail-model-breast-cancer-risk). Although the ideal mammographic screening interval is not clear, the American Cancer Society and US Preventive Services Task Force recommendations, as well as results from large studies done in the United Kingdom and Europe (eg, EUROSCREEN), continue to support the life-saving value of mammography.

Other modalities available for breast cancer screening include ultrasonography, digital mammography, and MRI. Because MRI of the breast is more sensitive but less specific than other methods, it should be used primarily in high-risk younger patients. Women with known mutations in the breast cancer 1 gene *(BRCA1)* or *BRCA2* gene are at dramatically increased lifetime risk for breast and ovarian cancer and require more intensive counseling and surveillance, including yearly mammography and breast MRI.

DeSantis CE, Ma J, Goding Saur A, Newman LA, Jemal A. Breast cancer statistics, 2017, racial disparity in mortality by state. *CA Cancer J Clin.* 2017;67(6):439–448.

Cervical cancer

Cervical cancer is the most common gynecologic cancer in patients between 15 and 34 years of age. Overall, approximately 12,000 cases of invasive cancer of the cervix (about 4000 resulting in death) and 45,000 cases of carcinoma in situ occur each year in the United States. Worldwide, approximately 86% of the 450,000 cervical cancer cases diagnosed each year occur in developing countries. Despite advances in the diagnosis and treatment of cervical cancer, approximately half the women with the disease worldwide will die. In many developed countries (including the United States), mortality has been reduced by more than 50% due to the implementation of cytologic screening. Cervical cancer is the eighth most common cause of cancer mortality in the United States. The incidence of cervical cancer in the nations of the European Union (EU) varies widely; the highest incidence is in Romania and the lowest is in Finland. As of 2017, screening for cervical cancer is recommended in 22 EU countries.

The risk factors for cervical cancer include the presence of high-risk serotypes of HPV, the number of lifetime sexual partners, low socioeconomic status, positive smoking history, use of corticosteroid contraceptive hormones, and a history of other sexually transmitted infections. More than 99% of all cervical cancers are positive for HPV.

Early detection and appropriate treatment markedly reduce the morbidity and mortality from invasive cancer of the cervix. Cervical cancer is asymptomatic when it occurs in situ, and the most effective screening technique remains the Papanicolaou test ("Pap smear"). HPV can be detected with polymerase chain reaction assay techniques, and patients aged 30–65 years should consider receiving HPV testing at the time of their Papanicolaou test ("dual testing"). Vaccines to prevent HPV infection and its sequelae are discussed later in this chapter.

Curry SJ, Krist AH, Owens DK, et al; US Preventive Services Task Force. Screening for cervical cancer: US Preventive Services Task Force recommendation statement. *JAMA.* 2018;320(7):674–686.

Kahn JA. HPV vaccination for the prevention of cervical intraepithelial neoplasia. *N Engl J Med.* 2009;361(3):271–278.

Colorectal cancer

Colorectal cancer is a major killer in developed countries, second only to lung cancer in incidence and mortality. In the United States, the cumulative lifetime probability of developing colon cancer is roughly 4.5%, and approximately one-third of affected individuals will die from this disease. Although the overall incidence of colorectal cancer in the United States has been declining since 1980, there has been a steady increase in the incidence of colorectal cancer in individuals under the age of 50.

Most authorities accept the theory that colorectal cancer develops from an initially benign polyp in a mitotic process that occurs over approximately 10 years. Colonoscopic removal or ablation of all polyps has become the standard of care where facilities and trained personnel are available. Factors associated with a higher risk of development of colon cancer include increased size and number of polyps, high-grade dysplasia or villous features on biomicroscopy, and sessile polyps only partially removed during a previous colonoscopy. Increased dietary fiber intake and reduced dietary fat intake have been associated with reduced risk of colorectal cancer. Also, calcium supplementation, multivitamins containing folic acid, and the use of aspirin and other nonsteroidal anti-inflammatory drugs (NSAIDs) are associated with a moderate reduction in the risk of recurrent colorectal adenomas.

It is estimated that the mortality rate of colorectal cancer could be reduced by more than 50% with widespread adoption of screening studies, for example, the guaiac-based fecal occult blood test (gFOBT), fecal immunochemical test (FIT), flexible sigmoidoscopy, and colonoscopy, with aggressive follow-up of patients with positive test results. Another stool-based screening test, fecal DNA testing, can detect molecular tumor markers associated with colorectal cancer. FIT and fecal DNA testing are easier to use and more sensitive than gFOBT, so patient adherence may be better.

Flexible sigmoidoscopy (every 5 years) and home gFOBT (annually) have been recommended in asymptomatic adults between 50 and 75 years of age. Recommendations remain controversial because of a lack of randomized trials. FIT, fecal DNA testing, and gFOBT are now accepted screening modalities by the American Cancer Society. Sigmoidoscopy offers good specificity but misses proximal cancers. Home gFOBT has been shown to decrease the mortality rate of colon cancer by up to 40%. For this test, 3 gFOBT cards are completed at home; a single gFOBT completed at the time of an annual physical examination is not sufficient.

Colonoscopy has been increasingly used as a screening test for asymptomatic patients older than 50 years. When results are negative in low-risk patients, the test is repeated every 10 years. Many of the lesions discovered with colonoscopy would not be detected with sigmoidoscopy. Yearly colonoscopy has been advocated in populations at very high risk, such as patients with familial polyposis and first-degree relatives of patients with colon cancer. The disadvantages of colonoscopy are its higher cost when compared with other screening methods, the number of trained personnel required to conduct the procedure, and the risks associated with intravenous sedation and of colonic perforation (approximately 0.2%). Colonoscopy's advantage is its detection of suspicious polyps, which can then be removed, preventing progression to cancer.

CT colonography, another screening tool, may be able to screen out patients without neoplasia. Colonoscopy could then be reserved for only those patients with significant lesions. CT colonography may be preferable for those patients who are not healthy enough to undergo colonoscopy.

For persons older than 50 years, current American Cancer Society guidelines recommend a variety of screening tests, the exact method to be determined following discussion between the physician and the patient (see Table 12-1). In 2012, the European Council recommended only gFOBT screening for individuals between the ages of 50 and 74 years.

Lansdorp-Vogelaar I, von Karsa L; International Agency for Research on Cancer. European guidelines for quality assurance in colorectal cancer screening and diagnosis. First Edition—Introduction. *Endoscopy.* 2012;44(Suppl 3):SE15–30.

Yang DX, Gross CP, Soulos PR, Yu JB. Estimating the magnitude of colorectal cancers prevented during the era of screening: 1976 to 2009. *Cancer.* 2014;120(18):2893–2901.

Gastrointestinal cancer

Accounting for 80%–90% of cases, the primary risk factors for squamous cell carcinoma of the esophagus are tobacco use and alcohol consumption. The main risk factors for adenocarcinoma of the esophagus are gastroesophageal reflux disease (GERD), obesity, and a history of Barrett esophagus (a complication resulting from long-standing GERD). Treatment for esophageal cancer has poor results; thus, prevention or elimination of the risk factors is worthwhile. The incidence of adenocarcinoma of the esophagus is increasing in developed countries, but squamous cell carcinoma remains dominant in developing areas. Currently, no effective preventive screening programs are available, and most patients present with advanced or metastatic disease.

Gastric cancer appears to be associated with certain geographic areas (Japan, China, Central and South America, Eastern Europe, and parts of the Middle East), high ingestion of nitrates, loss of gastric acidity, lower socioeconomic status, and blood type A. It remains the second most frequent and lethal malignancy worldwide. Although routine endoscopic screening is not cost-effective, widespread screening for and treatment of *Helicobacter pylori* infection in high-incidence populations could be an effective strategy for reducing gastric cancer in these groups. Further testing is recommended only for individuals in high-risk groups.

Pancreatic cancer is 2–3 times more common in heavy smokers than in nonsmokers, and it has also been associated with chronic pancreatitis, diabetes mellitus, and obesity. Familial pancreatic cancer represents only about 5%–10% of all cases but carries a higher mortality rate than sporadic pancreatic cancer. Several genetic mutations have been identified that are responsible for a small percentage of familial cases.

Hepatocellular cancer is more common in persons with preexisting liver disease, especially cirrhosis and hepatitis B and C.

Lung cancer

Lung cancer is the leading cause of cancer-related deaths in men and women in the United States. Worldwide, there were 1.6 million deaths due to lung cancer in 2012. Among male patients with lung cancer in the United States, 85% are smokers. The number and percentage of cases in women have risen with the increased incidence of smoking in women. Fortunately, with the decreasing incidence of smoking, the incidence of and death rate from lung cancer in the United States have been declining. The usefulness of chest radiography and sputum cytologic screening in the general population is generally considered to be low. In high-risk patient groups, screening protocols effect a higher yield. In the US National Lung Screening Trial, lung cancer mortality in high-risk patients decreased when these patients were screened annually with low-dose helical chest CT. Positron emission tomography is a promising tool for identifying early malignant changes in the central airways; fluorescent bronchoscopy may also be useful for this purpose. New molecular markers detected in sputum and serum show promise in the future of lung cancer screening. Prevention through smoking cessation remains the most effective way to decrease lung cancer mortality.

Church TR, Black WC, Aberle DR, et al; National Lung Screening Trial Research Team. Results of initial low-dose computed tomographic screening for lung cancer. *N Engl J Med.* 2013;368(21):368:1980–1991.

Melanoma

Melanoma is the deadliest form of skin cancer, and its incidence is increasing faster than that of all other cancers. In the United States, about 1 in 75 persons will develop melanoma during his or her lifetime. According to the American Cancer Society, an estimated 91,270 new melanoma cases and 9320 related deaths were predicted in the United States in 2018.

Most melanomas probably arise from dysplastic nevi. Risk factors for melanoma include history of melanoma or atypical moles, presence of more than 50 moles, positive melanoma family history, history of previous nonmelanoma skin cancer, giant congenital nevus (>20 cm), xeroderma pigmentosum, treatment with UV-A and psoralens, frequent tanning with UV-A light, and a history of 3 or more severe (blistering) sunburns. Other, less significant risk factors are light complexion of the hair and eyes, freckles, inability to tan, indoor occupation with outdoor hobbies, and proximity to the equator.

UV damage probably causes most melanomas. Intense intermittent exposures are directly related to melanoma, whereas other skin cancers are more associated with cumulative exposure. UV radiation causes DNA damage, which is usually corrected by DNA repair enzymes; however, these DNA repair processes degrade with increasing age.

A pigmented lesion with any of the following characteristics, easily remembered by the *ABCDE* mnemonic, is suggestive of melanoma: *a*symmetrical lesions, *b*order (irregular), *c*olor (variable), *d*iameter (≥6 mm), and *e*volving (change in size, shape, or color). Other characteristics suggestive of melanoma are pruritus, bleeding, changing morphology, and new lesions or scalp lesions. Everyone should perform periodic self–skin examinations; suspicious lesions require referral to a dermatologist and possible biopsy. Avoiding the sun during peak hours and using sunblock can reduce the risk of melanoma and other skin cancers. In addition to providing simple visualization, when conducted by skilled examiners, dermoscopy (epiluminescence microscopy) can increase the specificity of clinical examination for the detection of melanomas.

American Cancer Society. Melanoma skin cancer: About and key statistics. www.cancer.org/cancer/melanoma-skin-cancer/about/key-statistics.html. Last medical review: January 12, 2021. Accessed September 10, 2021.

Urologic cancer

In the United States, approximately 16% of new cancer cases per year are found in the prostate, bladder, kidney, and testes, with most of the common malignancies occurring in middle-aged and older men. Approximately 164,690 new cases of prostate cancer and nearly 29,430 related deaths are expected in 2018 in the United States. Although prostate cancer can sometimes be detected early by digital rectal examination (DRE) of the prostate, no effect on mortality has been demonstrated, so annual DRE is no longer recommended. Serum prostate-specific antigen (PSA) screening remains controversial, and data suggest that this screening does not affect mortality. The PSA false-negative rate varies between 15% and 38%, and only about 30% of patients with elevated PSA levels truly have prostate carcinoma. A trend of increasing PSA levels is a more sensitive indicator of prostate cancer than is an individual elevated PSA level. Because of the high rate of false-negatives, minimal disease identified by PSA screening, and the potentially significant adverse effects of treating minimal disease, routine yearly serum PSA screening is no longer recommended except for higher-risk individuals, such as African American men and those with a positive family history of prostate cancer. Instead, in 2017, the US Preventive Services Task Force recommended individualized discussion of the risks and benefits of prostate cancer screening for men between the ages of 55 and 69; this guidance is similar to that given by the European Society for Medical Oncology.

Although prostate cancer is a potentially lethal illness, many detectable prostate cancers are of little threat to life. Some studies suggest that more than 75% of men with screen-detected localized disease may not even need treatment. Some men with low-grade prostate cancer receive curative treatment, even though their disease may not require treatment. More specific screening methods are needed to allow differentiation between potentially lethal and nonlethal cancers.

Grossman DC, Curry SJ, Owens DK, et al; US Preventive Services Task Force. Screening for prostate cancer: US Preventive Services Task Force recommendation statement. *JAMA*. 2018;319(18):1901–1913.

Infectious Diseases

The major public health screening efforts in the United States have been for tuberculosis and sexually transmitted infections (syphilis, chlamydia, gonorrhea, HIV, and herpes simplex virus). Hepatitis screening is used primarily for blood donation, institutionalized populations, and health care workers rather than for the general population. These disorders are discussed in more detail in Chapter 14.

Tuberculosis

One-third of the world's population is infected with *Mycobacterium tuberculosis (TB)*. The prevalence of TB has recently increased in the United States, reversing decades of steady decline. Thus, TB skin testing should be performed on individuals in high-risk groups, and positive results should prompt chest radiography and consideration of chemoprophylaxis. Some experts advocate regular skin testing of all persons younger than 35 years at the time of routine health examination (for detection as well as for baseline data). The US Occupational Safety and Health Administration recommends that all health care facilities conduct a TB risk assessment, with testing performed if indicated; routine testing is no longer recommended. In addition to TB skin testing, an interferon-gamma release assay (IGRA) can be used to screen for TB exposure. This blood test may be more specific in some clinical situations, including screening for TB in patients who previously received the BCG vaccine. Although acid-fast smears and histopathology remain the most common approach for confirming a diagnosis of TB, a number of nucleic acid amplification assays are also now available.

Several candidate vaccines for TB are currently being investigated; they include subunit; recombinant BCG; and inactivated whole-cell vaccines. The current BCG vaccine can also provide limited protection to newborns in endemic areas.

Kaufmann SH, Weiner J, von Reyn CF. Novel approaches to tuberculosis vaccine development. *Int J Infec Dis.* 2017;56:263–267.

Syphilis

The incidence of syphilis is increasing in the United States, particularly among men who have sexual intercourse with other men. Syphilis is almost always transmitted sexually; congenital disease transmitted in utero still occurs but is rare (600 cases in the United States in 2016). The incidence of congenital syphilis has dropped 90% since the 1940s because of required premarital screening and pregnancy screening. Better prenatal care and increased syphilis screening during pregnancy improve the likelihood of detecting infants at risk for congenital syphilis, thus allowing early maternal treatment.

Latent, untreated cases of syphilis in which the primary or secondary mucocutaneous lesion is no longer present can be detected only by screening. It is important to detect early latent disease: in approximately 25% of cases, infectious mucocutaneous lesions reemerge spontaneously in the first 2 years. Late latent disease should be detected and treated because of the long-term destructive effects on the central nervous system, the aorta, and the skeletal system.

Screening is generally performed with the more sensitive, but less specific, nontreponemal antigen tests (VDRL, RPR, TRUST). Positive results are then confirmed with treponemal antigen tests (FTA-ABS, MHA-TP, TPPA, TP-EIA), which were more expensive in the past; automation of these treponemal antigen tests has decreased their costs, and these tests are now sometimes used for the initial screening.

Bibbins-Domingo K, Grossman DC, Curry SJ, et al; US Preventive Services Task Force (USPSTF). Screening for syphilis infection in nonpregnant adults and adolescents: US Preventive Services Task Force recommendation statement. *JAMA*. 2016;315(21): 2321–2327.

Immunization

The development of immunization as a means of preventing the spread of infectious disease began in 1796, when Edward Jenner injected cowpox virus, which causes a mild disease, into a child to prevent smallpox, a severe, potentially fatal illness. Immunization today still relies on Jenner's inoculation methods to protect against disease. There are 2 types of immunization: active and passive.

In *active immunization,* the recipient develops an acquired immune response to inactivated or killed viruses, viral subtractions, bacterial toxoids or antigens, or synthetic vaccines. Once the immune response to a particular pathogen has developed, it protects the host against infection. The persistence of acquired immunity depends on the perpetuation of cell strains responsive to the target antigenic stimulus; for certain immunogens, booster inoculations may be required.

In general, live, attenuated vaccines produce longer-lasting immunity; however, they are contraindicated in immunocompromised persons or pregnant women because the pathogen can potentially replicate in the host. Ideally, active immunization should be completed before exposure; however, life-saving postexposure immunity can be developed by combining active and passive immunization.

Passive immunization depends on the transfer of immunoglobulin in serum from a host with active immunity to a susceptible host. Passive immunity does not result in active immunity and sometimes even blocks the development of active immunity. Passive immunity is short-lived and does not confer long-term immunity; however, it confers immediate protection on the recipient who has been exposed to the pathogen. Pooled human globulin, antitoxins, and human globulin with high antibody titers for specific diseases are the usual products available for passive immunization.

The current recommended US immunization schedules, developed by the Advisory Committee on Immunization Practices—including immunization schedules for persons aged 0–18 years, the catch-up schedule for individuals aged 4 months to 18 years, and the adult schedule—can be found on the CDC website (www.cdc.gov/vaccines/schedules/index.html). The catch-up protocols are for children who have missed some of the recommended immunization doses.

Immunization should be avoided in persons who have allergic reactions to the vaccine or its components. Idiopathic autoantibody or cross-reacting antibody development may occur after vaccination, resulting in systemic disease such as Guillain-Barré syndrome, a rare but devastating complication of vaccination. Immunization should be avoided during a febrile illness. Multidose immunization schedules that are interrupted can be resumed; however, doses given outside the schedule should not be counted toward completion of the vaccination sequence.

For patients who are pregnant, immunization against tetanus, diphtheria, and influenza is indicated; immunization against other diseases (hepatitis, pneumococcal or meningococcal disease) is indicated if a patient is at high risk of exposure. Additional immunizations may be considered but must be weighed against rare potential risks to the fetus.

The following sections are based on the more extensive recommended immunization schedules in the United States. In other parts of the world, immunizations are performed based on World Health Organization (WHO) guidelines, national programs, or recommendations by multinational organizations such as the European Centre for Disease Prevention and Control (ECDC). As a general rule, national immunization schedules for children are quite similar, but recommended immunizations for adults vary widely between countries (Table 12-2 lists a sampling). For more information on the immunization schedules of EU nations, see the ECDC website (https://vaccine-schedule.ecdc.europa.eu).

Chlibek R, Anca I, André F, et al. Adult vaccination in 11 Central European countries—calendars are not just for children. *Vaccine.* 2012;30(9):1529–1540.

Robinson CL, Romero JR, Kempe A, Pellegrini C, Szilagyi P. Advisory Committee on Immunization Practices recommended immunization schedule for children and adolescents aged 18 years or younger—United States, 2018. *MMWR Morb Mortal Wkly Rep.* 2018;67(5):156–157.

US Centers for Disease Control and Prevention. Recommended immunization schedules for adults aged 19 years or older, United States 2021. www.cdc.gov/vaccines/schedules/hcp/imz/adult.html. Updated February 3, 2020. Accessed September 10, 2021.

Hepatitis

There are 3 main types of hepatitis viruses. Infection with *hepatitis A virus* (HAV) is the leading cause of viral hepatitis in the United States. HAV is usually transmitted orally and may be acquired from contaminated water supplies and unwashed or undercooked foods. Vaccination against HAV infection is recommended for children aged 12–23 months and for persons at high risk of exposure to HAV (eg, travelers to endemic areas, patients with blood clotting factor disorders, military personnel, drug abusers, family contacts of infected patients, laboratory workers exposed to the virus). In the United States, 2 preparations are available (Vaqta, Havrix), each consisting of viral antigens purified from human cell cultures.

Approximately 250,000 cases of *hepatitis B* occur annually in the United States. Between 6% and 10% of adult patients with hepatitis B become carriers, and chronic active hepatitis occurs in 25% of these carriers. Of the patients with chronic active disease, 20% will die of cirrhosis and 5% will die of hepatocellular carcinoma. Worldwide, 250 million persons are chronic carriers.

In the United States, the available recombinant vaccines based on the hepatitis B virus (HBV) surface antigen are Engerix-B and Recombivax HB. In adults, HBV vaccine is usually administered in a series of 3 doses, and 90% of recipients develop protective antibody

Table 12-2 2017 National Adult Immunization Recommendations: A Sampling[a]

Vaccine	United States	United Kingdom	Finland	Germany	France	Spain
Influenza	Annually ≥6 months	Annually ≥65 years	Annually ≥65 years	Annually >60 years	Annually >65 years	Annually >65 years
Tetanus, diphtheria	Tdap once 19–64 years of age, then Td booster every 10 years	Catch-up only	Tetanus and diphtheria boosters	Tetanus and diphtheria boosters	Tetanus and diphtheria boosters	Tetanus and diphtheria boosters
Pertussis	Pertussis as Tdap	Expectant mothers	Pertussis by age 15 years	Once as adult	Once as adult	–
Human papillomavirus (HPV)	Males and females, 3 doses	Females only	High-risk groups	Females only	Females and men who have sexual intercourse with other men	–
Varicella-zoster	2 doses, ≥60 years	1 dose, >70 years	–	–	–	–
Measles/mumps/rubella (MMR)	1–2 doses	Catch-up only	–	Catch-up only	Catch-up only	–
Pneumococcal	1 dose, >65 years	1 dose, >65 years	1 dose, >65 years	1 dose, >60 years	–	High-risk groups

Td = tetanus and diphtheria toxoid vaccine; Tdap = tetanus toxoid, diphtheria, and acellular pertussis vaccine.

[a]Recommendations as of August 9, 2017.

Data from the European Centre for Disease Prevention and Control website, https://vaccine-schedule.ecdc.europa.eu/. Accessed September 10, 2021.

levels (>10 milli-international units/ml [mIU/mL]), which persist for at least 3 years and may be protective for up to 30 years. Booster injections are advised for persons whose antibody levels are less than 10 mIU/mL. A second vaccination results in the development of protective antibodies in 50% of the initial nonresponders.

Vaccination before exposure to HBV is recommended and cost-effective for all infants and children and for individuals in certain high-risk groups: health care workers, hemodialysis patients, diabetic adults over age 60, residents and staff of long-term care facilities, household and sexual contacts of chronic carriers of HBV, hemophiliacs, users of illicit injectable drugs, prison inmates, sexually active homosexual men, and HIV-seropositive individuals. Vaccination can be combined with passive immunization for postexposure prophylaxis without affecting the development of active immunity. The incorporation of the vaccine into childhood immunization schedules has resulted in a decrease in the number of new hepatitis B cases reported annually, and there has also been a significant reduction in the number of hepatocellular carcinoma cases reported in children. Some of the available combination vaccines protect against not only hepatitis B, but also hepatitis A, diphtheria, pertussis, tetanus, and polio.

Postexposure prophylaxis with hepatitis B immunoglobulin should be considered when there is perinatal exposure of an infant born to a carrier, accidental percutaneous or permucosal exposure to blood that is positive for the HBV surface antigen, or sexual exposure (within 14 days) to a carrier of HBV. Hepatitis B immunoglobulin should be given as soon as possible after exposure; the recombinant HBV vaccine should be concurrently administered in an accelerated dosing schedule.

Patients with chronic hepatitis B infection and evidence of liver disease may improve after treatment with antiviral medications. If indicated, Interferon or nucleos(t)ide analogues (tenofovir or entecavir) are effective and have a lower incidence of viral resistance than lamivudine.

Hepatitis C is the leading indication for liver transplantation in the United States. The CDC has recommended that all adults in the United States born between 1945 and 1965 have a one-time test for hepatitis C. Early intervention in chronically infected individuals, including treatment and alcohol counseling, can slow the progression of disease. Vaccines against hepatitis C and E are being developed. See Chapter 14 for additional discussion of hepatitis C and other forms of the hepatitis virus.

Smith BD, Morgan RL, Beckett GA, Falck-Ytter Y, Holtzman D, Ward JW. Hepatitis C virus testing of persons born during 1945–1965: recommendations from the Centers for Disease Control and Prevention. *Ann Intern Med.* 2012;157(11):817–822.

Terrault NA, Bzowej NH, Chang KM, et al; American Association for the Study of Liver Diseases. AASLD guidelines for treatment of chronic hepatitis B. *Hepatology.* 2016;63(1): 261–283.

Influenza

Although influenza is usually a self-limited disease with rare sequelae, it can be associated with severe morbidity and mortality in older persons or those with chronic diseases.

Influenza vaccines produce long-lasting immunity. However, antigenic shifts, primarily in type A rather than type B influenza virus, require yearly reformulation of the vaccine to contain the antigens of strains considered most likely to cause disease. Protection is correlated with the development of antihemagglutinin and antineuraminidase antibodies, which decrease the patient's susceptibility and the severity of the disease. The influenza vaccine is as effective in HIV-seropositive patients as it is in HIV-seronegative patients, regardless of the individual's $CD4^+$ T-cell counts. In the United States, annual vaccination is recommended for all adults and for children older than 6 months. The influenza vaccine is well tolerated, and there has been no increased risk of neurologic complications with the vaccines administered after 1991. Trivalent and quadrivalent *inactivated influenza vaccines (IIVs)* are available, as well as a recombinant influenza vaccine. A live-attenuated influenza vaccine (LAIV) is also available but may not be as effective as the IIV. Pregnant women may safely receive the IIV. Health care workers working with severely immunocompromised patients should receive the IIV. The IIV and LAIV should not be administered to persons with anaphylactic hypersensitivity to eggs, but the recombinant vaccine (Flublok) may be used. A high-dose vaccine for patients older than 65 years is also available. Antiviral agents may be indicated to treat influenza in high-risk patients who are more likely to have serious sequelae from influenza (eg, elderly individuals, pregnant women, individuals with certain chronic conditions). The CDC (and others) suggest treatment with neuraminidase inhibitors (zanamivir, oseltamivir, peramivir) due to emerging resistance to amantadine and rimantadine.

Grohskopf LA, Sokolow LZ, Broder KR, et al. Prevention and control of seasonal influenza with vaccines: recommendations of the Advisory Committee on Immunization Practices—United States, 2017–18 influenza season. *MMWR Recomm Rep.* 2017;66(2):1–20.

Varicella-Zoster

Varivax, an approved live, attenuated varicella-zoster vaccine, is recommended in the United States for immunocompetent pediatric patients older than 12 months with no history of previous infection with varicella-zoster virus (VZV). A second dose is given when the child is between 4 and 6 years of age. For patients older than 13 years, 2 doses of vaccine are given 4–8 weeks apart. Health care workers who have not been exposed to chickenpox (varicella) should also be vaccinated. Varivax is safe and provides immunity for up to 20 years. Data from the CDC confirmed a dramatic decline (87%) in the incidence of varicella in the United States from 1995 to 2000.

Shingrix, an inactivated recombinant zoster vaccine given in 2 doses, is recommended by the FDA for adults aged 50 or older to reduce the incidence of VZV infection. This vaccine, approved in 2017, decreases the risk of VZV by 90% and may be safe to use in immunocompromised patients. Zostavax was previously recommended to reduce the risk of VZV infection and postherpetic neuralgia. However, Zostavax appears to be less effective than Shingrix, and it cannot be used in adults receiving high-level immunosuppressive therapy. Neither Zostavax nor Shingrix may be used in place of Varivax in younger persons. Zostavax is no longer available in the United States as of November 2020. Also see Chapter 14.

Ophthalmic considerations The incidence of varicella-zoster virus (VZV) infection increases with increasing age; it has a rate of 11 cases per 1000 person-years for patients in their 80s. In the United States, 1.2 million new cases of varicella-zoster infections are diagnosed each year in adults, 20% of which have ophthalmic involvement. Ophthalmologists should encourage their patients over age 50 to receive the new VZV vaccine (Shingrix) even if they previously received the Zostavax vaccine.

Cornea Society and American Academy of Ophthalmology Secretariat, Hoskins Center for Quality Eye Care. Clinical Statements. *Recommendations for Herpes Zoster Vaccine for Patients 50 Years of Age and Older—2018.* San Francisco: American Academy of Ophthalmology; 2018. www.aao.org/clinical-statement/recommendations-herpes-zoster-vaccine-patients-50-. Accessed September 10, 2021.

Measles

Vaccination has dramatically reduced the incidence of measles, along with its associated encephalitis and mortality. Introduced in 1963, the initial vaccine was based on an inactivated virus that did not provide a long duration of protection. In 1967, a live, attenuated vaccine providing long-lasting immunity was introduced. Vaccination with the attenuated strain should be routine not only for individuals aged 15 months but also for persons born between 1957 and 1967 who were neither vaccinated nor infected and for persons who received the inactivated viral vaccine. Individuals born before 1957 are considered immune by virtue of natural infection. The vaccine is contraindicated for persons with allergic or previous anaphylactic reactions to gelatin or neomycin but is safe for patients with hypersensitivity to eggs. Measles-mumps-rubella (MMR) vaccination is recommended for all children and is usually given first at about 15 months and again when the child is between the ages of 4 and 6, but the second dose can be given sooner if necessary. The preservative thimerosal is no longer used in this vaccine, and multiple studies have refuted previous concerns about an association between MMR vaccines and autism. For nonimmunized persons exposed to measles, postexposure prophylaxis with immunoglobulin should be given within 6 days of exposure.

Mumps

The number of reported cases of mumps in the United States has decreased steadily since the introduction of a live mumps vaccine in 1967. Although mumps is generally self-limited, meningeal signs may appear in up to 15% of cases and orchitis in up to 20% of clinical cases in postpubertal males. Other possible complications include permanent deafness and pancreatitis. Mumps vaccination is indicated for all children and susceptible adults, such as child care workers. Revaccination should be considered for patients who originally received only a single dose of the vaccine, particularly students entering college, health care workers, and individuals traveling to endemic areas. A third prophylactic dose reduced the incidence of outbreaks of clinical mumps on college campuses by 78%.

Rubella

Rubella immunization is intended to prevent fetal infection and consequent congenital rubella syndrome, which can occur in up to 80% of fetuses of mothers infected during the first trimester of pregnancy. The number of reported cases of rubella in the United States has decreased steadily from more than 56,000 in 1969, the year the rubella vaccine was licensed, to 10 cases in 2005. Rubella was declared eliminated from the United States in 2004, and from the Americas in 2010, although rare outbreaks still occur elsewhere in the world.

Rubella vaccine is recommended for adults, particularly women, unless proof of immunity is available (documented rubella vaccination on or after the first birthday or a positive serologic test result) or the vaccine is specifically contraindicated. A single subcutaneously administered dose of live, attenuated rubella vaccine provides long-term (probably lifetime) immunity in approximately 95% of persons vaccinated. Because of the theoretical risk to the fetus, women of childbearing age should receive the vaccine only if they are not pregnant.

Polio

Before the introduction of the first polio vaccine in 1955, polio (poliomyelitis) caused thousands of cases of paralysis. Despite widespread immunization with oral vaccine since 1962, polio persists in some nations in Asia and Africa. There are 2 forms of the vaccine: an oral form containing live, attenuated poliovirus (oral poliovirus vaccine [OPV], Sabin vaccine); and an injectable form containing killed virus (inactivated poliovirus vaccine [IPV], Salk vaccine), which is administered subcutaneously. To eliminate the risk of vaccine-associated paralytic poliomyelitis, a condition that has been associated more often with OPV than with IPV, only IPV is used in the United States. Because OPV is cheaper and easier to distribute and because it transmits the virus to unimmunized contacts of those who are vaccinated, helping the former develop immunity, the WHO suggests that OPV be used for immunization in developing countries. The currently used bivalent OPV is less likely to cause vaccine-associated polio than the older trivalent form. OPV is contraindicated in pregnant women or immunosuppressed patients, who should receive only the inactivated virus vaccine.

Tetanus and Diphtheria

The combined tetanus and diphtheria toxoid vaccine (Td) is highly effective; it is used for both primary and booster immunization of adults. The pediatric vaccine, diphtheria-tetanus-pertussis (DTP), has been replaced with the newer pediatric vaccine, DTaP (diphtheria and tetanus toxoid with acellular pertussis). Tdap, which contains a lower concentration of diphtheria toxoid and acellular pertussis than does DTaP, is recommended in the United States as a one-time booster for all adults aged 19–64 years, and particularly for all health care professionals and anyone caring for infants younger than 12 months. Young adults should also receive a booster dose of Td every 10 years. If serious doubt exists about the completion of a primary series of immunizations, 2 doses of the combined toxoids should be given intramuscularly at monthly intervals, followed by a third dose 6–10 months later. Thereafter, a booster dose of 0.5 mL should be given at 10-year intervals.

In wound management of tetanus, previously immunized persons with severe wounds should receive a booster if more than 5 years has elapsed since the last injection. The management of previously unimmunized patients with severe wounds should include tetanus immunoglobulin as well as Td. Although tetanus is uncommon, more than 60% of cases occur in persons older than 60 years. Therefore, older adults should be given a single booster at age 65. Pregnant women should receive one dose of Tdap during each pregnancy.

Rotavirus

Rotavirus, a double-stranded RNA virus, is the most common cause of severe acute gastroenteritis in children and infants worldwide. In the United States, 2 live-attenuated oral rotavirus vaccines are available: 1 based on a bovine rotavirus strain, and 1 an attenuated human rotavirus. Three oral doses of the bovine strain are given to infants at 2, 4, and 6 months of age; alternately, 2 doses of the attenuated human vaccine are given at 2 and 4 months of age. The vaccine is not recommended in children with a history of intussusception or children receiving high-level immunosuppressive therapies.

Cortese MM, Parashar UD, Centers for Disease Control and Prevention. Prevention of rotavirus gastroenteritis among infants and children: recommendations of the Advisory Committee on Immunization Practices (ACIP). *MMWR Recomm Rep.* 2009;58(RR-2):1–25.

Pneumococcal Pneumonia

Pneumococcal pneumonia is the most serious and prevalent of the community-acquired respiratory tract infections. Although pneumococcal disease affects children and adults, the incidence of pneumococcal pneumonia increases in persons older than 40 years. Since 1974, penicillin-resistant pneumococci have emerged. The mortality rate from bacteremic pneumococcal infection exceeds 25% despite treatment with antibiotics.

The current unconjugated pneumococcal vaccine contains polysaccharide antigens from the 23 serotypes of *Streptococcus pneumoniae* most commonly found in bacteremic pneumococcal disease. The 23-valent pneumococcal polysaccharide vaccine (PPSV23) has been designed to induce a protective level of serum antibodies in immunocompetent adults and is highly effective in healthy young adults aged 19–64. Adults aged 65 years and older may receive the PPSV23 either alone or in combination with PCV13 (see discussion in the following paragraph), particularly if they are in a high-risk group (eg, a history of cardiac or respiratory disease, sickle cell disease, splenic dysfunction, renal and hepatic disease, or immunodeficiency). Those who receive pneumococcal vaccine before age 65 years should be revaccinated at age 65 if more than 5 years has passed since the initial vaccination. PPSV23 is not effective for children under the age of 2.

A pneumococcal conjugate vaccine (PCV) is recommended in the United States for all children younger than 5 years. In the United States, a 13-valent conjugate vaccine (PCV13) is typically used, while in Europe a 10-valent vaccine is more commonly used. PCV13 is administered in 4 intramuscular doses, given at 2, 4, 6, and 12–15 months of age. The vaccine provides coverage for approximately 80% of the invasive pneumococcal diseases in children in the United States. PCV is recommended for all infants and toddlers younger than 2 years, all children between 2 and 5 years of age who have chronic cardiopulmonary disorders or immune suppression, and some adults older than 65 years.

The duration of protection afforded by primary vaccination with pneumococcal vaccine seems to be 9 years or more.

Haemophilus influenzae

A vaccine against *Haemophilus influenzae* type b (Hib) is recommended for all children before age 24 months. The vaccine has significantly reduced the number of infections caused by encapsulated Hib. In the past, meningitis comprised approximately 60% of Hib infections, amounting to about 10,000 cases each year in the United States. The type b capsule enhances the invasive potential of *H influenzae;* thus, the presence or absence of serum antibodies to these capsular antigens is a critical factor that determines an individual's susceptibility to systemic Hib infection.

The vaccine significantly reduces the risk of contracting Hib-related epiglottitis, meningitis, and orbital cellulitis. The vaccine is available as a conjugated protein between the capsular polysaccharide PRP and other agents that increase the immunologic response (PRP-OMP and PRP-T). It is also available in combination with other vaccines, such as DTaP or meningococcus (Hib-MenCY), for increased patient convenience and adherence. The vaccine is administered in 3 or 4 doses, with the first dose given at age 2 months and the final dose after age 12 months. When the full series is given, the vaccine is more than 95% effective.

Meningococcus

For the prevention of meningococcal meningitis, there are 3 meningococcal conjugate vaccines (Hib-MenCY, Men ACWY-D, and Men ACWY-CRM) and 1 unconjugated vaccine (MPSV4) available; these vaccines are recommended for use in all adolescents aged 11–18 as well as military personnel, college students living in dormitories, travelers to endemic areas (such as sub-Saharan Africa), close contacts of infected patients, new outbreaks, and high-risk patients (especially splenectomized and complement-deficient patients). The Men-ACWY vaccines are recommended for high-risk patients aged 2–10 or 19–55 years. These vaccines are approximately 85% effective in preventing the spread of group C meningococcal infections, but they will not prevent infection from strains of meningococcus not represented in the vaccine. Immunity may wane over time, so revaccination may be required.

MacNeil JR, Rubin L, Folaranmi T, Ortega-Sanchez IR, Patel M, Martin SW. Use of serogroup B meningococcal vaccines in adolescents and young adults: recommendations of the Advisory Committee on Immunization Practices, 2015. *MMWR Morb Mortal Wkly Rep.* 2015;64(41):1171–1176.

Human Papillomavirus

The human papillomavirus (HPV) is a sexually transmitted virus that causes anal and genital warts (condylomata). More importantly, HPV is present in 90% of all cervical cancers in women and is a leading cause of penile and anal cancer in men. It is hoped that preventing HPV infection will significantly reduce the incidence of cervical and other gynecologic cancers. HPV vaccines do not eradicate existing viral disease, so they are most effective if given before the patient becomes sexually active. The 9-valent HPV vaccine is given in a series of 3 doses over a 6-month period, beginning at age 11–12 years in boys and girls. Catch-up doses can be given up to age 21 years in men or age 26 years in women or in men who have sexual intercourse with other men.

Travel Immunizations

Precise travel vaccination recommendations depend on the geographic destinations, duration of travel, consumption of local food and untreated water, and likelihood of close contact with local populations. Health information for travelers, including updated immunization and prevention recommendations for various regions of the world, can be found on the CDC website (www.cdc.gov/travel) and the WHO website (www.who.int/health-topics/travel-and-health).

Routine childhood vaccinations should be reviewed in all travelers and updated as needed. Children older than 6 months should be immunized against measles (MMR) prior to travel abroad. Yellow fever vaccination may be required for anyone going to or through a yellow fever endemic area or, to prevent introduction of the disease, for travelers returning from an endemic area. Immunization against hepatitis B should be considered in travelers who expect to have close contact with local populations known to have high rates of hepatitis B transmission. Emergency and relief workers should consider cholera vaccination. Meningococcus vaccination is required in order to obtain a visa to Saudi Arabia and is recommended for those planning to visit sub-Saharan Africa. Immunization for tick-borne encephalitis is available in Europe and Australia but not in the United States. Japanese encephalitis vaccine should be offered to those whose travel plans include prolonged trips to rural areas in Southeast Asia or the Indian subcontinent during the endemic season. Typhoid fever and hepatitis A immunizations are recommended for travelers who may be exposed to potentially contaminated food and water sources. Pre-exposure rabies vaccination should be considered for travelers whose plans include a prolonged visit in a remote area or for those whose activities might involve working near animals. See the WHO website for emergency treatment recommendations following a bite from a suspected rabid animal.

Travelers planning to visit areas endemic for malaria should consult the CDC or WHO websites to determine appropriate chemoprophylaxis for the region. *Plasmodium falciparum* is almost always resistant to chloroquine and sulfadoxine/pyrimethamine, so these drugs are no longer recommended. The drugs used for malaria prevention include atovaquone/proguanil, hydroxychloroquine, doxycycline, mefloquine, and primaquine. All these medications may cause serious adverse effects.

Freedman DO, Leder K. Immunizations for travel. www.uptodate.com. Accessed September 19, 2017.

New and Future Vaccines

New vaccines are now available for typhoid fever *(Salmonella typhi),* anthrax, and rabies. Vaccines undergoing investigation include those for HIV, dysentery *(Shigella), Campylobacter, Clostridium difficile,* respiratory syncytial virus, Ebola virus, Zika virus, malaria, cytomegalovirus, herpes simplex type 2, Epstein-Barr virus, TB, *Pseudomonas aeruginosa, Helicobacter pylori, Staphylococcus, Propionibacterium acnes* (now *Cutibacterium*), parainfluenza virus, and leishmaniasis. Some vaccines, such as those for smallpox and plague (Yersinia), are in development largely in anticipation of a future bioterrorism attack using these disease vectors.

Passive immunization with human hyperimmunoglobulin is currently available to treat or prevent rabies, tetanus, cytomegalovirus, hepatitis A, hepatitis B, hepatitis C, herpesvirus, and varicella-zoster infections. Respiratory syncytial virus immune globulin is no longer available, but new monoclonal antibodies show promise.

Considering the worldwide impact of infectious diseases, there is great interest in developing new vaccines for the treatment of gonorrhea, syphilis, leprosy, trachoma, and other infectious diseases. It is hoped that ongoing research will lead to the development of safe and effective vaccines for many or all of these illnesses.

Centers for Disease Control and Prevention website; www.cdc.gov.

European Centre for Disease Prevention and Control website; www.ecdc.europa.eu.

Kanoi BN, Egwang TG. New concepts in vaccine development in malaria. *Curr Opin Infect Dis*. 2007;20(3):311–316.

World Health Organization website; www.who.int/health-topics/vaccines-and-immunization.

CHAPTER 13

Cancer

Highlights

- Biologic therapies continue to play a major role in the treatment of cancer.
- Advances in stem cell biology may alter therapeutic strategies for cancer.
- Genetic profiling of tumors and patients can contribute significantly to treatment and identify patients at risk for cancer.
- More precise molecular targets for cancer increase the effectiveness and reduce the toxicity of systemic therapies.

Introduction

Cancer is the second-leading cause of death in the United States; approximately 23% of all US deaths are due to cancer. In 2015, 1.6 million new cases were diagnosed in the United States, and 595,919 deaths occurred. In 2016, more than 15.5 million Americans had a history of cancer; it is estimated that cancer will develop in approximately 38% of US men and women during their lifetimes. Worldwide, in 2012, there were 14 million new cases and 8.2 million deaths due to cancer. Developing countries are disproportionately affected, accounting for 60% of all new cases and 70% of all deaths due to cancer.

Cancer is the term used to refer to a group of related diseases; discussions of etiology, prevention, and cure must therefore address the specific types of tumors. Nonmelanotic skin cancers, including squamous cell and basal cell carcinomas, are the most common tumors, but these cancers are rarely a cause of death. After skin cancer, the most common forms of cancer in adult Americans (in decreasing order of incidence) are breast, lung, prostate, and colorectal. Approximately 80% of adult cancers arise from the epithelial tissues.

Cancer is the second-leading cause of death in children younger than 15 years in the United States, trailing only accidental death. Nevertheless, death rates have dropped, and survival rates have risen sharply. The 5-year survival rate for all childhood cancers combined has improved in the United States, from approximately 51% in 1973 to over 80% today.

Etiology

Cancer is caused by mutations in genes that control cell division. Some of these genes, called *oncogenes,* stimulate cell division; others, called *tumor suppressor genes,* slow this process. In the normal state, both types of genes work together, enabling the body to replace dead cells and repair damaged ones. Mutations in these genes cause cells to proliferate out of control; these cells grow and divide without regard for cell death. The cell cycle is regulated biochemically, and 2 important groups of enzymes are involved in this process: cyclin-dependent kinases (CDKs) and cyclin-dependent phosphatases. (An example of CDK function involves the p53 tumor suppressor gene, which upregulates the p21 inhibitor of CDK function.)

Gene mutations can be inherited or can result from damage to DNA caused by environmental exposures. Cancer causes, therefore, are explained on the basis of chemical, radiation-related, or viral conditions that occur in a complex milieu, including the host's genetic composition and immunobiologic status. Epidemiologic data suggest that as many as 80% of the cases of cancer in humans may be due to exogenous or environmental chemical exposure. If these chemicals could be properly identified, a major proportion of human cancers could be prevented by reducing host exposure or by protecting the host.

The general population is exposed to both naturally occurring ionizing radiation and man-made ionizing radiation. Man-made sources include medical diagnostic equipment and technologically altered natural sources (such as phosphate fertilizers and building materials containing small amounts of radioactivity). The carcinogenic effects of radiation exposure result from molecular lesions caused by random interactions of radiation with atoms and molecules. Most molecular lesions induced in this way are of little consequence to the affected cell. However, DNA is not repaired with 100% efficiency, and mutations and chromosomal aberrations accrue with increasing radiation doses. Parameters that influence the response of the target tissue include the total radiation dose, the dose rate, the quality of the radiation source, the characteristics of certain internal emitters (such as radioiodine), and individual host factors.

The role of viruses in the etiology of cancer has been studied extensively. For example, researchers have inoculated laboratory animals with specific viruses to see whether tumor development is induced. Several human cancers show a definite correlation with viral infection and the presence and retention of specific virus nucleic acid sequences and virus proteins in the tumor cells. Table 13-1 lists several viruses and their associated cancers.

All the DNA virus groups have been associated with cancer, except the parvovirus family. This is notable because all the DNA viruses associated with cancer contain double-stranded DNA, whereas the parvoviruses contain only single-stranded DNA. Of the 9 RNA virus groups, only 1, the retrovirus group, is associated with oncogenicity. The papillomavirus of the papovavirus group has been associated with squamous cell carcinoma, cervical cancer, and laryngeal papilloma in humans. A vaccine against human papillomavirus (HPV) is now available. Immunization against HPV may prevent most cases of cervical cancer in women; see Chapter 12 for additional discussion.

Finally, cancers may aggregate in a nonrandom manner in certain families. These cancers may be of the same type or dissimilar. In such cancer-cluster families, several children may have soft tissue sarcoma and relatives may have a variety of cancers, especially breast cancer in young women. Multiple endocrine neoplasia types 1 and 2 are yet other examples of hereditary cancer syndromes. The recognition of familial cancer syndromes permits early detection that may be life-saving.

Table 13-1 Virus-Associated Cancers

Type of Virus	Systemic Findings	Associated Cancers
DNA virus		
Cytomegalovirus	Cytomegalovirus disease, transfusion mononucleosis, interstitial pneumonia, congenital defects	Carcinoma of the bladder and uterine cervix, Kaposi sarcoma, prostate cancer
Epstein-Barr virus	Infectious mononucleosis	Burkitt lymphoma, nasopharyngeal carcinoma
Hepatitis B virus	Cirrhosis	Hepatocellular carcinoma
Herpes simplex virus type 1	Gingivostomatitis, encephalitis, keratoconjunctivitis, neuralgia, labialis	Carcinoma of the lip and oropharynx
Herpes simplex virus type 2	Genital herpes, disseminated neonatal herpes, encephalitis, neuralgia	Cancer of the kidneys, nasopharynx, uterine cervix, vulva
Human papillomavirus	Cutaneous verrucae, laryngeal papilloma	Cervical cancer, squamous cell carcinoma
RNA virus		
Hepatitis C virus	Cirrhosis	Hepatocellular carcinoma
Human T lymphotropic virus type 1	Arthropathy, myopathy, polyneuropathy, Sjögren syndrome, uveitis	Adult T-cell leukemia

Radiation Therapy

Radiation therapy, which uses ionizing radiation to kill cancer cells and shrink tumors, is part of the treatment plan for many patients with cancer. Ionizing radiation interacts with tissues via an energy transfer and a chemical reaction, in which free radicals are released and water molecules decompose into hydrogen, hydroxyl, and perhydroxyl ionic forms. These ionic forms break atomic and molecular bonds, which in turn break the double-stranded DNA structure and cause cellular death. Consequent cell death occurs in both normal tissue and malignant lesions. In radiotherapy, biochemical recovery and biologic repair occur in the normal host cells, maintaining the integrity of vital systems.

In radiation oncology, *therapeutic ratio* refers to a fundamental concept in which the risks and benefits to the targeted cancer cells and the surrounding tissues must be weighed. Lymphocytes are damaged by 1 gray (Gy) of radiation and central nervous system tissue by 50 Gy. Table 13-2 lists some examples of the effects of radiation on ocular and nonocular tissues.

Radiation can be delivered through external beam radiotherapy (EBRT; most common) or internal placement (brachytherapy); radiation can also be administered systemically (eg, radioactive substance bound to a monoclonal antibody). In EBRT, high-energy x-ray beams generated either by linear accelerators, which produce photons or electrons, or by cobalt machines, which use radioactive decay of an element such as cobalt 60, are aimed at the tumor site. Planning for EBRT involves not only localizing the tumor, but also determining the proper dose of radiation: one that will kill the malignant cells while

Table 13-2 Radiation Damage to Ocular and Nonocular Tissues

Type of Tissue	Damage Produced by Radiation	Amount of Radiation, in Gy
Ocular tissues		
Cornea	Dry eye syndrome	60
Lens	Hastened cataract formation	2
Optic nerve	Neuropathy	60
Retina	Retinopathy	50
Nonocular tissues		
Central nervous system	Tissue damage	50
Lymphocytes	Cell damage	1
Fetus	Congenital abnormalities	0.5
Skin	Erythema	10

Gy = gray.

minimizing damage to the surrounding noncancerous tissue. There are many other methods of EBRT, including particle therapy and stereotactic radiosurgery.

In brachytherapy (also called *internal radiation therapy*), radioactive material is implanted within or adjacent to the tumor, delivering radiation while minimizing damage to the surrounding normal tissue. The term *brachytherapy* refers to various types of procedures, one example of which is seed implantation, used in the treatment of prostate cancer and some uveal melanomas. See BCSC Section 4, *Ophthalmic Pathology and Intraocular Tumors,* for more on brachytherapy and uveal melanomas.

For some conditions, monoclonal antibodies are available as a vector to deliver radiation directly to the target tissue; these antibodies are discussed later in this chapter in the section Biologic Therapies.

Jeganathan VS, Wirth A, MacManus MP. Ocular risks from orbital and periorbital radiation therapy: a critical review. *Int J Radiat Oncol Biol Phys.* 2011;79(3):650–659.

Ophthalmic considerations The ocular effects of irradiation depend not only on total dose, fractionation, and treatment portal size but also on the presence of any associated systemic diseases such as diabetes mellitus and hypertension. Concomitant chemotherapy has an additive effect.

The lens is the most radiosensitive structure in the eye, followed by the cornea, the retina, and the optic nerve. The orbit is completely included in the treatment portal in diseases such as large retinoblastomas; it is partially included in tumors of adjacent structures, such as the maxillary antrum, nasopharynx, ethmoid sinus, and nasal cavity. Usual radiation doses range from 20 to 100 Gy. The total dose is usually fractionated into smaller doses during the treatment. In brachytherapy, a low-energy isotope such as radioactive iodine delivers a high dose of radiation within a few millimeters of the tumor but does not penetrate deep into it. This allows for radioactive episcleral implants to deliver a dose of 100 Gy to the apex of a tumor but a much lower dose to the rest of the eye. The sclera can tolerate doses up to 400–800 Gy.

Doses to the lens as low as 2 Gy in a single fraction may cause cataract formation. However, cataracts caused by low doses may be asymptomatic and may not progress. Cataracts resulting from higher doses (7–8 Gy) may continue to progress, resulting in considerable vision loss. The average latent period for the development of radiation-induced cataracts is 2–3 years.

The clinical picture of radiation retinopathy resembles that of diabetic retinopathy. The usual interval between radiation therapy and the development of radiation-induced retinopathy is 2–3 years. Radiation retinopathy may develop earlier in patients with diabetes mellitus or in those undergoing chemotherapy. The earliest clinical manifestation of radiation retinopathy is usually cotton-wool spots. After several months, these spots fade away, leaving areas of capillary nonperfusion. Telangiectatic vessels grow from the retina into these areas. Microaneurysms may also develop. These ischemic changes may cause neovascularization of the iris, which in turn may lead to neovascular glaucoma. The capillary endothelial cell is the first type of cell to be damaged, followed closely by the pericytes and then the endothelial cells of the larger vessels. The new intraretinal telangiectatic vessels have thick collagenous walls. There may be spotty occlusion of the choriocapillaris. Panretinal photocoagulation or injection with anti–vascular endothelial growth factor (anti-VEGF) agents are effective treatments for radiation retinopathy. See BCSC Section 12, *Retina and Vitreous,* for more on this topic.

Radiation optic neuropathy may present with optic nerve head pallor with splinter hemorrhages. Injury to the more proximal part of the optic nerve resembles retrobulbar optic neuropathy. Affected patients may report unilateral headaches and ocular pain; the optic nerve head may not reveal edema or hemorrhage. With doses of 60–70 Gy, dry eye syndrome sometimes develops. This syndrome usually develops within a year and occasionally progresses to corneal ulceration and severe pain. For more on radiation optic neuropathy, see BCSC Section 5, *Neuro-Ophthalmology.*

Ocular manifestations of fetal irradiation in the first trimester include microphthalmos, congenital cataracts, and retinal dysplasia.

Chemotherapy

The goal of cancer chemotherapy is to damage or destroy cancer cells without killing normal cells. The type of chemotherapy treatment used depends on the treatment goals for the type and extent of the cancer being treated. *Curative chemotherapy* is used to eliminate cancer cells and to achieve a permanent cure for the patient. *Adjuvant chemotherapy* is given after surgical resection of the cancer to eliminate undetectable microscopic cancer cells. This method lowers recurrence rates in these patients. The goal of *neoadjuvant chemotherapy* is to shrink large tumors that would be too large for total resection, potentially creating a less invasive surgical procedure. *Palliative chemotherapy* is used when it is no longer possible to remove all the cancer cells; this option can provide the patient with

Table 13-3 Antineoplastic Drugs

Drug Class	Mechanism of Action	Drug Generic Name[a]
Alkylating agents	Act directly on DNA to prevent cell division, causing cross-linking of DNA strands, abnormal base pairing, or DNA strand breaks	Busulfan, carboplatin, chlorambucil, cyclophosphamide, melphalan, thiotepa
Angiogenesis inhibitors	Interfere with tumor angiogenesis; inhibit endothelial proliferation and other signaling pathways	Tyrosine kinase inhibitors (bosutinib, dasatinib, imatinib), aflibercept, bevacizumab
Antimetabolites	Interfere with metabolic pathways, thereby causing cell death. Cell-cycle specific; most effective in cells undergoing synthesis of new DNA in the synthesis phase of the cell cycle	Metabolic antagonists to folate (methotrexate), purine (6-mercaptopurine), and pyrimidine (5-fluorouracil)
Antitumor antibiotics	Disrupt cell survival; are not cell-cycle specific. Bind with DNA to prevent RNA synthesis, stopping protein synthesis	Anthracyclines (daunorubicin, doxorubicin), bleomycin, mitomycin-c, mitoxantrone
Hormones	Bind to androgen or estrogen receptors	Estramustine, Flutamide, leuprorelin, tamoxifen
Inorganic ions	Inhibit uncoiling of DNA	Cisplatin
Mitotic inhibitors/plant alkaloids	Cytotoxic drugs that stop cell division, thereby causing cell death. Bind to tubulin, inhibiting microtubule formation during the mitotic phase of the cell cycle	Estramustine, paclitaxel, vinblastine, vincristine, vinorelbine
Nitrosoureas	Alkylate DNA, restricting DNA uncoiling and replication	Carmustine, lomustine
Topoisomerase inhibitors	Interfere with enzymes (topoisomerases) involved in DNA copying	Etoposide, teniposide, topotecan

[a]These are examples of drugs within each class; lists of drugs are not all-inclusive.

symptomatic relief, slow the progression of tumor growth, and help avoid complications from the tumor.

Natural products, meaning agents that either are naturally occurring or have been synthetically modified, have played a significant role in cancer chemotherapy and include a variety of agents, the most common of which are alkylating agents, antimetabolites, plant alkaloids, and antitumor antibiotics (Table 13-3).

Angiogenesis Inhibitors

Angiogenesis is important to the growth and spread of cancers, as new blood vessels are critical to tumor formation. In animal studies, angiogenesis inhibitors have successfully stopped the formation of new blood vessels, causing tumors to shrink and die. Various angiogenesis inhibitors have been evaluated in human clinical trials. Participants in these studies include patients with cancers of the breast, prostate, brain, pancreas, lung, stomach, ovary, and cervix; patients with certain leukemias and lymphomas; and those with AIDS-related Kaposi sarcoma.

Antibodies against vascular endothelial growth factor (VEGF), which promotes vascular proliferation, have proved effective in cancer therapy. Bevacizumab, a humanized monoclonal antibody directed against VEGF-A, was the first angiogenesis inhibitor approved for the treatment of cancer in the United States. It has demonstrated clinical efficacy in the treatment of colorectal and other solid tumors and, on an off-label basis, in the treatment of neovascular ("wet") age-related macular degeneration (AMD). Bevacizumab is also effective in the treatment of optic nerve gliomas in children. Tyrosine kinase inhibitors (TKIs), including pazopanib, have also shown promise in antitumor activity use; TKIs interfere with the modulation of growth factor signaling and thus inhibit angiogenesis. Aflibercept is a recombinant fusion protein that functions as a decoy receptor for VEGF. This agent inactivates VEGF-A, VEGF-B, and placental growth factor and is effective in the treatment of colorectal cancer and neovascular AMD.

Avery RA, Hwang EI, Jakacki RI, Packer RJ. Marked recovery of vision in children with optic pathway gliomas treated with bevacizumab. *JAMA Ophthalmol.* 2014;132(1):111–114.

Biologic Therapies

Biologic therapies (sometimes called *immunotherapy, biotherapy,* or *biologic response modifier therapy*) do not target cancer cells directly but rather harness the immune system, either directly or indirectly, to fight cancer or to lessen the adverse effects that may be caused by some cancer treatments. Further, because cancer may develop when the immune system breaks down or is not functioning adequately, biologic therapies are designed to repair, stimulate, or enhance the immune system's responses.

Cells in the immune system secrete 2 types of proteins: antibodies and cytokines. Cytokines are nonantibody proteins produced by some immune system cells to communicate with other cells. Types of cytokines include lymphokines, interferons, interleukins, and colony-stimulating factors. Some antibodies and cytokines, called *biologic response modifiers,* can be used in the treatment of cancer. Other biologic response modifiers include monoclonal antibodies, which can also be used to treat cancer, and vaccines.

Interleukins occur naturally in the body and can also be made in the laboratory. Many interleukins have been identified; interleukin-2 has been the most widely studied for use in cancer treatment. Interleukin-2 stimulates the growth and activity of many immune cells (eg, lymphocytes) that can destroy cancer cells. The FDA has approved interleukin-2 for the treatment of metastatic kidney cancer and metastatic melanoma.

Colony-stimulating factors (sometimes called *hematopoietic growth factors*) usually do not directly affect tumor cells but instead stimulate bone marrow production. Colony-stimulating factors allow doses of anticancer drugs to be increased without increasing the risk of infection or need for transfusion.

Monoclonal antibodies (mAbs) are produced by a single type of cell and are specific for a particular antigen. Researchers continue to examine ways to create mAbs that are specific for the antigens found on the surface of cancer cells being treated. Some examples of mAbs currently used in cancer treatment are rituximab and trastuzumab; note that the suffix for the names of all monoclonal antibodies is "-mab."

Therapeutic mAbs are made by injecting human cancer cells into mice, which stimulates an antibody response. The cells producing antibodies are then removed and fused with laboratory-grown cells to create hybrid cells called *hybridomas.* Hybridomas can produce large quantities of these mAbs indefinitely.

Monoclonal antibodies have many potential uses in cancer treatment; for example, they could be linked to anticancer drugs, radioisotopes, other biologic response modifiers, or other toxins. When these antibodies attach to cancer cells, they are able to deliver these poisons directly to the cells. One example of this is ado-trastuzumab emtansine, which uses trastuzumab to deliver a cytotoxic microtubule inhibitor. Another is tositumomab radioconjugate, which delivers specifically targeted radiotherapy to tumors. Monoclonal antibodies carrying radioisotopes may also prove useful in the diagnosis of certain cancers, such as colorectal, ovarian, and prostate cancer.

Cancer treatment vaccines are being developed to help the immune system recognize cancer cells. These vaccines are designed to be injected after the disease is diagnosed rather than before it develops, in contrast to the vaccines against HPV or hepatitis B, which are aimed at cancer prevention. The cancer treatment vaccines may help the body reject tumors and prevent recurrence. The first treatment vaccine, which was approved in 2010, was customized to each patient for the treatment of metastatic prostate cancer. In 2015, an oncolytic virus treatment vaccine was approved to treat melanoma that cannot be surgically removed.

Other biologic approaches to cancer therapy include *genetic profiling* of certain tumors. Current management of lung cancer and melanoma is based on such profiling. Genetic profiling may also prove more helpful and effective than classifying tumors by their organ of origin. An example of this is the differentiation between those tumors with a normal tumor suppressor gene p53 from those with an abnormal tumor suppressor gene p53. Tumor cells with normal p53 genes are far more sensitive to chemotherapy than those with mutant p53.

Dharmadhikari N, Mehnert JM, Kaufman HL. Oncolytic virus immunotherapy for melanoma. *Curr Treat Options Oncol.* 2015;16(3):326.

Ophthalmic considerations The eye and its adnexa are frequently involved in systemic malignancies as well as in extraocular malignancies that extend into ocular structures (including local malignancies of the skin, bone, and sinuses). Breast and lung cancers frequently metastasize to the eye and are the most common intraocular tumors in adults. Acute myelogenous and lymphocytic leukemias often have uveal and posterior choroidal infiltrates as part of their generalized disease. In children, these manifestations are often signs of central nervous system involvement and suggest a poor prognosis. Although malignant lymphomas do not usually involve the uveal tract, histiocytic lymphoma often involves the vitreous and presents as uveitis. The retina and choroid may also be involved.

Tumors of the eye and adnexa are discussed in several other BCSC volumes, including Section 4, *Ophthalmic Pathology and Intraocular Tumors;* Section 6, *Pediatric Ophthalmology and Strabismus;* Section 7, *Oculofacial Plastic and Orbital Surgery;* and Section 8, *External Disease and Cornea.*

American Cancer Society website; www.cancer.org.
European Society for Medical Oncology website; www.esmo.org.
UpToDate; www.uptodate.com.

CHAPTER 14

Infectious Diseases

Highlights

- Vancomycin-resistant strains of enterococci and staphylococci are a significant cause of life-threatening infection in hospitalized patients.
- DNA probes using polymerase chain reaction (PCR) provide more sensitive diagnostic tools for detecting gonorrhea, syphilis, and Lyme disease, as well as chlamydial, mycobacterial, fungal, and many viral infections.
- Treatment of patients in the early stages of HIV infections has improved. All individuals between the ages of 15 and 65 years should be screened for HIV.
- The treatment of cytomegalovirus (CMV) retinitis consists of intravitreal ganciclovir or foscarnet and oral valganciclovir.
- Newer antibiotics such as ansamycin, ceftaroline, ceftobiprole, daptomycin, delafloxacin, evernimicin, linezolid, teicoplanin, telithromycin, and quinupristin/dalfopristin provide expanded antimicrobial coverage over previous antibiotics and offer treatment options for multidrug-resistant infections. Teixobactin appears to represent an entirely new class of antibiotic.
- Zika virus and Ebola virus have emerged recently as causes of significant ocular disease.

General Microbiology

Despite formidable immune and mechanical defense systems, the human body harbors an extensive, well-adapted population of microorganisms on the skin and in the gastrointestinal, vaginal, and upper respiratory tracts. The organisms maintain their foothold on these epithelial surfaces chiefly by adherence, and they indirectly benefit the host by excluding pathogenic bacterial colonization and by priming the immune system. If antimicrobial agents alter this host–microbe interplay by eliminating the normal flora, the host's susceptibility to normally excluded pathogenic microorganisms is increased. When the mechanical defenses of the epithelial layers are breached and normally sterile areas are exposed, or if a critical component of the immune system that usually prevents microbial invasion fails, severe infections can result from the normal microbial flora.

The components of the immune system of multicellular organisms are sorted into 2 categories. The first, *innate immunity,* is present in nearly all multicellular organisms and includes humoral and cellular immune receptors that have broad specificity. The innate immune response is usually immediate; there is no immune memory of prior exposure.

The second category, *adaptive immunity,* is found only in vertebrates and does involve immune memory of prior exposure. Pathogens are recognized by many randomly generated B-lymphocyte and T-lymphocyte receptors, each of which has a very narrow specificity, that can recognize a particular antigen (epitope). Adaptive immune response is initially slower (days), because the clones of responding immune cells take time to proliferate. After the first encounter, the adaptive immune response is faster and stronger, because of immunologic memory.

However, even when both the mechanical and immune defense systems are intact, pathogenic microbes can cause infections by means of specific virulent characteristics that allow the microbes to invade and multiply. These virulent traits vary among different species and include attachment, polysaccharide encapsulation, blocking of lysosomal fusion, antigenic surface variation, immunoglobulin A protease, endotoxins, exotoxins, and biofilm formation.

The immune system, which makes possible the host's adaptive response to colonization and infection, is classically divided into the humoral and cellular immune systems. The *humoral immune system,* composed of cells derived from the B lymphocytes, is responsible for antibody-mediated opsonization, complement-mediated bacterial killing, antitoxin, and mediation of intracellular infections. The *cellular immune system,* determined by the T lymphocytes, is responsible for interaction with and stimulation of the humoral immune system, direct cytotoxicity, release of chemical messengers, and control of chronic infections. The successful interplay between the humoral and cellular immune systems mitigates and usually eradicates infections, allowing for repair and healing. Also see BCSC Section 9, *Uveitis and Ocular Inflammation.*

Staphylococcus

Staphylococcus aureus colonizes the anterior nares and other skin sites in 15% of community isolates. Of the tertiary care hospital isolates, more than 25% are resistant to all β-lactam antibiotics. The increasing prevalence of methicillin-resistant *S aureus* (MRSA) in tertiary referral hospitals appears to be related to the population of high-risk patients at such centers. Unfortunately, MRSA is now an increasingly common cause of serious infection in primary care settings as well.

Acute serious staphylococcal infections require immediate intravenous antibiotic therapy. A penicillinase-resistant penicillin or first-generation cephalosporin is normally used, pending the results of susceptibility tests.

Since 1997, infections due to strains of *S aureus* with reduced susceptibility to vancomycin (glycopeptide-intermediate *S aureus*) have been identified, and their frequency is increasing throughout the world. Some reported cases have been successfully treated with various forms of combination therapy, and newer antibiotics including daptomycin, evernimicin, linezolid, ceftaroline, and quinupristin/dalfopristin.

Staphylococcus epidermidis is an almost universal inhabitant of the skin; it is present in up to 90% of skin cultures. It can cause infection when local defenses are compromised. Its characteristic adherence to prosthetic devices makes it the most common cause of prosthetic heart valve infections, and it is a common infectious organism of intravenous catheters and cerebrospinal fluid shunts.

Most isolates are resistant to methicillin and cephalosporins; therefore, the drug of choice is vancomycin, occasionally in combination with rifampin or gentamicin. Unfortunately, there have also been reports of vancomycin-resistant infections caused by coagulase-negative *Staphylococcus.* In addition to antibiotic therapy, management usually involves removal of the infected prosthetic device or vascular catheter.

Ophthalmic considerations The ongoing Antibiotic Resistance Monitoring in Ocular Microorganisms (ARMOR) study is a nationwide surveillance program of antibiotic resistance among ocular pathogens. The study has demonstrated the prevalence of methicillin resistance among staphylococcal isolates from ocular infections, as well as a high probability of concurrent resistance to fluoroquinolones, aminoglycosides, or macrolides. All staphylococcal isolates were susceptible to vancomycin, and overall ocular resistance did not increase during the 5-year study period.

Asbell PA, Sanfilippo CM, Pillar CM, DeCory HH, Sahm DF, Morris TW. Antibiotic resistance among ocular pathogens in the United States: five-year results from the Antibiotic Resistance Monitoring in Ocular Microorganisms (ARMOR) Surveillance Study. *JAMA Ophthalmol.* 2015;133(12):1445–1454.

Gould IM. Treatment of bacteraemia: meticillin-resistant *Staphylococcus aureus* (MRSA) to vancomycin-resistant *S. aureus* (VRSA). *Int J Antimicrob Agents.* 2013;42(Suppl):S17–21.

Streptococcus

Group A β-hemolytic streptococci *(Streptococcus pyogenes)* cause a variety of acute suppurative infections via droplet transmission. Suppurative streptococcal infections in humans include pharyngitis, impetigo, pneumonia, erysipelas, wound and burn infections, puerperal infections, and scarlet fever. Rapid identification with antigen detection tests allows prompt treatment of patients with pharyngitis due to this strain of *Streptococcus* and can reduce the risk of spread of infection.

Streptococcus pyogenes remains highly susceptible to penicillin G; however, in the presence of allergy, erythromycin or (if no cross-allergy exists) a cephalosporin is substituted. Macrolide-resistant and clindamycin-resistant strains of group A β-hemolytic streptococci have been reported.

Streptococcus pneumoniae are lancet-shaped diplococci that cause α-hemolysis on blood agar. Although 10%–30% of the general population carry 1 or more serologic types of pneumococci in the throat, the incidence of and mortality from pneumococcal pneumonia increase sharply after 50 years of age, with a fatality rate approaching 25%.

Besides pneumonia, conditions caused by *S pneumoniae* include sinusitis, meningitis, otitis media, and peritonitis. Pneumococci are usually highly susceptible to penicillin, other β-lactams, erythromycin, or the newer fluoroquinolones. Routine susceptibility testing should be performed on patients with meningitis, bacteremia, or other life-threatening infections. Penicillin-resistant strains of *S pneumoniae* have been reported with increasing frequency. Treatment of highly resistant strains may require vancomycin or meropenem. Prophylaxis is available through use of the 23-valent pneumococcal conjugate vaccine for adults and the 13-valent vaccine for children (see Chapter 12 in this volume).

Between 10% and 35% of cases of community-acquired infectious endocarditis are caused by α-hemolytic streptococci, while *S aureus* accounts for 30%–50% of cases. *S aureus* also accounts for 60%–80% of cases of nosocomial endocarditis, with the majority due to MRSA. Prophylaxis for infectious endocarditis is usually not considered necessary for routine ocular surgery but can be considered for surgery involving the nasolacrimal drainage system, the sinuses, or for surgical repair of orbital trauma, if the patient has a high risk of adverse outcome from endocarditis (Table 14-1). These include patients with prosthetic cardiac valves or prosthetic material used to repair cardiac valves, previous endocarditis, certain types of congenital heart disease, and cardiac transplantation with valve regurgitation.

Grabenstein JD, Musey LK. Differences in serious clinical outcomes of infection caused by specific pneumococcal serotypes among adults. *Vaccine.* 2014;32(21):2399–2405.

Table 14-1 SBE Prophylaxis Regimens for Dental and Incisional Nasolacrimal Procedures

		Regimen: Single Dose 30 to 60 min Before Procedure	
Situation	**Agent**	**Adults**	**Children**
Oral	Amoxicillin	2 g	50 mg/kg
Unable to take oral medication	Ampicillin	2 g IM or IV	50 mg/kg IM or IV
	OR cefazolin or ceftriaxone	1 g IM or IV	50 mg/kg IM or IV
Allergic to penicillins or ampicillin—oral	Cephalexin[ab]	2 g	50 mg/kg
	OR clindamycin	600 mg	20 mg/kg
	OR azithromycin or clarithromycin	500 mg	15 mg/kg
Allergic to penicillins or ampicillin and unable to take oral medication	Cefazolin or ceftriaxone[b]	1 g IM or IV	50 mg/kg IM or IV
	OR clindamycin	600 mg IM or IV	20 mg/kg IM or IV

IM = intramuscular; IV = intravenous; SBE = subacute bacterial endocarditis.

[a] Or other first- or second-generation oral cephalosporin in equivalent adult or pediatric dosage.

[b] Cephalosporins should not be used in an individual with a history of anaphylaxis, angioedema, or urticaria with penicillins or ampicillin.

Modified with permission from Wilson W, Taubert KA, Gewitz M, et al. Prevention of infective endocarditis. Guidelines from the American Heart Association: a guideline from the American Heart Association Rheumatic Fever, Endocarditis, and Kawasaki Disease Committee; Council on Cardiovascular Disease in the Young; and the Council on Clinical Cardiology; Council on Cardiovascular Surgery and Anesthesia; and the Quality of Care and Outcomes Research Interdisciplinary Working Group. *Circulation.* 2007;116(15):1736–1754, Table 5. Full online text available at: www.ahajournals.org/doi/full/10.1161/circulationaha.106.183095.

Habib G, Lancellotti P, Antunes MJ, et al; ESC Scientific Document Group. 2015 ESC Guidelines for the management of infective endocarditis: the Task Force for the Management of Infective Endocarditis of the European Society of Cardiology. *Eur Heart J.* 2015;36(44):3075–3128.

Nishimura RA, Otto CM, Bonow RW, et al. 2017 AHA/ACC focused update of the 2014 AHA/ACC guideline for the management of patients with valvular heart disease: a report of the American College of Cardiology/American Heart Association Task Force on Clinical Practice Guidelines. *J Am Coll Cardiol.* 2017;70(2):252–289.

Clostridium difficile

Clostridium difficile is an endemic anaerobic gram-positive bacillus that is part of the normal gastrointestinal flora. It has acquired importance because of its role in the development of pseudomembranous enterocolitis following the use of antibiotics. In these cases, fever and diarrhea develop 1–14 days after the start of antibiotic therapy. The diarrhea occasionally becomes bloody and typically contains a cytopathic toxin that is elaborated by *C difficile.*

Enzyme immunoassay and PCR tests allow for rapid detection. The most frequently implicated antibiotics include clindamycin, ampicillin, chloramphenicol, tetracycline, erythromycin, and the cephalosporins. New, hypervirulent strains of *C difficile* have emerged recently in the United States, Europe, and Japan. Initial treatment includes discontinuing the causative antibiotic and administering metronidazole for 10 days. Vancomycin should be used only in patients who cannot tolerate or have not responded to metronidazole, or in situations in which metronidazole use is contraindicated, such as during the first trimester of pregnancy. Bezlotoxumab, a human monoclonal antibody against *C difficile* toxin B, is associated with a rate of recurrent infection that is 38% lower than that associated with standard-of-care therapy alone.

Bagdasarian N, Rao K, Malani PN. Diagnosis and treatment of *Clostridium difficile* in adults: a systematic review. *JAMA.* 2015;313(4):398–408.

Khanna S, Pardi DS. *Clostridium difficile* infection: management strategies for a difficult disease. *Therap Adv Gastroenterol.* 2014;7(2):72–86.

Wilcox MH, Gerding DN, Poxton IR, et al; the MODIFY I and MODIFY II Investigators. Bezlotoxumab for prevention of recurrent *Clostridium difficile* infection. *N Eng J Med.* 2017;376(4):305–317.

Haemophilus influenzae

Haemophilus influenzae, a small pleiomorphic gram-negative coccobacillus, is a common inhabitant of the upper respiratory tract in 20%–50% of healthy adults and 80% of children. *H influenzae* is 1 of the 3 organisms responsible for most cases of bacterial meningitis. Roughly 14% of patients with meningitis develop significant neurologic damage. Other infections caused by this organism include orbital cellulitis, epiglottitis, arthritis, otitis media, bronchitis, pericarditis, sinusitis, and pneumonia. A DNA PCR probe assay can be used for rapid diagnosis of the most virulent strain, *H influenzae* type b (Hib) infections.

Treatment of acute *H influenzae* infections has been complicated by the emergence of β-lactamase strains, with an incidence approaching 50% in some geographic areas. Current recommendations are to treat with third-generation cephalosporins, which are highly effective against *H influenzae* infections. Alternative treatments include meropenem or ampicillin and chloramphenicol. Nearly all isolates of *H influenzae* are resistant to macrolides. Serious or life-threatening infections should be treated with an intravenous third-generation cephalosporin with known activity against *H influenzae,* such as ceftriaxone or cefotaxime, pending results of sensitivity testing.

Hib conjugate vaccines are available for use in infants and have shown their effectiveness in protecting infants and older children against meningitis and other invasive diseases caused by Hib infection. The incidence of meningitis, orbital cellulitis, and other infections caused by Hib has been reduced significantly since Hib conjugate vaccines became available. However, it is important to remember that immunized patients are still susceptible to infections caused by strains of *H influenzae* other than type b.

Davis S, Feikin D, Johnson HL. The effect of *Haemophilus influenzae* type B and pneumococcal conjugate vaccines on childhood meningitis mortality: a systematic review. *BMC Public Health.* 2013;13(Suppl 3):S21.

Neisseria

The common pathogenic *Neisseria* species are meningococci and gonococci. Meningococci can be cultured in up to 15% of healthy persons in nonepidemic periods. Virulence is determined by the polysaccharide capsule and the potent endotoxic activity of the cell wall, which can cause cardiovascular collapse, shock, and disseminated intravascular coagulation. Persons who are complement deficient or asplenic are at risk for serious clinical infections. Diagnostic testing may include Gram stain, blood and cerebrospinal fluid cultures, enzyme-linked immunosorbent assay (ELISA), and PCR. An automated fluorescent multiplex PCR assay that can simultaneously detect *N meningitidis, H influenzae,* and *S pneumoniae* can be used to evaluate patients with suspected meningitis. This test provides extremely high sensitivity and a specificity of 100% for each organism.

The range of meningococcal infections includes meningitis, mild to severe upper respiratory tract infections, and, less often, endophthalmitis, endocarditis, pericarditis, arthritis, and purpura fulminans. *Neisseria meningitidis* serogroup B is the most common cause of bacterial meningitis in children and young adults. Meningitis with a petechial or purpuric exanthem is the classic presentation, although each may occur in isolation.

Historically, the treatment of choice for meningococcal meningitis has been high-dose penicillin or, in the case of allergy, chloramphenicol or a third-generation cephalosporin. Rifampin or minocycline is used as chemoprophylaxis for family members and intimate personal contacts of the infected individual. Polysaccharide vaccines are most effective in older children and adults.

Among women with gonococcal infections, 50% are asymptomatic, whereas 95% of men with gonococcal infections are symptomatic. Asymptomatic patients are infectious for several months, with a transmissibility rate of 20%–50%. Nonsexual transmission is rare. The key to prevention is identification and treatment of asymptomatic carriers and their sexual contacts.

The range of gonococcal infections includes cervicitis; urethritis; pelvic inflammatory disease; pharyngitis; conjunctivitis; ophthalmia neonatorum; and disseminated gonococcal disease with fever, polyarthralgias, and rash. *Chlamydia trachomatis* coexists with gonorrhea in 25%–50% of women with gonococcal cervicitis and 20%–33% of men with gonococcal urethritis. Diagnosis of gonococcal infections, as well as infections caused by many other bacteria, mycobacteria, viruses, and *Mycoplasma,* has been aided by the development of highly sensitive DNA probes that use PCR techniques.

Because penicillin-resistant and tetracycline-resistant gonococcal strains have become common in many areas of the United States, treatment should be tailored to their local prevalence. Tetracycline is effective for patients who are infected by susceptible strains, are allergic to penicillin, or have concurrent chlamydial infections. Ceftriaxone (via intramuscular injection) is the drug of choice for penicillinase-resistant strains; thus far, reduced susceptibility to this antibiotic has been extremely rare. Alternatives include oral cefixime, cefuroxime, azithromycin, and the fluoroquinolones. The macrolides and fluoroquinolones have the added benefit of excellent activity against concomitant *C trachomatis* infection. However, gonococcal isolates with reduced sensitivity to macrolides and fluoroquinolones have been reported with increasing frequency, and the US Centers for Disease Control and Prevention (CDC) recommends that clinicians no longer use fluoroquinolones as a first-line treatment for gonorrhea, leaving cephalosporins as the only class of antimicrobials available for treatment of gonorrhea in the United States.

Grad YH, Harris SR, Kirkcaldy RD, et al. Genomic epidemiology of gonococcal resistance to extended-spectrum cephalosporins, macrolides, and fluoroquinolones in the United States, 2000–2013. *J Infec Dis.* 2016; 214(10):1579–1587.

Pseudomonas aeruginosa

Pseudomonas aeruginosa is a gram-negative bacillus found in moist environments. Together with *Serratia marcescens, P aeruginosa* is 1 of the 2 most consistently antimicrobial-resistant pathogenic bacteria. The virulence of pseudomonas is related to extracellular toxins, endotoxin, and a polysaccharide protection from phagocytosis. Usual sites of infection include the respiratory system, skin, eyes, urinary tract, bone, and wounds. Systemic infections caused by a resistant organism carry a high mortality rate and are usually associated with depressed immunity, often in a hospital setting.

More than half of *P aeruginosa* isolates are now resistant to aminoglycosides. Ceftazidime has been the most effective cephalosporin for treatment of pseudomonal infections. Piperacillin-tazobactam, imipenem, and meropenem also remain highly effective against most isolates, but resistance to the carbapenems and fluoroquinolones has been increasing gradually. The initial choice of antimicrobials depends on local susceptibility prevalence and should be guided by susceptibility testing.

The use of vaccines incorporating multiple *P aeruginosa* serotypes is under investigation for the treatment of patients with severe burns, cystic fibrosis, or immunosuppression.

Theuretzbacher U. Global antimicrobial resistance in gram-negative pathogens and clinical need. *Curr Opin Microbiol.* 2017;39:106–112.

Treponema pallidum

He who knows syphilis knows medicine.
Sir William Osler

Syphilis, caused by the bacterium *Treponema pallidum,* is spread by either sexual contact or transmission from a pregnant woman to her fetus. The course of the disease is divided into 4 stages: primary, secondary, latent, and tertiary (late). Initial inoculation occurs through intact mucous membranes or abraded skin and, within 6 weeks, results in a small ulcerated, painless papule called a *chancre.* The spirochetes readily enter the lymphatic system and bloodstream. The chancre heals spontaneously, and signs of dissemination appear after a variable quiescent period of several weeks to months.

The secondary stage is heralded by a truncal rash that may spread over the entire body. Fever, malaise, adenopathy, and hair loss may occur. Meningitis, uveitis, optic neuritis, and hepatitis may also occur, but are less common. The secondary lesions may resolve in a few weeks or may relapse in the first year. Without treatment, the disease enters the latent stage.

Latent syphilis, which is characterized by positive serologic test results in a patient without clinical signs, is divided into 2 stages. The *early latent stage* occurs within 1 year of infection. During this time, the disease is potentially transmissible, because relapses associated with spirochetemia are possible. The *late latent stage* is associated with immunity to relapse and resistance to infectious lesions.

Tertiary manifestations can occur many years after the initial untreated infection. Up to one-third of untreated cases of latent disease progress to this stage; the remaining two-thirds either are subclinical or resolve spontaneously. *Tertiary disease* is characterized by destructive granulomatous lesions with a typical endarteritis that can affect the skin, bones, joints, oral and nasal cavities, parenchymal organs, cardiovascular system, eyes, meninges, and central nervous system (CNS).

On pathologic examination, obliterative endarteritis with a perivascular infiltrate of lymphocytes, monocytes, and plasma cells is a feature of all active stages of syphilis. Gummata are a form of granuloma that can develop on the skin, bones, or other organs during tertiary syphilis.

Ocular syphilis and neurosyphilis can occur at any stage of syphilis. Ocular syphilis manifests most commonly as posterior uveitis or panuveitis, but it can also present with interstitial keratitis, anterior uveitis, optic neuropathy, and retinal vasculitis.

Diagnosis

Most cases of syphilis are diagnosed serologically. *Nontreponemal tests* such as the VDRL test or rapid plasma reagin (RPR) test are usually positive during the early stages of the disease, uniformly positive during the secondary stage, and progressively nonreactive in the later stages. Nontreponemal test results become predictably negative after successful therapy and can be used to assess the efficacy of treatment; however, in patients with a variety of autoimmune diseases, false-positive results can occur, especially in patients with systemic lupus erythematosus and antiphospholipid syndrome (see Chapter 9 in this volume).

Treponemal tests include the fluorescent treponemal antibody absorption (FTA-ABS) test, the hemagglutination treponemal test for syphilis (HATTS), the *T pallidum* hemagglutination assay (TPHA), and the microhemagglutination test for *T pallidum* (MHA-TP). Treponemal antibody detection tests are more specific than nontreponemal tests, and should be considered confirmatory, especially in cases in the later stages of disease. False-positive results of treponemal tests can occur in 15% of patients with systemic lupus erythematosus, in patients with other treponemal infections or Lyme disease, and, in rare instances, in patients who have lymphosarcoma or who are pregnant.

The ELISA, Western blot, and DNA PCR techniques may allow more rapid and accurate diagnosis of congenital syphilis and neurosyphilis.

Management

Treatment of syphilis is determined by disease stage and by CNS involvement. *Treponema pallidum* is exquisitely sensitive to penicillin, which remains the treatment of choice for all stages. In pregnant women, penicillin is the only treatment option. Acceptable alternatives to penicillin include erythromycin, azithromycin, chloramphenicol, tetracycline, doxycycline, and the cephalosporins.

Treatment of ocular syphilis and neurosyphilis is either aqueous crystalline penicillin G IV or procaine penicillin IM with probenecid for 10–14 days. Per the CDC, cases of ocular syphilis should be reported to the local or state health department.

Lumbar puncture should be performed to determine cerebrospinal fluid involvement in several circumstances, namely in cases of latent syphilis of more than 1 year's duration, suspected neurosyphilis, treatment failure, HIV coinfection, high RPR titers (>1:32), and evidence of other late manifestations (cardiac involvement, gummata). Either penicillin G or a single oral dose of azithromycin has been recommended for treatment of patients who were recently exposed to a sexual partner with infectious syphilis.

Many reports have described an accelerated clinical course of syphilis in HIV-infected patients; furthermore, such patients may experience an incomplete response to standard therapy. A patient coinfected with HIV and syphilis often requires a longer and more intensive treatment regimen, ongoing follow-up to assess for recurrence, and a complete neurologic workup with an aggressive cerebrospinal fluid investigation for evidence of neurosyphilis. Ceftriaxone compares favorably with intravenous penicillin for the treatment of neurosyphilis in HIV-coinfected patients. Patients with any stage of clinical syphilis should be tested for HIV serostatus.

Cantor AG, Pappas M, Daeges M, Nelson HD. Screening for syphilis: updated evidence report and systematic review for the US Preventive Services Task Force. *JAMA*. 2016;315(21):2328–2337.

Centers for Disease Control and Prevention. Sexually transmitted disease surveillance 2019. Atlanta: US Department of Health and Human Services; 2020. https://www.cdc.gov/std/statistics/2019/. Accessed September 10, 2021.

Ghanem KG, Workowski KA. Management of adult syphilis. *Clin Infect Dis*. 2011;53(Suppl 3):S110–128.

Borrelia burgdorferi

Borrelia burgdorferi, a large plasmid-containing spirochete, is transmitted to humans and domestic animals through the bite of the *Ixodes* genus of ticks. The illness caused by this transmission, which was first recognized in 1975, is called Lyme disease and is the most common vector-borne infection in the United States. Although cases have been reported in nearly all states, clusters are apparent in the northeast Atlantic, the upper Midwest, and the Pacific southwest areas, corresponding to the distribution of the *Ixodes* tick population. The range of the disease extends throughout Europe and Asia. Two other tick-borne zoonoses, babesiosis and human granulocytic ehrlichiosis, can be cotransmitted with Lyme disease.

Stages

Lyme disease usually occurs in 3 stages following a tick bite:

- *Localized (stage 1):* present in 86% of infected patients. It is characterized by skin involvement, initially a red macule or papule, which later expands in a circular manner, usually with a bright red border and a central clear indurated area, known as *erythema chronicum migrans.*
- *Disseminated (stage 2):* can occur within days to weeks. It manifests as a flulike illness with headaches, fatigue, and musculoskeletal aches.
- *Persistent (stage 3):* more profound symptoms occur during this stage, as the infection localizes to the nervous, cardiovascular, and musculoskeletal systems.

Neurologic complications such as meningitis, encephalitis, cranial neuritis (including Bell palsy), radiculopathy, and neuropathy occur in 10%–15% of patients.

Late persistent manifestations are usually confined to the nervous system, skin, and joints. Late neurologic signs include encephalomyelitis as well as demyelinating and psychiatric syndromes. Joint involvement includes asymmetric pauciarticular arthritis; skin involvement is characterized by acrodermatitis chronica atrophicans or localized lesions resembling those of systemic sclerosis.

Other systemic manifestations during the initial dissemination or the late persistent state include uveitis, conjunctivitis, keratitis, neuritis, lymphadenopathy, orbital myositis, hematuria, and orchitis. In some studies, serologic testing of patients with chronic fatigue syndrome has shown an increased incidence of positive results for *B burgdorferi* antibodies.

Diagnosis

The serologic tests most commonly used to aid in the diagnosis of Lyme disease are the immunofluorescence antibody assay or the more sensitive ELISA. The ELISA is 50% sensitive during the early stages of the disease, and almost all symptomatic patients test seropositive during the later disseminated and persistent phases of the infection. These tests should be used only to support a clinical diagnosis of Lyme disease, not as the primary basis for making diagnostic or treatment decisions. Positive IgG and IgM ELISA results are usually confirmed with Western immunoblot testing. Serologic testing is not as useful for individuals who are early in the course of Lyme disease because of the low sensitivity. Serologic testing is more helpful in later disease, when the sensitivity and specificity are greater. False-positive results can occur in patients with syphilis, Rocky Mountain spotted fever, yaws, pinta, *Borrelia recurrentis* infection, and various rheumatologic disorders. PCR has been used to detect *B burgdorferi* DNA in serum and cerebrospinal fluid. Although patients with Lyme disease may test positive on the FTA-ABS test for syphilis, their VDRL test result should be nonreactive.

Management

Treatment of *B burgdorferi* infection depends on the stage and severity of the infection. Early Lyme disease is typically treated with oral doxycycline, amoxicillin, cefuroxime, or erythromycin. Mild disseminated disease is treated with oral doxycycline or amoxicillin. Serious disease (with cardiac or neurologic manifestations) is typically treated with ceftriaxone or high-dose penicillin G for up to 6 weeks. Infections that do not respond to the initial regimen may require alternate or combination therapy.

Klempner MS, Baker PJ, Shapiro ED, et al. Treatment trials for post-Lyme disease symptoms revisited. *Am J Med.* 2013;126(8):665–669.

Schwartz AM, Hinckley AF, Mead PS, Hook SA, Kugeler KJ. Surveillance for Lyme disease—United States 2008–2015. *MMWR Surveill Summ.* 2017;6622:1–12.

Chlamydia trachomatis

Transmitted by close contact, *Chlamydia trachomatis* is the causative agent of a common sexually transmitted infection, with 200,000 new cases per year in the United States. More than 15% of pregnant women and 10% of men with chlamydial infections are asymptomatic. Chlamydia can be transmitted by a pregnant woman to her newborn during delivery, resulting in pneumonia or conjunctivitis in the infant.

Chlamydial infections in humans include trachoma, inclusion conjunctivitis, nongonococcal urethritis, epididymitis, mucopurulent cervicitis, proctitis, salpingitis, infant pneumonia syndrome, and lymphogranuloma venereum. Genital *C trachomatis* infection can cause pelvic inflammatory disease, tubal infertility, and ectopic pregnancy. Diagnostic techniques include culture, direct immunofluorescence antibody testing of exudates, enzyme immunoassay, and DNA PCR probe assay.

Chlamydial infections are readily treated with tetracycline, erythromycin, or one of the quinolones or macrolides. Although single-dose azithromycin therapy for urethritis and cervicitis has proved effective in some studies, it is usually recommended that patients continue treatment for at least 7 days to ensure complete eradication. Sexual partners of patients with chlamydial infections or other sexually transmitted infections should be examined and counseled for consideration of antibiotic treatment as well.

Neonatal chlamydial conjunctivitis is treated with oral erythromycin (50 mg/kg divided, 4 times daily) for 14 days. See BCSC Section 8, *External Disease and Cornea,* for more information.

LeFevre ML; US Preventive Services Task Force. Screening for chlamydia and gonorrhea: US Preventive Services Task Force recommendation statement. *Ann Intern Med.* 2014;161(12):902–910.

Workowski KA, Bolan GA; Centers for Disease Control and Prevention. Sexually transmitted diseases treatment guidelines, 2015. *MMWR Recomm Rep.* 2015; 64(RR-03):1–137.

Mycoplasma pneumoniae

Mycoplasma pneumoniae can cause multiple disorders, including pharyngitis, otitis media, tracheobronchitis, pneumonia, endocarditis, nephritis, encephalitis, meningitis, optic neuritis, and facial nerve palsy; it has also been implicated in some cases of chronic fatigue and fibromyalgia syndromes. Serious *M pneumoniae* infections requiring hospital admission can occur in both adults and children and may involve multiple organ systems. Recent evidence suggests that *M pneumoniae* may play a contributory role in chronic lung disorders such as asthma.

PCR assays have been adapted for the direct detection of *M pneumoniae* organisms, but in clinical practice, sensitive serologic tests are usually used initially to detect antibodies. Since mycoplasma lack a cell wall, they are unaffected by antibiotics that target cell wall synthesis.

Initial treatment of *M pneumoniae* infections typically involves use of a macrolide, tetracycline, or fluoroquinolone.

Atkinson TP, Balish MF, Waites KB. Epidemiology, clinical manifestations, pathogenesis and laboratory detection of *Mycoplasma pneumoniae* infections. *FEMS Microbiol Rev.* 2008;32(6):956–973.

Mycobacteria

Mycobacteria include a range of pathogenic and nonpathogenic species distributed widely in the environment. *Mycobacterium tuberculosis* is one of the top 10 causes of death globally, causing 1.7 million deaths each year. Most cases, and resulting deaths, occur in developing countries, with the largest number of new cases occurring in Asia and Africa. Hansen disease (leprosy) is caused by *Mycobacterium leprae* and *Mycobacterium lepromatosis.*

Nontuberculous mycobacteria (NTM) consist of the other mycobacteria that can cause lung disease resembling tuberculosis, lymphadenitis, skin disease, and bacteremia. Multidrug-resistant NTM, also known as *Mycobacterium abscessus* complex, are more difficult to treat because of their resistance to standard antituberculous regimens.

Tuberculosis

Infection with *M tuberculosis* usually occurs through inhalation of infective droplets and, in rare cases, by way of the skin or gastrointestinal tract. Infection mainly involves the lungs but can spread systemically and involve any organ system.

The purified protein derivative (PPD) tuberculin skin test measures delayed hypersensitivity to tuberculoprotein. A positive PPD reaction is defined as a 10 mm or greater area of induration in the area of intradermal injection of 0.1 milliliter (mL) of PPD, read 48–72 hours after the injection. A false-positive test may occur in patients who have been vaccinated with the BCG vaccine. Therefore, blood tests are used in patients who have received the BCG vaccine; they are also used in patients who are high risk and have a negative skin test. These tuberculosis (TB) blood tests include the Interferon-γ release assay tests (eg, the QuantiFERON-TB Gold and the T-SPOT.TB tests). Following positive skin test results, chest x-ray, chest computed tomography, and sputum samples aid in diagnosis.

Treatment of active TB infection consists of intensive therapy with daily isoniazid (INH), rifampin (RIF), pyrazinamide (PZA), and ethambutol (EMB) for 8 weeks. EMB may be discontinued following confirmation of drug regimen susceptibility. The intensive therapy is followed by continuation therapy with daily INH and rifampin for 18 weeks, or thrice weekly INH and rifampin for 18 weeks.

All currently used agents have toxic adverse effects, especially hepatic and neurologic; patients should be carefully monitored during the course of therapy. INH and EMB can cause optic neuropathy in a small percentage of patients, and rifampin may cause pink-tinged tears and blepharoconjunctivitis.

Outbreaks of nosocomial and community-acquired multidrug-resistant TB (MDRTB; meaning TB that is resistant to INH and RIF) have increased, particularly in the presence of concurrent HIV infection. MDRTB in HIV-infected patients is associated with widely disseminated disease, poor treatment response, and substantial mortality. MDRTB infection has also been documented in health care workers exposed to these patients. Treatment of MDRTB involves using at least 3 agents from the following medications or classes of medications: a fluoroquinolone (eg, levofloxacin, ciprofloxacin, ofloxacin), an injectable aminoglycoside (eg, amikacin, kanamycin, streptomycin, capreomycin), PZA, EMB, cycloserine, para-aminosalicylic acid, terizidone, a thioamide (eg, ethionamide, prothionamide), and the newer agent bedaquiline. These agents are used for at least 18–24 months following sputum culture conversion.

Ophthalmic considerations For patients taking ethambutol at doses greater than 15 mg/kg/day, screening recommendations have been established. The initial baseline examination should include visual acuity testing, color vision testing, Amsler grid testing, dilated fundus examination, and formal visual field testing. The patient should be examined monthly, and if there is any change in vision, loss of color vision, or visual field loss, the medication should be adjusted or discontinued, in concordance with the prescribing physician. Optical coherence tomography (OCT) imaging and visual evoked potential testing may help to identify optic neuropathy in its early stages.

There are no standard screening recommendations for patients taking ethambutol at doses less than 15/mg/kg/day; however, these patients should be screened regularly, including formal visual field testing. Informed consent that explains the risk of potentially irreversible loss of vision associated with any dose of ethambutol should be obtained prior to initiating care of the patient taking ethambutol.

Chamberlain PD, Sadaka A, Berry S, Lee AG. Ethambutol optic neuropathy. *Curr Opin Ophthalmol.* 2017;28(6):545–551.
Menon V, Jain D, Saxena R, Sood R. Prospective evaluation of visual function for early detection of ethambutol toxicity. *Br J Ophthalmol.* 2009;93(9):1251–1254.

Sollai S, Galli L, de Martino M, Chiappini E. Systematic review and meta-analysis on the utility of interferon-gamma release assays for the diagnosis of *Mycobacterium tuberculosis* infection in children: a 2013 update. *BMC Infect Dis.* 2014;14(Suppl 1):S6.
World Health Organization (WHO). Guidelines for treatment of drug-susceptible tuberculosis and patient care (2017 update). www.who.int/publications/i/item/9789241550000. Published April 2017. Accessed September 10, 2021.
World Health Organization (WHO). WHO treatment guidelines for isoniazid-resistant tuberculosis: Supplement to the WHO treatment guidelines for drug-resistant tuberculosis. www.who.int/publications/i/item/9789241550079. Published 2018. Accessed September 10, 2021.
Zumla AI, Gillespie SH, Hoelscher M, et al. New antituberculosis drugs, regimens, and adjunct therapies: needs, advances, and future prospects. *Lancet Infect Dis.* 2014;14(4):327–340.

Fungal Infections

Candida albicans is a yeast that is present in the mouth and gastrointestinal tract in 40%–60% of healthy adults. In individuals with disrupted local defenses or depressed immunity, overgrowth and parenchymal invasion can occur, with the potential for systemic spread. Associated infections include oral lesions (thrush) and vaginal, skin, esophageal, and urinary tract involvement. Chronic mucocutaneous lesions may occur in persons with specific T-lymphocyte defects. Disseminated disease can involve any organ system, most commonly the kidneys, brain, heart, and eyes, and is more common in immunocompromised patients and those with indwelling vascular catheters.

Other important invasive fungal infections are cryptococcosis, histoplasmosis, blastomycosis, aspergillosis, and coccidioidomycosis. Invasive fungal infections are a major problem in immunocompromised patients. Fungal PCR assays allow more rapid diagnosis of serious fungal infections and offer higher sensitivity compared with fungal cultures.

Treatment of serious systemic infections has traditionally involved the use of intravenous amphotericin B, sometimes combined with flucytosine or an imidazole. Lipid complex and liposome-encapsulated formulations of amphotericin B were developed to reduce the nephrotoxic and myelosuppressive effects of this drug. Imidazoles, such as fluconazole, itraconazole, and voriconazole, are less toxic and better-tolerated alternatives. Please see the section Antifungal Agents later in this chapter.

Toxoplasma

Toxoplasmosis is caused by infection with the protozoan parasite *Toxoplasma gondii,* which infects up to one-third of the world's population. Although acute infections may be asymptomatic in pregnant women, the infection can be transmitted to the fetus and cause severe complications, including cognitive impairment, blindness, and epilepsy. As many as 4000 new cases of congenital toxoplasmosis occur each year in the United States. Of the nearly 750 US deaths attributed to toxoplasmosis each year, approximately half are believed to be caused by eating contaminated undercooked or raw meat. *Toxoplasma gondii* can also be transmitted to humans by ingestion of oocysts, an environmentally resistant form of the organism, through exposure to cat feces, water, or soil containing the parasite or from eating unwashed contaminated fruits or vegetables.

Infection can be prevented in large part by cooking meat to a safe temperature, peeling or thoroughly washing fruits and vegetables before eating, and cleaning cooking surfaces and utensils after they have come into contact with raw meat. Pregnant women should avoid changing cat litter and handling raw or undercooked meat. Also, pet owners should keep cats indoors, where they are less likely to eat infected prey and subsequently acquire *T gondii.*

Primary infection is usually subclinical, but cervical lymphadenopathy or ocular disease can be present in some patients. The ocular manifestations include uveitis and chorioretinitis with macular scarring. The clinical picture and histopathology of toxoplasmosis reflect the immune response. In immunocompromised patients, reactivation of latent disease can cause life-threatening encephalitis.

Diagnosis of toxoplasmosis can be established by direct detection of the parasite or by serologic techniques. Real-time PCR is a very sensitive technique for diagnosing infection caused by *T gondii* and for determining the precise genotype of the organism. In the past, the most commonly used therapeutic regimen was pyrimethamine combined with sulfadiazine and folinic acid. Recently, this regimen has been largely replaced by trimethoprim-sulfamethoxazole (TMP-SMX), which is more readily available and less expensive. Other drugs with activity against *T gondii* include azithromycin, atovaquone, and clindamycin. See BCSC Section 12, *Retina and Vitreous,* for more details on the treatment of ocular toxoplasmosis.

Villard O, Breit L, Cimon B, et al; French National Reference Center for Toxoplasmosis Network. Comparison of four commercially available avidity tests for *Toxoplasma gondii*-specific IgG antibodies. *Clin Vaccine Immunol.* 2013;20(2):197–204.

Herpesvirus

As a class, viruses are strictly intracellular parasites, relying on the host cell for their replication. Herpesviruses, which are large-enveloped, double-stranded DNA viruses, are some of the most common human infectious agents and are responsible for a wide spectrum of acute and chronic diseases. Herpesviruses of interest to the ophthalmologist are the herpes simplex viruses (HSV-1 and HSV-2), varicella-zoster virus (VZV), cytomegalovirus (CMV), and Epstein-Barr virus (EBV). There are 9 recognized types of human herpesviruses. Type 1 is HSV-1; type 2 is HSV-2; type 3 is VZV; type 4 is EBV; type 5 is CMV; human herpesvirus types 6A, 6B, and 7 are known as HHV-6A, HHV-6B, and HHV-7, respectively; and type 8 (HHV-8) is associated with Kaposi sarcoma.

Herpes Simplex

Herpes simplex virus (HSV) types 1 and 2 are members of the Herpesviridae family. HSV type 1 and 2 infections differ in severity and clinical manifestation; many persons with HSV antibodies are asymptomatic. Latent infection of sensory and autonomic ganglia can occur. Reactivation of HSV from the trigeminal ganglia may be associated with asymptomatic excretion or with the development of mucosal herpetic ulceration. Serologic testing, DNA PCR testing, and viral culture can help diagnose difficult cases, particularly CNS infections.

HSV-1 is associated with mucocutaneous infections of the pharynx, skin, oral cavity, vagina, eye, and brain. Ophthalmic infection most often manifests as corneal dendritic or stromal disease but may present as acute retinal necrosis. (The ocular manifestations of HSV infection are discussed in more detail in BCSC Section 8, *External Disease and Cornea,* and Section 9, *Uveitis and Ocular Inflammation.*) Herpes encephalitis carries a 10%–20% mortality rate. *HSV-2* infection is an important sexually transmitted disease that is associated with genital infections, aseptic meningitis, and congenital infection. *Neonatal herpes infection* affects around 1 in 3500 babies born in the United states and is defined by vertical transmission from mother to infant within the first 28 days of life. Neonatal herpes infection involves multiple systems and, if untreated, has a mortality rate around 25%.

The drug of choice for treating acute systemic infections is acyclovir. Localized disease can be treated with oral acyclovir. Topical treatment of skin or mucocutaneous lesions with acyclovir ointment decreases the healing time. Oral acyclovir can also be used prophylactically for severe and recurrent genital herpes. Long-term suppressive oral acyclovir (400 mg twice a day) also reduces the recurrence of herpes simplex epithelial keratitis and stromal keratitis. Intravenous acyclovir is used to treat herpes encephalitis.

Famciclovir and valacyclovir are also approved in the United States for the treatment of herpes zoster and herpes simplex infections. Compared with acyclovir, these agents have better bioavailability, achieve higher blood levels, and require less frequent dosing. HSV is also sensitive to vidarabine. Cidofovir or foscarnet can also be used to treat acyclovir-resistant herpes simplex.

Cernik C, Gallina K, Brodell RT. The treatment of herpes simplex infections: an evidence-based review. *Arch Intern Med.* 2008;168(11):1137–1144.

Chau Tran TH, Cassoux N, Bodaghi B, Lehoang P. Successful treatment with combination of systemic antiviral drugs and intravitreal ganciclovir injections in the management of severe necrotizing herpetic retinitis. *Ocul Immunol Inflamm.* 2003;11(2):141–144.

Varicella-Zoster

Varicella-zoster virus, also sometimes referred to as *herpes zoster,* produces infection in a manner similar to that of HSV. After a primary infection, VZV remains latent in dorsal root ganglia; host cellular immune interaction inhibits reactivation. Primary infection usually occurs in childhood in the form of *chickenpox (varicella),* a generalized vesicular rash accompanied by mild constitutional symptoms. Reactivation may be heralded by pain in a sensory nerve distribution, followed by a unilateral vesicular eruption occurring over 1 to 3 dermatomic areas. New crops of lesions appear in the same area within 7 days.

Resolution of the lesions may be followed by postherpetic neuralgia. Other neurologic sequelae following VZV reactivation include segmental myelitis, Guillain-Barré syndrome, and Ramsay Hunt syndrome. The incidence of VZV is 2 or 3 times higher in patients older than 60 years. Postherpetic neuralgia occurs after VZV infection in approximately 50% of patients older than 50 years. The pain of postherpetic neuralgia can be severe and debilitating and may persist for months or even years. Immunosuppressed persons experience recurrent lesions and an increased incidence of disseminated disease.

For immunocompetent adults with cutaneous VZV infection, recommended 7-day treatment regimens include famciclovir (500 mg twice a day), valacyclovir (1000 mg 3 times a day), and acyclovir (800 mg 5 times a day). Treatment of acute infection in immunocompromised patients or those with visceral involvement may include acyclovir, famciclovir, or valacyclovir. Newer drugs being evaluated for resistant VZV strains or concomitant HIV infection include sorivudine, brivudine, fialuridine, fiacitabine, netivudine, lobucavir, foscarnet, and cidofovir.

Varivax, a live attenuated varicella-zoster vaccine, is available for use in children for prevention of primary disease. The CDC recommends Shingrix, a recombinant zoster vaccine given in 2 doses separated by 2 to 6 months, for the prevention of shingles in immunocompetent adults aged 50 years and older. Please see Chapter 12 in this volume for further discussion of varicella zoster vaccines.

In some patients, tricyclic antidepressants, pregabalin, gabapentin, and topical capsaicin cream reduce the pain of postherpetic neuralgia. For refractory cases, transcutaneous electronic nerve stimulation, nerve blocks, or intrathecal glucocorticoid injections may be helpful.

Finnerup NB, Attal N, Haroutounian S, et al. Pharmacotherapy for neuropathic pain in adults: a systematic review and meta-analysis. *Lancet Neurol.* 2015;14(2):162–173.

Cytomegalovirus

Cytomegalovirus is a ubiquitous human virus: 50% of adults in developed countries harbor antibodies, which are usually acquired during the first 5 years of life. The virus can be isolated from all body fluids, even in the presence of circulating neutralizing antibodies, for up to several years after infection. Serologic and PCR testing is available to assist in the diagnosis of CMV infection. The pp65 antigen assay is a sensitive and specific test used to guide antiviral therapy in transplant recipients and detect subclinical disease in high-risk patients.

Congenital CMV disease carries a 20% incidence of hearing loss or cognitive impairment and a 0.1% incidence of various other severe congenital disorders, including jaundice, hepatosplenomegaly, anemia, microcephaly, and chorioretinitis. Infections in adults include heterophile-negative mononucleosis, pneumonia, hepatitis, and Guillain-Barré syndrome. In immunocompromised patients, CMV interstitial pneumonia carries a 90% mortality rate. Disseminated spread to the gastrointestinal tract, CNS, and eyes is common in patients with AIDS. Latent infection within leukocytes causes transfusion-associated disease. CMV retinitis has been reported following intravitreal corticosteroid injections.

Allice T, Cerutti F, Pittaluga F, et al. Evaluation of a novel real-time PCR system for cytomegalovirus DNA quantitation on whole blood and correlation with pp65-antigen test in guiding pre-emptive antiviral treatment. *J Virol Methods.*2008;148(1–2):9–16.

Ophthalmic considerations The FDA has approved several systemic treatments for CMV retinitis: oral valganciclovir, intravenous ganciclovir, intravenous foscarnet, and intravenous cidofovir. Oral valganciclovir is usually the first-line therapy. These medications are administered at high doses for 3 weeks for induction therapy and then at maintenance doses afterward to prevent relapse of retinitis. Intravitreal injections of ganciclovir, foscarnet, or cidofovir can be used to supplement treatment.

Epstein-Barr Virus

Epstein-Barr virus antibodies are found in over 90% of all adults. Childhood infections are usually asymptomatic, while EBV infection in young adults results in infectious mononucleosis. Lymphoproliferative disorders may develop in transplant recipients taking cyclosporine and in patients with AIDS. EBV is epidemiologically associated with Burkitt lymphoma, Hodgkin lymphoma, non-Hodgkin lymphoma, and nasopharyngeal carcinoma, and has also been reported in EBV-associated hemophagocytic lymphohistiocytosis (EBV-HLH), also known as *EBV-associated hemophagocytic syndrome.* This disease develops mostly in children and young adults and may be fatal. EBV has also been reported as a cause of pediatric acute renal failure. A highly sensitive PCR assay is available for detecting primary EBV infection and infectious mononucleosis.

Treatment of acute disease is largely supportive, although the EBV DNA polymerase is sensitive to acyclovir and ganciclovir, which decrease viral replication in tissue culture. No vaccine is currently available against EBV, but research is ongoing; it is estimated that an EBV vaccine could prevent 2% of cancers worldwide.

Young LS, Yap LF, Murray PG. Epstein-Barr virus: more than 50 years old and still providing surprises. *Nat Rev Cancer.* 2016;16(12):789–802.

Influenza

See Chapter 12 in this volume for a discussion of influenza and immunization.

Hepatitis

Hepatitis A and B

See Chapter 12 for discussion of hepatitis A and B and immunization.

Hepatitis C and Other Forms of Hepatitis

Approximately 20%–40% of acute viral hepatitis cases reported in the United States are of the non-A, non-B type; of this group, most cases are caused by the hepatitis C virus (HCV). The prevalence of chronic HCV infection in the United States is 3.5 million individuals; the worldwide prevalence is approximately 71 million individuals. Risk factors for the transmission of HCV include parenteral drug use, hemodialysis, occupational exposure to HCV-infected blood, blood transfusion or organ transplant prior to 1992, receiving clotting factor concentrates prior to 1987, and incarceration. Persons born between 1945 and 1965 have the highest incidence of hepatitis C infection. Although the role of sexual activity in the transmission of HCV remains to be fully elucidated, this mode is not a predominant source of transmission.

Of all the hepatitis viruses, HCV causes the most damage in immunocompetent hosts because of direct hepatocyte cytotoxicity. It may cause cirrhosis, fulminant hepatitis, and hepatocellular carcinoma. At present, hepatitis C is the most common cause of liver cancer and the most common indication for liver transplantation in the United States.

A sensitive enzyme immunoassay has been developed for the detection and quantification of total HCV core antigen in anti-HCV-positive or anti-HCV-negative sera. In addition, a 1-step PCR assay is available to detect HCV RNA and provide HCV genotyping.

Treatment of acute HCV infection with interferon-α_{2a} reduces the rate of acute infections converting to chronic HCV infections. Spontaneous resolution of acute HCV infection may occur in up to 50% of patients. Ledipasvir/sofosbuvir has demonstrated a 94%–99% sustained virologic response in patients with or without prior treatment, with or without cirrhosis, and with prior liver transplant.

Other hepatitis viruses include:

- *Hepatitis D:* causes chronic delta hepatitis, a severe form of chronic liver disease. Interferon-α_{2a} and lamivudine have been found to be beneficial in treating chronic hepatitis D infection.
- *Hepatitis E:* causes sporadic as well as epidemic acute viral hepatitis and is prevalent in many developing countries. In patients with preexisting chronic liver disease, acute hepatitis E infection has a protracted course, with high morbidity and mortality.
- *Hepatitis G:* often occurs as a coinfection with hepatitis B virus or HCV, but it usually does not increase their pathogenicity.
- *Transfusion-transmitted virus (TTV):* identified in a small percentage of patients with posttransfusion hepatitis. TTV has been implicated as a potential cause of 30%–50% of cases of lymphoma and Hodgkin disease.

American Association for the Study of Liver Diseases; Infectious Diseases Society of America (AASLD-IDSA). Recommendations for testing, managing, and treating hepatitis C. www.hcvguidelines.org. Accessed September 10, 2021.

European Association for the Study of the Liver. EASL Recommendations on treatment of hepatitis C 2016. *J Hepatol.* 2017;66(1):153–194.

Human Papillomavirus

Human papillomavirus (HPV) infection is highly prevalent and is closely associated with condylomata (genital warts), cervical intraepithelial neoplasia, cervical cancer (>99% of all cervical cancers are positive for HPV), conjunctival intraepithelial neoplasia, and some cases of head and neck squamous cell carcinoma. HPV has a possible etiologic role in some cases of lung adenocarcinoma as well. More than 50% of all persons are infected with HPV during their lifetimes, via either intrauterine or sexually transmitted infection. HPV can be detected with PCR assay techniques, and women at high risk for HPV should receive HPV testing at the time of the Papanicolaou (Pap) test. Please see Chapter 12 for further discussion of HPV vaccination and cervical cancer.

Harper DM, DeMars LR. HPV vaccines—A review of the first decade. *Gynecol Oncol.* 2017; 146(1):196–204.

Ebola Virus

Ebola virus disease (EVD) was first discovered in 1976 when cases of hemorrhagic fever occurred near the Ebola River in the Democratic Republic of Congo. The West Africa Ebola outbreak of 2013–2016 involved over 28,000 reported cases and over 11,000 recorded deaths, mainly in the countries of Guinea, Liberia, and Sierra Leone. The Ebola virus is believed to be transmitted by fruit bats and affects humans and nonhuman primates. Of the 5 known viruses belonging to the *Ebolavirus* genus, 4 are known to cause disease in humans, and all are members of the Filoviridae family of single-stranded RNA viruses.

The Ebola virus can be contracted through contact with the blood, body fluid, or tissue of infected bats, primates, or humans. The virus can penetrate broken skin or mucous membranes, and infection can occur when touching infected blood, body fluids, or contaminated objects. Early symptoms of infection appear 2–21 days after exposure to the virus and include fever, chills, muscle aches, headache, and weakness. Hemorrhagic conjunctivitis is a known presentation of infection. Later symptoms include rash, nausea, emesis, diarrhea, bruising, and bleeding, with eventual multisystem organ failure and death.

Infection of blood or body fluids can be confirmed by PCR, ELISA, or *Ebolavirus* immunoglobulin testing.

Post-Ebola virus syndrome in patients who have recovered from EVD includes joint, muscle, and chest pain, neurological problems, and ocular complications.

Ophthalmic considerations The most common ocular manifestation of Ebola virus disease (EVD) is uveitis, which may lead to impaired vision or loss of vision. Other known sequelae include cataract, retinal scarring, optic neuropathy, hypotony, and phthisis bulbi. The CDC recommends taking the highest-level precautions when treating patients with EVD. Ophthalmologists working in endemic areas should suspect Ebola virus infection when encountering patients with hemorrhagic conjunctivitis. The ophthalmologist treating patients with EVD or post-Ebola virus syndrome should assume the virus remains active in the eye for months following the initial infection and should consult the CDC for the most current guidelines.

Shantha JG, Crozier I, Yeh S. An update on ocular complications of Ebola virus disease. *Curr Opin Ophthalmol.* 2017;28(6):600–606.

Van Gelder RN, Margolis TP. Ebola and the ophthalmologist. *Ophthalmology.* 2015;122(11):2152–2154.

Varkey JB, Shantha JG, Crozier I, et al. Persistence of Ebola virus in ocular fluid during convalescence. *N Engl J Med.* 2015;372(25):2423–2427.

Zika Virus

The Zika virus (ZIKV) was first isolated in 1947 from a rhesus macaque monkey from the Zika forest in Uganda. It is a single-stranded RNA virus belonging to the virus family Flaviviridae and the genus *Flavivirus*, and is related to the dengue, yellow fever, chikungunya, and West Nile viruses. Its vector of transmission is the female *Aedes aegypti* mosquito. Transmission between humans can occur through sexual intercourse; blood transfusion; and mother-to-child vertical transmission via pregnancy, delivery, or breast milk.

The first evidence of human infection was discovered in Uganda in 1952. Few cases were identified until an outbreak in Yap, Micronesia, in 2007. Subsequently, the virus was documented in the Americas via the Pacific Islands when an outbreak occurred in Brazil in 2015. Since then, over 1.5 million individuals have been infected with ZIKV in Brazil.

The symptoms of Zika virus infection in adults are mild and self-limited; many individuals infected with ZIKV are asymptomatic. Symptoms include nonspecific fever, joint and muscle pain, conjunctivitis, and rash.

In northeastern Brazil, a sharp rise in the number of infants born with microcephaly (head circumference < 32 cm) occurred 6 months after the onset of the Zika outbreak. The Zika virus is identified via PCR and serologic testing, which was not readily available in parts of Brazil. Therefore, the association between ZIKV and microcephaly was presumptive. In 2015, 29 infants with microcephaly and a presumed diagnosis of congenital ZIKV infection underwent ophthalmologic examination. The most common vision-threatening ocular abnormalities identified were focal pigment mottling of the retina, chorioretinal atrophy, optic nerve abnormalities, bilateral iris coloboma, and lens subluxation.

Since the 2015 Brazil outbreak, vector-borne transmission of ZIKV infection has been reported in 84 countries, territories, or subnational areas. Recently, the term congenital Zika syndrome (CZS) was coined to describe the devastating ophthalmological, neurological, skeletal, and audiological effects the virus exacts on the developing fetus. The most common ocular findings in infants with CZS are chorioretinal atrophy and pigment mottling in the macula similar to that seen in eyes with toxoplasmosis. Zika virus vaccines are currently in development; it remains unknown whether an approved vaccine will protect against CZS. Therefore, when examining microcephalic infants in affected areas, ophthalmologists should be aware of the ocular manifestations of suspected congenital ZIKV infection.

de Paula Freitas, B, de Oliveira Dias JR, Prazeras J, et al. Ocular findings in infants with microcephaly associated with presumed Zika virus congenital infection in Salvador, Brazil. *JAMA Ophthalmol.* 2016;134(5):529–535.
Marquezan MC, Ventura CV, Sheffield JS, et al. Ocular effects of Zika virus—a review. *Surv Ophthalmol.* 2018;63(2):166–173.

Human Immunodeficiency Virus

In June 1981, the CDC's Morbidity and Mortality Weekly Report highlighted 5 homosexual men in Los Angeles, California, who had biopsy-confirmed *Pneumocystis jirovecii* (formerly called *Pneumocystis carinii*) pneumonia. In 1982, the CDC used the term AIDS for the first time and released the first case definition; by the next year the major routes of transmission for AIDS were identified. In 1983, HIV, a newly recognized retrovirus, was identified as the cause of AIDS.

HIV is a blood-borne virus and is transmitted via sexual intercourse, shared intravenous drug paraphernalia, blood transfusion, and from mother to child during birth or breastfeeding. Although HIV infection may be transmitted via blood or blood products, the risk of transmission by accidental needle-stick appears quite low (less than 0.5%).

The CDC estimated that as of the end of 2015, 1.1 million persons aged 13 years and older were living with HIV infection in the United States. The most affected population for new HIV diagnosis in the United States in 2016 was Black men who have sex with men. Worldwide, more than 70 million people have been infected with HIV, and 35 million people have died from HIV infection. At the end of 2016, 36.7 million people worldwide had HIV, with the majority in sub-Saharan Africa; 2.1 million of the infected individuals were children younger than 15 years of age.

Etiology and Pathogenesis

HIV belongs to a family of viruses known as *retroviruses*. A retrovirus encodes its genetic information in RNA and uses a unique viral enzyme named *reverse transcriptase* to copy its genome into DNA. HIV has 2 subtypes, HIV-1 and HIV-2. HIV-1 is further classified into several groups, including M, N, and O. Thus far, there are 9 known serotypes of HIV-1 group M, and 1 each of HIV-1 groups N and O. In the United States, HIV-1 group M, serotype B is the most common form of HIV. HIV-2, another human T-lymphotropic retrovirus, has been isolated in West African individuals and is closely related to simian immunodeficiency virus.

HIV preferentially infects T lymphocytes, especially helper T ($CD4^+$) lymphocytes. The virus infects mature T lymphocytes in vitro, although other cells can serve as targets. CD4 is the phenotypic marker for this subset and is identified by monoclonal antibodies OKT4 and Leu-3.

The hallmark of the immunodeficiency in AIDS is a depletion of the $CD4^+$ helper-inducer T lymphocytes. HIV selectively infects these lymphocytes as well as macrophages; with HIV replication, the helper T lymphocytes are killed. Because the helper T lymphocytes are central to the immune response, loss of this subset results in a profound immune deficiency, leading to the life-threatening opportunistic infections indicative of AIDS.

This selective depletion of $CD4^+$ helper T lymphocytes leads to the characteristic inverted $CD4^+/CD8^+$ ratio (also known as the *T4/T8 ratio*), where the ratio drops to less than 1.0, in comparison to the normal $CD4^+/CD8^+$ ratio, which is around 2. Years may pass between the initial HIV infection and the development of these immune abnormalities.

In addition to cellular immunodeficiency, patients with AIDS have abnormalities of B-lymphocyte function. These patients are unable to mount an antibody response to novel T lymphocyte–dependent B-lymphocyte challenges, although they have B-lymphocyte hyperfunction with polyclonal B-lymphocyte activation, hypergammaglobulinemia, and circulating immune complexes. This B-lymphocyte hyperfunction may be a direct consequence of HIV infection: studies have demonstrated that polyclonal activation can be induced in vitro by adding HIV to B lymphocytes.

HIV has also been documented to infect macrophages in the brains of patients with AIDS. It is thought that HIV infection of the brain is responsible for the HIV encephalopathy syndrome.

Clinical Syndromes

HIV infection has 3 phases: acute seroconversion, asymptomatic infection, and AIDS. In the acute seroconversion phase, viremia is high and the $CD4^+$ helper T lymphocyte cell count falls rapidly. Symptoms, including fever, rash, lymphadenopathy, and malaise, typically occur within 2 to 4 weeks after infection. The second phase of infection can be asymptomatic or present with persistent generalized lymphadenopathy. Viral replication occurs and the $CD4^+$ lymphocyte count steadily declines. This chronic or latent phase can last more than a decade. The final stage, AIDS, is defined by a $CD4^+$ lymphocyte count below 200 cells/microliter of blood or by development of opportunistic infections or malignancy.

Diagnosis

The CDC recommends that every individual between the ages of 13 and 64 be tested for HIV at least once, and that persons at high risk for HIV infection be screened at least annually. The American College of Physicians encourages testing of all persons. The US Preventive Services Task Force recommends screening for adolescents and adults at increased risk for HIV infection, and for all pregnant women.

Risk factors for exposure to HIV include unprotected sexual intercourse, large number of sexual partners, history of sexually transmitted infection, blood transfusion, needlestick injury, sharing of intravenous drug paraphernalia, mucosal contact with infected blood, and mother-to-child vertical transmission.

An ELISA test is used for screening. A positive immunoassay should be followed by confirmatory Western blot testing. A rapid detection combination antigen/antibody test is available. The $CD4^+$ lymphocyte count is used for classification and to monitor for opportunistic infection. The viral load in peripheral blood is used to guide therapy; the rate of progression to AIDS and death is related to viral load.

The workup of a patient with newly diagnosed HIV infection should include an ophthalmologic examination and testing for TB, CMV, syphilis, hepatitis A–C, *Toxoplasma*, chlamydia, and gonococcus.

Centers for Disease Control and Prevention (CDC). Detection of acute HIV infection in two evaluations of a new HIV diagnostic testing algorithm—United States, 2011–2013. *MMWR Morb Mortal Wkly Rep.* 2013;62(24):489–494.

Joyce MP, Kuhar D, Brooks JT. Notes from the field: occupationally acquired HIV infection among health care workers—United States, 1985–2013. *MMWR Morb Mortal Wkly Rep.* 2015;63(53):1245–1246.

Treatment

It is recommended that all patients with early HIV infection begin antiretroviral therapy (ART) as soon as possible; initiation of ART soon after the initial HIV infection may be associated with a greater chance of immune reconstitution to normal or near-normal $CD4^+$ lymphocyte levels. The goals of ART include durable suppression of HIV viral load to less than 50 copies/mL, restoration of immune function (as indicated by the $CD4^+$ lymphocyte count), prevention of HIV transmission, prevention of drug resistance, and improvement in quality of life. ART regimens for treatment-naive patients are composed of a "base" medication and a "backbone" regimen. The base is either an integrase strand transfer inhibitor, a nonnucleoside reverse transcriptase inhibitor (NNRTI), or a protease inhibitor (PI). The backbone typically consists of 2 nucleoside reverse transcriptase inhibitors (NRTIs). Treatment is based on adverse-effect profiles, comorbidities, potential drug interactions, results of drug resistance testing, virologic efficacy, allergy history, pregnancy status, pill burden, and dosing frequency.

ART has been shown to dramatically reduce the HIV viral load, increase $CD4^+$ lymphocyte counts, delay disease progression, reduce the number of opportunistic infections, decrease the number of hospital admissions, and prolong survival. Some statistics show up to an 82% decline in the number of opportunistic infections in patients on ART. These advantages translate into improved survival and enhanced quality of life for HIV-infected patients.

A small percentage of the population appears to be naturally immune to HIV infection. These persons have defective genes for CCR5, a surface receptor that HIV requires to attach to T lymphocytes. Also, approximately 50% of long-term survivors of HIV infection are heterozygous for the CCR5 defect. This finding has led to speculation concerning the possibilities for genetic therapy, in which anti-HIV genes could be "injected" into a patient's chromosomes with a harmless viral vector.

Pre-exposure prophylaxis (PrEP) with tenofovir-emtricitabine can be considered in high-risk individuals. When taken consistently, and when used in combination with condoms and other preventive methods, PrEP can reduce the risk of HIV infection in high-risk patients. For post-exposure prophylaxis (PEP), ART is taken within 72 hours after possible exposure to HIV. Efforts continue to develop a safe and effective HIV vaccine.

Günthard HF, Saag MS, Benson CA, et al. Antiretroviral drugs for treatment and prevention of HIV infection in adults: 2016 Recommendations of the International Antiviral Society—USA panel. *JAMA.* 2016; 316(2):191–210.

World Health Organization. *Consolidated Guidelines on the Use of Antiretroviral Drugs for Treating and Preventing HIV Infection: Recommendations for a Public Health Approach.* 2nd ed. Geneva, Switzerland: World Health Organization; 2016.

Immune Reconstitution Inflammatory Syndrome

Some patients starting ART develop new or worsening opportunistic infections or malignancies despite improvements in the clinical markers of HIV infection. These examples of paradoxical clinical worsening, known as immune reconstitution inflammatory syndrome (IRIS), occur in patients with previous opportunistic infections or low $CD4^+$ T-lymphocyte levels. IRIS results from an inflammatory response to reemergence of the immune system's ability to recognize pathogens or from tumor antigens that were previously present but asymptomatic. With the increased availability of ART, more cases and more new forms of IRIS are likely to be recognized. Immune recovery uveitis (IRU) occurs in nearly 10% of HIV-infected patients with immune recovery and a history of CMV retinitis. Of these IRU patients, 46% develop significant cystoid macular edema and 49% develop epiretinal membrane.

Ophthalmic considerations The ocular manifestations of HIV infection and AIDS are discussed in BCSC Section 9, *Uveitis and Ocular Inflammation.* HIV has been found in tears, conjunctival epithelial cells, corneal epithelial cells, aqueous humor, and the retina, including retinal vascular endothelium. Although transmission of HIV infection via ophthalmic examinations or ophthalmic equipment has not been documented, several precautions are recommended for clinicians.

Health care professionals performing eye examinations or other procedures involving contact with tears should wash their hands immediately after the procedure and between patients. The use of gloves is advisable when the hands have cuts, scratches, or dermatologic lesions.

Any instrument that comes into direct contact with external surfaces of the eyes should be wiped clean and disinfected by a 5- to 10-minute exposure to one of the following:

- a fresh solution of 3% hydrogen peroxide
- a fresh solution containing 5000 parts per million (ppm) free available chlorine—a one-tenth dilution of common household bleach (sodium hypochlorite)
- 70% ethanol
- 70% isopropanol

The device should be thoroughly rinsed in tap water after disinfection and dried before use.

Diluted bleach provides effective disinfection of tonometer tips to prevent the transmission of HSV, adenovirus, and severe acute respiratory syndrome coronavirus 2 (SARS-CoV-2) and is recommended by the CDC and most tonometer manufacturers.

Contact lenses used in trial fittings should be disinfected between fittings with a commercially available hydrogen peroxide contact lens–disinfecting system or with the standard heat disinfection regimen (78°–80°C for 10 minutes). The demonstration of HIV in corneal epithelium has led to the recommendation that all corneal donors be screened for antibodies to HIV and that all potential donor corneas from HIV antibody–positive persons be discarded.

For more specific recommendations, see the American Academy of Ophthalmology's Clinical Statement, "Infection Prevention in Eye Care Services and Operating Areas and Operating Rooms—2012," available at www.aao.org/clinical-statement/infection-prevention-in-eye-care-services-operatin.

Centers for Disease Control and Prevention website; www.cdc.gov.
European Centre for Disease Prevention and Control website; www.ecdc.europa.eu/en.
Junk AK, Chen PP, Lin SC, et al. Disinfection of tonometers: a report by the American Academy of Ophthalmology. *Ophthalmology.* 2017;124(12):1867–1875.

Update on Antibiotics

For more than 60 years, the main trends in the management of infectious diseases have been the evolution and refinement of antibiotic therapy. Factors that have stimulated the development of new antibiotics include the continuous emergence of resistant bacteria, economics, and the desire to eliminate adverse effects. During the past 25 years, emphasis has gradually shifted from aminoglycosides to β-lactams and the development of new classes of antibiotics such as carbapenems and monobactams. In addition, vancomycin, TMP-SMX, erythromycin, and rifampin have enjoyed a resurgence in popularity and new applications. Quinolones offer the possibility of treating serious infections on an outpatient basis.

Antibacterial Agents

Antibacterial agents can be separated into groups according to their specific targets on or within bacteria:

- β-Lactams and glycopeptides inhibit cell-wall synthesis.
- Polymyxins distort cytoplasmic membrane function.
- Quinolones and rifampicins inhibit nucleic acid synthesis.
- Macrolides, aminoglycosides, and tetracyclines inhibit ribosome function.
- Trimethoprim and sulfonamides inhibit folate metabolism.

All antibiotics facilitate the growth of resistant bacteria consequent to the destruction of susceptible bacteria. Although the wide use of antimicrobial agents for veterinary and agricultural purposes has contributed to the emergence of multiresistant microorganisms, the excessive use of antibiotics, especially in hospitals, has been the most significant catalyst for resistance. Bacteria resist antibiotics by inactivation of the antibiotic, decreased accumulation of the antibiotic within the microorganism, or alteration of the target site on the microbe. For example, resistance to penicillins and cephalosporins is initiated by β-lactamase enzymes that hydrolyze the β-lactam ring, thus destroying the antibiotic's effectiveness. Resistance can be mediated by chromosomal mutations or by the presence of extrachromosomal DNA, also known as *plasmid resistance.* Plasmid resistance is important from an epidemiologic point of view because it is transmissible and usually highly stable, confers resistance to many different classes of antibiotics simultaneously, and is often associated with other characteristics that enable a microorganism to colonize and invade a susceptible host.

Resistance-conferring plasmids have been identified in virtually all bacteria. Plasmids can pick up chromosomal genes for resistance and transfer them to species that are not currently resistant. Bacteria that have acquired chromosomal and plasmid-mediated resistance can neutralize or destroy antibiotics in 3 different ways (they can use 1 or more of these mechanisms simultaneously):

- by preventing the antibacterial agent from reaching its receptor site
- by modifying or duplicating the target enzyme so that it is insensitive to the antibacterial agent
- by synthesizing enzymes that destroy the antibacterial agent or modify the agent to alter its entry or receptor binding

Antimicrobial susceptibility testing permits a rational choice of antibiotics, although correlation of in vivo and in vitro susceptibility is not always precise. Disk-diffusion susceptibility testing has provided qualitative data about the inhibitory activity of commonly used antimicrobials against an isolated pathogen, and these data are usually sufficient. For serious infections, it is useful to quantify the drug concentrations that inhibit and kill the pathogen. The lowest drug concentration that prevents the growth of a defined inoculum of the isolated pathogen is the *minimal inhibitory concentration (MIC)*; the lowest concentration that kills 99.9% of an inoculum is the *minimal lethal concentration (MLC)*. For bactericidal drugs, the MIC and MLC are usually similar.

β-Lactam antibiotics

The β-lactam group includes the penicillins, cephalosporins, and monobactams, all of which possess a β-lactam ring that binds to specific microbial binding sites and interferes with cell-wall synthesis. Although the carbapenems and carbacephems are often grouped with β-lactams, they have a slightly different ring structure. Most new agents have been created by side-chain manipulation of the β-lactam ring, which has improved resistance to enzymatic degradation. However, some of the newer antibiotics (such as third-generation cephalosporins) show diminished potency against gram-positive cocci, especially staphylococci.

Penicillins The first *natural penicillins,* types G and V, were degraded by the enzyme penicillinase. The *penicillinase-resistant penicillins,* such as methicillin, nafcillin, oxacillin, and cloxacillin, were developed for treating resistant *Staphylococcus* species and were effective except against strains of methicillin-resistant *S epidermidis.* The next generation of penicillins included the *aminopenicillins,* ampicillin and amoxicillin, which were created by placing an amino group on the acyl side chain of the penicillin nucleus. This change broadened their effectiveness to include activity against *H influenzae, Escherichia coli,* and *Proteus mirabilis.* The next advance was development of the *carboxypenicillins,* carbenicillin and ticarcillin, which are active against aerobic gram-negative rods such as *P aeruginosa,*

Enterobacter species, and indole-positive strains of *Proteus.* The fourth-generation penicillins, known as *acyl ureidopenicillins,* include azlocillin, mezlocillin, and piperacillin. Because of the possibility of emergence of resistance, the newer penicillins are usually administered in combination with an aminoglycoside.

Allergic reactions are the chief adverse effects encountered in using the penicillins. Among antimicrobial agents, the penicillins are the leading cause of allergy; symptoms range from mild rashes to anaphylaxis.

Cephalosporins The cephalosporins also belong to the β-lactam group of antibiotics, and cross-allergenicity may occur in 3%–5% of patients with penicillin allergies. The cephalosporins and their characteristics are outlined in Table 14-2.

Polenakovik HM, Pleiman CM. Ceftaroline for methicillin-resistant *Staphylococcus aureus* bacteraemia: case series and review of the literature. *Int J Antimicrob Agents.* 2013;42(5):450–455.

Yang, MS, Kang DY, Seo B et al; Drug Allergy Work Group of KAAACI. Incidence of cephalosporin-induced anaphylaxis and clinical efficacy of screening intradermal tests with cephalosporins: a large multicenter retrospective cohort study. *Allergy.* 2018;73(9):1833–1841.

Monobactams *Monobactams* are a monocyclic class of antibiotics that use only the β-lactam ring as their core structure. *Aztreonam,* the first approved monobactam antibiotic, has an

Table 14-2 Cephalosporins

Drugs	Characteristics/Comments
First generation (eg, cefazolin, cephalexin)	Active against β-lactamase gram-positive cocci and gram-negative bacilli Usually ineffective against *Bacillus, Pseudomonas, Enterobacter,* and methicillin-resistant *Staphylococcus aureus* (MRSA) Do not cross the blood–brain barrier well
Second generation (eg, cefamandole, cefoxitin, cefaclor, cefuroxime)	Expanded coverage against gram-negative bacilli and *Haemophilus*
Third generation (eg, cefotaxime, ceftriaxone, ceftazidime)	More effective against gram-negative bacilli Less effective against gram-positive cocci (eg, staphylococci) and Enterobacteriaceae Cross blood–brain barrier, more effective for treatment of meningitis Ceftriaxone effective against Lyme disease, gonorrhea; represents the best all-purpose drug of the third-generation cephalosporins
Fourth generation (eg, cefepime, cefpirome)	Good coverage against most gram-negative and gram-positive organisms and anaerobes Expensive
Fifth generation (eg, ceftaroline, ceftobiprole, ceftolozone)	Ceftobiprole effective against pseudomonas Ceftolozone used for treatment of complicated intra-abdominal infections or complicated urinary tract infections

excellent safety profile and good success rate in the treatment of infections caused by aerobic gram-negative bacilli, but has poor activity against gram-positive and anaerobic organisms. Aztreonam has the spectrum of an aminoglycoside antibiotic without the ototoxicity or nephrotoxicity.

Carbapenems *Carbapenems* are a class of antibiotics with a basic ring structure similar to that of penicillins. The antibacterial spectrum of the carbapenems is broader than that of any other existing antibiotic and includes *S aureus, Enterobacter* species, and *P aeruginosa,* although carbapenem resistance is an ongoing global public health problem. Carbapenems produce a postantibiotic killing effect against some organisms, with a delay in regrowth of damaged organisms similar to that observed with aminoglycosides.

Imipenem/cilastatin combines a carbapenem, *imipenem,* with an inhibitor of renal dehydropeptidase, *cilastatin.* Cilastatin has no antimicrobial activity and is present solely to prevent degradation of imipenem by dehydropeptidase. Imipenem/cilastatin is an appropriate compound for monotherapy for mixed infections. Up to 50% of patients who are allergic to penicillin are also allergic to imipenem.

Meropenem, biapenem, panipenem, ertapenem, faropenem, tomopenem, and *ritipenem* are newer penems that have increased stability against degradation by dehydropeptidases. *Doripenem* is a newer agent that appears to be most effective in treating carbapenem-resistant gram-negative bacilli and penicillin-resistant streptococci.

Loracarbef is an oral carbacephem, a type of antibiotic that is structurally similar to cephalosporins but possesses a broader spectrum due to higher stability against both plasmid and chromosomally mediated β-lactamases. Loracarbef provides good coverage for most gram-positive and gram-negative aerobic bacteria.

Clavulanic acid, sulbactam, and *tazobactam* are β-lactam molecules that possess little intrinsic antibacterial activity but are potent inhibitors of many plasmid-mediated class A β-lactamases. Currently, there are 4 combinations of β-lactam antibiotics plus β-lactamase inhibitors available in the United States: *Augmentin* (oral amoxicillin and clavulanic acid), *Timentin* (intravenous ticarcillin and clavulanic acid), *Unasyn* (intravenous ampicillin and sulbactam), and *Zosyn* (intravenous piperacillin and tazobactam). These drugs have excellent activity against β-lactamase–producing gram-positive and gram-negative bacteria as well as many anaerobes.

El-Gamal MI, Brahim I, Hisham N, Aladdin R, Mohammed H, Bahaaeldin A. Recent updates of carbapenem antibiotics. *Eur J Med Chem.* 2017;131:185–195.

Meletis, G. Carbapenem resistance: overview of the problem and future perspectives. *Ther Adv Infect Dis.* 2016;3(1):15–21.

Glycopeptides

Vancomycin has regained popularity because of the emergence of methicillin-resistant staphylococci and the recognition that *C difficile* is a cause of pseudomembranous colitis. This drug has excellent activity against *Clostridium* and against most gram-positive bacteria, including methicillin-resistant staphylococci, *Corynebacterium* species, and other diphtheroids. Vancomycin has been used alone to treat serious infections caused by methicillin-resistant staphylococci.

Vancomycin-resistant enterococcal infections have recently become more common. The CDC has issued recommendations regarding appropriate use of vancomycin to help counteract the problem of bacterial drug resistance.

Teicoplanin has several advantages over vancomycin, including longer half-life, lower nephrotoxicity, and no requirement for monitoring drug levels. Teicoplanin is effective for treatment of staphylococcal infections, including endocarditis, bacteremia, osteomyelitis, and septic arthritis. Teicoplanin may be preferable to vancomycin for surgical prophylaxis because of its excellent tissue penetration, lower toxicity, and long half-life, allowing single-dose administration in several surgical procedures. The antibacterial activity of teicoplanin is similar to that of vancomycin but with increased potency, particularly against *Streptococcus* and *Enterococcus.* Teicoplanin is active against many vancomycin-resistant organisms. The newer agents oritavancin and dalbavancin are also highly active against vancomycin-resistant infections.

Smith JR, Barber KE, Raut A, Aboutaleb M, Sakoulas G, Rybak MJ. β-lactam combinations with daptomycin provide synergy against vancomycin-resistant *Enterococcus faecalis* and *Enterococcus faecium. J Antimicrob Chemother.* 2015;70(6):1738–1743.

Yim J, Smith JR, Rybak MJ. Role of combination antimicrobial therapy for vancomycin-resistant *Enterococcus faecium* infections: review of the current evidence. *Pharmacotherapy.* 2017;37(5):579–592.

Quinolones

The introduction of a fluorine into the basic quinolone nucleus of nalidixic acid has produced compounds known as *fluoroquinolones,* which have excellent activity against gram-positive bacteria. The subsequent addition of piperazine produced compounds such as norfloxacin and ciprofloxacin, which have a broad spectrum of activity, encompassing staphylococci and most of the significant gram-negative bacilli, including *Pseudomonas.* Ciprofloxacin is available in both oral and parenteral forms and can be used to treat urinary tract infections, gonorrhea, and diarrheal diseases, as well as respiratory, skin, and bone infections. Other fluoroquinolones in the US market include ofloxacin, temafloxacin, lomefloxacin, enoxacin, levofloxacin, moxifloxacin, gemifloxacin, and besifloxacin.

The newer fluoroquinolones possess even greater activity against gram-positive and gram-negative bacteria. Either moxifloxacin or levofloxacin appears to be a good treatment choice for pneumococcal infections that are resistant to penicillin and the macrolides. Oral quinolones are an alternative form of therapy to β-lactams and aminoglycosides and have allowed physicians to treat more patients outside the hospital setting. Reported adverse effects include tendon rupture (especially in elderly patients), retinal detachment, and peripheral neuropathy. Of the quinolones, moxifloxacin carries the highest risk of dysglycemia.

Douros A, Grabowski K, Stahlmann R. Safety issues and drug-drug interactions with commonly used quinolones. *Expert Opin Drug Metab Toxicol.* 2015;11(1):25–39.

Macrolides

The macrolide *erythromycin* is often employed for the initial treatment of community-acquired pneumonia. This agent is effective against infections caused by pneumococci, group A streptococci, *M pneumoniae, Chlamydia,* and *Legionella.* Erythromycin is used to treat upper respiratory tract infections and sexually transmitted infections in patients who are allergic to penicillin.

Clarithromycin and *azithromycin* are macrolide antibiotics that are chemically related to erythromycin. Both are well-tolerated alternatives to erythromycin and may offer advantages in treating gonococcal and chlamydial infections and in treating *Mycobacterium avium* and other recalcitrant infections associated with AIDS and HIV infection. Clarithromycin and ethambutol are used to treat Mycobacterium avium-intracellulare complex (MAC) in an HIV-infected patient, and prophylactic therapy with azithromycin, clarithromycin, rifabutin, or combined therapy may help prevent disseminated MAC in AIDS patients. Azithromycin is subclassified as an *azalide,* and it causes far fewer drug interactions than erythromycin. There is increasing cross-resistance among the macrolides.

Clindamycin has a gram-positive spectrum similar to that of erythromycin and is also active against most anaerobes, including *Bacteroides fragilis.* Except for treating anaerobic infection, clindamycin is rarely the drug of choice, although it is well absorbed orally, and parenteral formulations are available. Its major adverse effect is diarrhea, which may progress to pseudomembranous enterocolitis in some patients. Macrolides, especially azithromycin, can increase the risk of cardiac arrhythmias.

Afghani T, Mansoor H, Nadeem M. Preventing long-term ocular complications of trachoma with topical azithromycin: a 3-year follow-up study. *Asia Pac J Ophthalmol (Phila).* 2017;6(1):8–12.

Aminoglycosides

The aminoglycoside antibiotics inhibit protein synthesis by binding to bacterial ribosomes. Gentamicin, tobramycin, amikacin, kanamycin, streptomycin, and netilmicin possess similar activity, pharmacology, and toxicity. Because of poor gastrointestinal absorption, parenteral administration is necessary to produce therapeutic levels.

Aminoglycosides are used to treat serious infections caused by gram-negative bacilli. They do not cross the blood–brain barrier. Aminoglycosides are not used for most gram-positive infections because the β-lactams are less toxic.

The major adverse effects of the aminoglycosides are nephrotoxicity and ototoxicity. Blood urea nitrogen, creatinine, and aminoglycoside peak and trough serum levels should be monitored, especially in patients with known renal disease. Combined administration of a loop diuretic such as furosemide with aminoglycosides has a synergistic ototoxic effect, potentially leading to permanent loss of cochlear function. Penicillins may decrease the antimicrobial effectiveness of parenteral aminoglycosides, particularly in patients with impaired renal function.

Poulikakos P, Falagas ME. Aminoglycoside therapy in infectious diseases. *Expert Opin Pharmacother.* 2013;14(12):1585–1597.

Tetracyclines

The tetracyclines are bacteriostatic agents that reversibly inhibit ribosomal protein synthesis. Although they are active against a wide range of organisms (including *Staphylococcus, Rickettsia, Chlamydia, Nocardia,* and *Actinomyces*), resistance is widespread, especially among *S aureus* and gram-negative bacilli. The principal clinical uses of tetracyclines are in the treatment of nongonococcal urethritis, Rocky Mountain spotted fever, chronic bronchitis, and sebaceous disorders such as acne rosacea. In addition, tetracyclines are an alternative for the penicillin-allergic patient with syphilis. Tetracyclines are well absorbed when taken on an empty stomach; however, their absorption is decreased when taken with milk, antacids, calcium, or iron. Tetracyclines are distributed throughout the extracellular fluid, but cerebrospinal fluid penetration is unreliable. Adverse effects include oral or vaginal candidiasis with prolonged use, gastrointestinal upset, photosensitivity, elevation of the blood urea nitrogen level, and idiopathic intracranial hypertension. Tetracyclines can prolong the international normalized ratio (INR) in patients taking warfarin, and they should not be administered to pregnant women or to children younger than 10 years because of the potential for harm to developing bone and teeth.

Grossman TH. Tetracycline antibiotics and resistance. *Cold Spring Harb Perspect Med.* 2016;6(4):a025387.

Miscellaneous antibacterial agents

Rifampin was originally developed as an anti-TB agent, but it is also used to treat several intractable bacterial infections. The drug is usually employed adjunctively because bacteria develop resistance to the drug when it is used as a single agent. It is effective in eradicating the carrier state of nasal *S aureus.* The drug is also effective prophylactically against *Neisseria meningitidis* and may be useful for treating oropharyngeal carriers of *H influenzae* type b.

Another oral antibiotic with potential for treating deep-seated infections is TMP-SMX. After a single oral dose, the mean serum levels of TMP-SMX are approximately 75% of the concentration that would be achieved via intravenous administration. In addition to its excellent pharmacokinetics, TMP-SMX has an extremely broad spectrum of activity, including effectiveness against Enterobacteriaceae and some organisms that are resistant to cephalosporins. Although there is a misconception that TMP-SMX has limited activity against gram-positive bacteria, in fact, most streptococci, staphylococci, and *Listeria monocytogenes* are susceptible to it. Beyond the broad-spectrum effect of TMP-SMX, the concomitant use of metronidazole creates an antibiotic combination with activity against microorganisms that surpasses that of a third-generation cephalosporin. TMP-SMX has been increasingly used in the treatment and prophylaxis of *Pneumocystis* infection and toxoplasmosis.

Chloramphenicol is a bacteriostatic agent that reversibly inhibits ribosomal protein synthesis. This drug is active against a wide variety of gram-negative and gram-positive organisms, including anaerobes. The major concern with this agent is hematopoietic toxicity, including reversible bone marrow suppression and irreversible aplasia. Aplastic anemia is an idiosyncratic late reaction to the drug and is usually fatal. Other adverse effects include hemolysis, allergy, and peripheral neuritis.

Future Directions

The World Health Organization (WHO) recently released a list that prioritizes antibiotic-resistant pathogens in order to guide research and development of new antimicrobial agents. The WHO's review determined that the antibiotics currently under development are insufficient to mitigate the threat of antibiotic resistance.

The WHO assigned the highest global priority for research and development of treatment of tuberculosis. The critical priority pathogens are carbapenem-resistant *Acinetobacter baumannii, P aeruginosa,* and Enterobacteriaceae. The high-priority pathogens include *Enterococcus faecium, S Aureus, Helicobacter pylori, Campylobacter, Salmonella,* and *Neisseria gonorrhoeae.* Medium priority has been assigned *to S pneumoniae, H influenzae,* and *Shigella. Clostridium difficile* was not listed as a priority pathogen, because the infection is addressed with infection prevention, control, and stewardship measures.

Pharmacologic research has provided entirely new classes of antibiotics that offer additional treatment options for emerging resistant bacterial strains. Most of these newer drugs are targeted against resistant strains of gram-positive bacteria.

World Health Organization (WHO). *Antibacterial Agents in Clinical Development: An Analysis of the Antibacterial Clinical Development Pipeline, Including Tuberculosis.* https://www.who.int/medicines/news/2017/IAU_AntibacterialAgentsClinicalDevelopment_webfinal_2017_09_19.pdf. Published September 2017. Accessed October 10, 2021.

Antifungal Agents

Imidazoles and triazoles function by inhibiting fungal cytochrome P-450–dependent enzymes, thereby blocking synthesis of the fungal cell membrane. The triazoles (fluconazole, itraconazole) offer a less-toxic alternative to amphotericin B for the treatment of cryptococcal meningitis and other invasive fungal diseases, and they may also play a role in the long-term suppression of *Cryptococcus* after remission of acute infection in severely immunocompromised patients. Ketoconazole is often less effective than the newer triazoles and carries a higher risk of hepatotoxicity. Voriconazole, a second-generation triazole, is available in both intravenous and oral formulations. It offers a better treatment option for invasive aspergillosis and other serious fungal infections. For more on antifungal agents, see Table 14-3.

Treatment of serious, deep-seated, systemic fungal infections may require the use of intravenous amphotericin B, sometimes in combination with either flucytosine or a triazole. Lipid complex and liposome-encapsulated formulations of amphotericin B are available to reduce the drug's toxicity. Nystatin, which is structurally similar to amphotericin B, is an antifungal agent administered topically, vaginally, or by mouth. *Terbinafine,* an allylamine oral antifungal agent, and *butenafine,* a benzylamine, are effective in controlling onychomycosis due to chronic dermatophyte infections.

Pappas PG, Kauffman CA, Andes DR, et al. Clinical practice guideline for the management of candidiasis: 2016 update by the Infectious Diseases Society of America. *Clin Infect Dis.* 2016;62(4):e1–50.

Zonios D, Yamazaki H, Murayama N, et al. Voriconazole metabolism, toxicity, and the effect of cytochrome P450 2C19 genotype. *J Infect Dis.* 2014;209(12):1941–1948.

Antiviral Agents

Acyclovir is a nucleoside analogue that is effective against HSV and VZV infections. It inhibits viral DNA replication. One phosphorylation step of acyclovir is catalyzed by the enzyme thymidine kinase. The virus-induced thymidine kinase is far more active than

Table 14-3 Antifungal Agents[a]

Class	Agents	Mechanism of Action	Spectrum
Echinocandins	Anidulafungin, caspofungin, micafungin	Damage cell wall by inhibiting synthesis of 1,3-β-D-glucan	Excellent against yeast, broad spectrum against molds
Fluorinated pyrimidine analog	Flucytosine	Inhibits fungal RNA and DNA synthesis	Use only in combination with other agents; relatively weak, rapid resistance
Imidazoles	Ketoconazole	Similar to triazoles	Fair against yeast, other azoles generally more effective
Polyenes	Amphotericin B, natamycin (pimaricin), nystatin	Bind to sterols and disrupt cell walls	Better against yeasts than molds, amphotericin B safer systemically in lipid formulation
Triazoles	Fluconazole, isavuconazole, itraconazole, posaconazole, voriconazole	Damage cell membrane through a cytochrome P-450–dependent enzyme	Fluconazole mostly effective against yeast: others are broad spectrum

[a] Not included in this table are butenafine and terbinafine. Terbinafine is an ergosterol synthesis inhibitor. Butenafine's exact mechanism of action has not been established.

the host cell thymidine kinase. Therefore, acyclovir is very active against viruses within infected host cells and yet is generally well tolerated.

Acyclovir has proved effective in treating a variety of herpetic infections. Oral acyclovir effectively treats acute severe genital herpes and can be used for long-term suppression in immunocompetent patients with frequently recurring genital herpes. Intravenous acyclovir is effective against herpes simplex encephalitis. Acyclovir in doses of 500 mg/M^2 every 8 hours has been used successfully in treating herpes zoster infections in immunocompromised patients.

Oral acyclovir may be used to treat herpes zoster ophthalmicus. Doses of 800 mg 5 times daily are usually effective in reducing the incidence of ocular complications of herpes zoster ophthalmicus. However, postherpetic neuralgia is not affected by this therapy. A randomized controlled study of acyclovir and oral corticosteroids demonstrated that the latter did not help to reduce the incidence of postherpetic neuralgia when added to oral acyclovir.

Famciclovir and *valacyclovir* are approved in the United States for the treatment of herpes zoster and herpes simplex infections, and studies have shown that they are effective against the latter. Both of these newer drugs allow less frequent dosing intervals (every 8–12 hours, depending on the indication). *Valganciclovir* is used for the prevention and treatment of CMV infections in patients who have undergone organ transplantation or who have AIDS, and it has also been found to be effective for treating acute retinal necrosis caused by VZV.

Adefovir is a nucleoside analogue and a potent inhibitor of many viruses, such as HIV, HSV, hepatitis B, HPV, and EBV. The nucleoside analogue *brivudine* appears to have a stronger antiviral effect against VZV than does acyclovir or penciclovir. The efficacy of brivudine has been documented in several clinical trials in patients with herpesvirus-related infections, particularly herpes zoster and herpes simplex infections.

Ganciclovir, foscarnet, and cidofovir are additional antiviral agents used for treating CMV infections, including retinitis. M2 protein inhibitors amantadine and rimantadine were used previously to treat influenza but are no longer recommended due to widespread resistance. Oseltamivir, peramivir, and zanamivir are oral neuraminidase inhibitors that are used to treat and prevent influenza.

Davies BE. Pharmacokinetics of oseltamivir: an oral antiviral for the treatment and prophylaxis of influenza in diverse populations. *J Antimicrob Chemother.* 2010;65(Suppl 2):ii5–ii10.

Dryden MS. Novel antibiotic treatment for skin and soft tissue infection. *Curr Opin Infect Dis.* 2014;27(2):116–124.

Fiore AE, Fry A, Shay D, et al; Centers for Disease Control and Prevention (CDC). Antiviral agents for the treatment and chemoprophylaxis of influenza—recommendations of the Advisory Council on Immunization Practices (ACIP). *MMWR Recomm Rep.* 2011;60(1):1–24.

Polenakovik HM, Pleiman CM. Ceftaroline for methicillin-resistant *Staphylococcus aureus* bacteraemia: case series and review of the literature. *Int J Antimicrob Agents.* 2013;42(5):450–455.

Rafailidis PI, Mavros MN, Kapaskelis A, Falagas ME. Antiviral treatment for severe EBV infections in apparently immunocompetent patients. *J Clin Virol.* 2010;49(3):151–157.

COVID-19

In December 2019, the WHO was notified of cases of atypical pneumonia of unknown etiology in Wuhan, China. In January 2020, the pathogen was identified by Chinese scientists as a novel coronavirus; in February 2020, the International Committee on Taxonomy of Viruses officially named the virus severe acute respiratory syndrome coronavirus 2 (SARS-CoV-2), which causes the disease coronavirus disease 2019 (COVID-19). An RNA virus, SARS-CoV-2 belongs to the *Betacoronavirus* genus and is of zoonotic origin. It is transmitted from human to human, primarily via respiratory droplets. The WHO declared COVID-19 a pandemic on March 11, 2020.

Common symptoms of COVID-19 infection include fever, cough, and shortness of breath. The known ocular manifestations of COVID-19 are follicular conjunctivitis with hyperemia, chemosis, light sensitivity, tearing, and discharge. Conjunctival swabs have yielded positive results for SARS-CoV-2 on reverse transcriptase–PCR testing. Therefore, the virus may be transmissible from contact with the ocular surface, tears, or fomites. Ophthalmologists should be aware of the possibility of conjunctivitis as a presenting sign of COVID-19 infection, and employ the use of eye protection, masks, and other personal protective equipment when examining patients who are potentially infectious. Additional information on COVID-19 and its impact on ophthalmic practice is available at www.aao.org/headline/alert-important-coronavirus-context.

Since December 2020, 3 vaccines to protect against COVID-19 infection have received emergency approval by the FDA: Pfizer-BioNTech COVID-19 Vaccine, Moderna COVID-19 Vaccine, and Johnson & Johnson/Janssen COVID-19 Vaccine. In August 2021, the FDA approved the Pfizer-BioNTech vaccine, now called Comirnaty, for the prevention of COVID-19 disease in individuals 16 years of age and older.

Cheema M, Aghazadeh H, Nazarali S, et al. Keratoconjunctivitis as the initial medical presentation of the novel coronavirus disease 2019 (COVID-19). *Can J Ophthalmol.* 2020;55(4):e125–e129.

Daruich A, Martin D, Bremond-Gignac D. Ocular manifestation as first sign of coronavirus disease 2019 (COVID-19): interest of telemedicine during the pandemic context. *J Fr Ophtalmol.* 2020;43(5):389–391.

Wu P, Duan F, Luo C, et al. Characteristics of ocular findings of patients with coronavirus disease 2019 (COVID-19) in Hubei Province, China. *JAMA Ophthalmol.* 2020;138(5):575–578.

CHAPTER 15

Perioperative Management in Ocular Surgery

Highlights

- Idarucizumab has been approved for reversal of the direct oral anticoagulant thrombin inhibitor dabigatran during emergency surgery.
- Perioperative prophylaxis with β-blockers in noncardiac surgery decreases the risk of acute myocardial infarction but may increase 30-day mortality rates and stroke risk.
- Malignant hyperthermia is a potentially lethal complication of anesthesia. Increased awareness about this complication, as well as rapid intraoperative recognition and treatment with dantrolene, has decreased patient mortality to less than 5%. A 24-hour hotline is available for expert medical advice and evaluation.

Introduction

Although morbidity and mortality rates associated with ocular surgery are generally considered to be low, the perioperative management of ophthalmic surgery patients can be challenging. Often, these patients are older and have numerous medical conditions. In addition, the ophthalmic condition requiring surgery is sometimes directly related to an underlying systemic disease, such as diabetes mellitus or thyroid disease. Finally, for some delicate surgical procedures there may be specific requirements about the patient's level of alertness during the operation, which in turn means that monitoring the level of sedation is particularly important for those patients. This chapter discusses some of the key issues to consider in the preoperative medical assessment and intraoperative management of the ocular surgery patient.

Preoperative Assessment

A complete history and physical examination are an essential part of the preoperative assessment of all patients. Determining a patient's perioperative risk status involves identifying any high-risk conditions and symptoms that may necessitate additional testing as well as specific consultation and management prior to elective ophthalmic surgery. Perioperative risk determination may also influence the decision as to whether the surgery should be performed in an ambulatory surgical center (ASC) versus a hospital outpatient setting.

The American Society of Anesthesiologists Physical Status (ASA-PS) is a classification system that defines a patient's overall health status prior to surgery; a higher ASA class (ASA III or higher) is associated with increased risk of complications, increased costs, unexpected hospital admission, and increased mortality, even after a low-risk surgery. Preoperative testing in a healthy patient or an asymptomatic stable patient, including electrocardiography and routine blood testing, is not necessary prior to ophthalmic surgery. Preoperative testing is performed only when indicated; that is, the tests would have been done even if surgery was not planned. Multiple clinical trials have failed to show a difference in perioperative adverse events in healthy patients undergoing elective eye surgery. The American Academy of Ophthalmology (AAO) advisory opinion on the responsibilities of the ophthalmologist, Appropriate Examination and Treatment Procedures, provides general guidance on determining the appropriateness and necessity of diagnostic procedures and perioperative treatment. Although ophthalmologists may delegate the acquisition of the data required for the preoperative history and the physical examination, the surgical planning and synthesis of information prior to surgery must be done by the operating ophthalmologist.

Avoiding surgical complications begins with the decision to operate. The risks and benefits of surgery, as well as any alternatives to it, are considered and the surgical plan is devised. Typically, the patient is involved in this process; informed consent is contingent on the patient's (or legal guardian's) receipt of a detailed, understandable explanation of the surgical plan. Open communication between the surgeon and the patient enhances patient education and ensures realistic expectations regarding the anesthesia depth, surgical procedure, anticipated recovery, and expected outcomes. If a patient is judged to have some level of cognitive impairment, an assessment should be made to evaluate the capacity of the patient to understand the treatment options and thereby provide informed consent. There are multiple instruments available to assess cognitive capacity. If the patient's level of cognitive impairment renders them unfit to provide consent, informed consent may be obtained from a legal proxy (power of attorney) designated to make treatment decisions for the patient (see Chapter 11 in this volume for more on informed consent).

A careful review of medication allergies, reactions to previous anesthetics, or family history of a reaction to anesthesia is critical in identifying patients at risk for malignant hyperthermia (see the section Malignant Hyperthermia later in this chapter). For a patient with an implantable cardioverter-defibrillator, the ophthalmologist should discuss the status and possible perioperative disabling of the device with the cardiologist before ocular surgery to avoid surgical complications, including possible electromagnetic interference with the pacemaker.

The operating physician typically provides postoperative eye care. Any transfer of management should be discussed and approved, ideally before surgery, by the referring physician, the physician assuming future care, and the patient.

American Academy of Ophthalmology. *Advisory Opinion of the Code of Ethics—Appropriate Examination and Treatment Procedures.* San Francisco: American Academy of Ophthalmology; 2016. www.aao.org/ethics-detail/advisory-opinion-appropriate-examination-treatment-2. Accessed September 10, 2021.

American Academy of Ophthalmology. *Advisory Opinion of the Code of Ethics—Pertinent Principles and Rules of the Code of Ethics Related to Delegation and Comanagement.* San

Francisco: American Academy of Ophthalmology; 2020. www.aao.org/ethics-detail/code-of-ethics--delegation-comanagement. Accessed September 10, 2021.

Apfelbaum JL, Connis RT, Nickinovich DG, et al; Committee on Standards and Practice Parameters, American Society of Anesthesiologists task force on preanesthesia evaluation. Practice advisory for preanesthesia evaluation: an updated report by the American Society of Anesthesiologists Task Force on Preanesthesia Evaluation. *Anesthesiology.* 2012;116(3):522–538.

Kristensen SD, Knuuti J, Saraste A, et al. 2014 ESC/ESA Guidelines on non-cardiac surgery: cardiovascular assessment and management: The Joint Task Force on Non-Cardiac Surgery: cardiovascular assessment and management of the European Society of Cardiology (ESC) and the European Society of Anesthesiology (ESA). *Eur Heart J.* 2014;35(35):2383–2431.

Children and Adolescents

If surgery is planned on a child who is healthy and does not routinely take prescribed medications, no laboratory tests are necessary, even when general anesthesia is to be used. There is no evidence that abnormalities in a complete blood count affect the choice of anesthetic management for asymptomatic children. However, African American patients should be screened for sickle cell disease or trait if they have not previously been tested, because some aspects of anesthetic management will change in patients with hemoglobinopathy. Routine pregnancy testing of female patients of childbearing age, prior to anesthesia, is a complex issue that may become even more complex in minors, because individual states may have statutes concerning parental notification of test results. Consent for a pregnancy test is required.

The decision whether to perform elective eye surgery in children with an upper respiratory tract infection requires judgment and should be made after careful consideration of the patient's overall health status. A child who is already ill will likely feel even worse after surgery, and the significance of a postoperative fever may be difficult to interpret. However, in the absence of high fever or findings that suggest a lower respiratory tract infection, many anesthesiologists elect to proceed if the child appears well except for a runny nose.

Management of Medical Conditions Associated with Increased Perioperative Risk

Cardiovascular Disease

Heart failure is one of the most common conditions requiring evaluation and treatment prior to noncardiac surgery. In stable asymptomatic patients undergoing low-risk surgery, preoperative assessment with electrocardiography (ECG), echocardiography, stress testing, chest radiographs, and cardiac catheterization is not necessary. Functional status is a reliable predictor of perioperative cardiac events; it can be assessed with a questionnaire such as the Duke Activity Status Index. If results from a recent stress test are not available, patients with good functional status are generally at low risk for a cardiac event in the perioperative period. However, if the patient shows clinical signs of decompensation, appropriate evaluation and management are indicated prior to surgery.

Coronary heart disease is a risk factor for perioperative myocardial ischemia, infarction, and death. However, even in patients with significant coronary heart disease, the risk of a major adverse cardiac event (MACE) is still low in patients undergoing low-risk surgery such as ophthalmic surgery. The goal of perioperative management of these patients is to minimize the risk of ischemic complications developing. Patients who have undergone percutaneous coronary intervention require treatment with dual antiplatelet therapy (DAT) with aspirin and $P2Y_{12}$ inhibitors (eg, clopidogrel) to prevent a recurrent occlusion of the stented artery. See Chapter 5 in this volume for further discussion of heart disease.

Although hypertension is associated with an increased risk of perioperative complications, whether there is any benefit of lowering blood pressure (BP) in terms of risk reduction is unproven. Optimal blood pressure is also unclear, but the joint guidelines from the Association of Anaesthetists of Great Britain & Ireland and the British and Irish Hypertension Society recommend a target BP below 160 mm Hg systolic and 100 mm Hg diastolic prior to elective surgery. The guidelines allow for patients with unknown preoperative blood pressures to undergo surgery with BP lower than 180 mm Hg systolic and lower than 110 mm Hg diastolic. In general, if patients are asymptomatic and have taken their BP medications, and their documented BP has typically been under 160/100 mm Hg prior to the day of surgery, then elective surgery may be performed regardless of the BP measurement on the morning of surgery. See Chapter 3 in this volume for further discussion of hypertension.

Atrial fibrillation is the most common sustained cardiac arrhythmia encountered in clinical practice. Atrial fibrillation increases the risk of death, heart failure, thromboembolic events, and hospital admissions. Patients with a history of stable atrial fibrillation do not require any preoperative specialized testing, but if the atrial fibrillation is newly onset, workup is recommended as well as delay of elective surgery. It is advisable to maintain medications for ventricular rate control, including their administration on the morning of surgery. If digoxin is used, obtaining preoperative blood levels is usually not necessary.

Diabetes Mellitus

Management of blood glucose is important in avoiding central nervous system dysfunction. Although no single regimen works for all patients, in general, insulin-dependent patients should undergo surgery early in the day whenever possible to minimize disruption of their metabolic status, and their glucose levels should be monitored postoperatively. For a diet-controlled diabetic patient undergoing a brief surgical procedure, management generally involves only monitoring of the blood glucose level immediately after surgery and every 3 hours until oral intake is resumed. It is imperative to provide close perioperative monitoring of glucose and electrolyte levels.

Respiratory Diseases

Pulmonary complications after surgery are a significant cause of perioperative morbidity and mortality. This is especially true in patients undergoing major intrathoracic and intra-abdominal surgery. Ophthalmic surgery is usually performed with the patient under local sedation, is of short duration relative to thoracic and abdominal surgery, and doesn't result in pain for the patient, obviating the need for postoperative opioids that increase pulmonary risks. Intravenous sedation under monitored anesthesia care (MAC) during eye surgery can result in hypoventilation, hypercapnia, hypoxia, and atelectasis in patients with chronic obstructive pulmonary disease (COPD). It is important for the ophthalmic surgeon to ensure that the patient's respiratory status is optimized preoperatively. If a patient's history and physical examination identifies a potential comorbidity that could impact pulmonary function and increase risk of administering preoperative sedation, then obtaining a chest x-ray and/or pulmonary function tests would be of value. Medical optimization may involve increasing the patient's inhaler regimen, administration of antibiotics (if infection is suspected), administration of corticosteroids to reduce inflammation, and/or chest physiotherapy to manage secretions. Patients who are on long-term steroid therapy should receive their usual dose on the day of the surgery; however, "stress-dose" glucocorticoid administration is generally unnecessary prior to ophthalmic surgery. Occasionally, general anesthesia with a laryngeal mask airway may be beneficial, for example, in patients with COPD who have severe dyspnea and cough in a supine position, are unable to lie still, or have high anxiety.

Fleisher LA, Fleischmann KE, Auerbach AD, et al; American College of Cardiology; American Heart Association. 2014 ACC/AHA guideline on perioperative cardiovascular evaluation and management of patients undergoing noncardiac surgery: a report of the American College of Cardiology/American Heart Association Task Force on practice guidelines. *J Am Coll Cardiol.* 2014;64(22):e77–137.

Rusk MH. Avoiding unnecessary preoperative testing. *Med Clin North Am.* 2016;100(5):1003–1008.

Perioperative Medication Management

Cardiac

In general, patients taking cardiac or blood pressure medications should continue their current medical regimen, including on the morning of surgery, to minimize the risk of rebound hypertension and ischemia. However, diuretics may be held the morning of surgery and resumed when the patient begins taking oral fluids postoperatively. Digoxin, which has a long half-life, may also be withheld the morning of surgery.

Guidelines for the use of prophylactic β-blockers in the perioperative period have been revised following the publication of the POISE-II (Perioperative Ischemic Evaluation) trial study and a subsequent meta-analysis of clinical trials. These trials demonstrated that although perioperative administration of β-blockers resulted in reduced incidence of acute myocardial infarction, the incidence of mortality and stroke increased within the first 30 days after surgery. The American College of Cardiology and the American Heart Association as well as the European Society of Cardiology currently recommend that β-blockers should be continued without interruption during the perioperative period in patients already taking them, but due to risk of harm, β-blocker prophylaxis therapy should *not* be initiated on patients undergoing low-risk surgery (eg, ophthalmic surgery).

Anticoagulants/antiplatelet agents

Whether to maintain or discontinue anticoagulants or antiplatelet agents in patients planning to undergo ocular surgery depends on the nature of surgery to be performed, the risk of ophthalmic bleeding, the potential effect of bleeding on postoperative outcome of proposed surgery, and the risk of a serious or fatal thrombotic event if the anticoagulant or antiplatelet agent is discontinued. In general, because cataract surgery is usually performed via a clear corneal approach using topical anesthesia, the potential benefit of stopping anticoagulants prior to surgery to prevent ophthalmic bleeding does not outweigh the potential risk. In a published meta-analysis of 11 clinical trials, when warfarin use was continued in patients undergoing cataract surgery, although there was an increased risk of ophthalmic bleeding, the bleeding events were minor and had no impact on vision. Similarly, continued use of aspirin or clopidogrel before cataract surgery did not result in an increased risk of ophthalmic bleeding events.

The success of other ocular surgeries, such as trabeculectomy or drainage implant surgery impact, could potentially be impacted by subconjunctival and scleral bleeding (although the bleeding is generally not life-threatening). Furthermore, patients with concomitant iris neovascularization are at high risk of developing postoperative hyphema. As a result, some surgeons prefer to stop therapy with antiplatelet agents, direct anticoagulants, and warfarin prior to filtering surgeries. In a study evaluating the risk of stroke, transient cerebral ischemia, myocardial infarction, or deep venous thrombosis, no difference was demonstrated in the number of thrombotic events experienced by continuous users of aspirin or warfarin versus users who discontinued these agents prior to cataract surgery.

In theory, the same idea should apply to patients who discontinue use of direct anticoagulants before surgery. However, in patients who are on *dual antiplatelet therapy* (aspirin *plus* clopidogrel), for example, patients who have had a recent coronary event or placement of a cardiac stent, the risk of thrombosis of the stented artery leading to a potentially fatal outcome after withdrawal of these agents warrants a 1-year delay of the elective ocular surgery. Surgery may be performed sooner in patients undergoing cataract surgery in whom cessation of anticoagulants is unnecessary. If a year's delay is not possible, surgery should be deferred at least 30 days after bare-metal stenting and at least 6 months after a drug-eluting stent is inserted.

A recent study showed a 20% lower risk of intraocular bleeding with the direct-acting anticoagulants during eye surgery when compared to warfarin. In an urgent situation in which it is necessary to reverse the effect of the thrombin inhibitor dabigatran, idarucizumab can reverse its effect within 15 minutes. Andexanet alfa was recently approved by the US Food and Drug Administration for reversal of direct factor Xa inhibitors rivaroxaban and apixaban (see Chapter 5 in this volume).

Diabetes Mellitus

Oral hypoglycemic medications are usually withheld the day of surgery. These medications have a relatively long duration of action, which could lead to hypoglycemia late in the day if the patient's oral caloric intake is inadequate. For patients with relatively well-controlled insulin-requiring diabetes mellitus and reasonable glucose control (<250 mg/dL), one option is to hold all short-acting insulin and give a portion (one-third or one-half) of the usual dose of intermediate-acting or long-acting insulin the morning of the surgery.

Pulmonary Medications

Theophylline should be held the night before surgery due to potential risk of arrhythmia. If the patient is currently taking corticosteroids, the usual dose of steroids is given on the morning of surgery, but stress-dose steroids are usually unnecessary.

Mahmoud KD, Sanon S, Habermann EB, et al. Perioperative cardiovascular risk of prior coronary stent implantation among patients undergoing noncardiac surgery. *J Am Coll Cardiol.* 2016;67(9):1038–1049.

Sun MT, Wood MK, Chan W, et al. Risk of bleeding with novel oral anticoagulants compared with warfarin: a systematic review and meta-analysis. *JAMA Ophthalmol.* 2017;135(8):864–870.

Wijeysundera DN, Duncan D, Nkonde-Price C, et al; ACC/AHA Task Force Members. Perioperative beta blockade in noncardiac surgery: a systematic review for the 2014 ACC/AHA guideline on perioperative cardiovascular evaluation and management of patients undergoing noncardiac surgery: a report of the American College of Cardiology/American Heart Association Task Force on practice guidelines. *Circulation.* 2014;130(24):2246–2264.

Perioperative Considerations

Preoperative Fasting

The purpose of preoperative fasting is to reduce the amount of particulate matter in the stomach and to lower the gastric fluid volume and acidity in case aspiration of stomach contents occurs. Gastric emptying times vary depending on the type and quantity of food consumed. Clear liquids (eg, water, coffee, pulp-free juice, and carbohydrate drinks) empty fastest, breast milk empties after 4 hours, nonhuman milk by 6 hours, and large meals that include meat or fatty substances empty by 8 hours after consumption. Small meals, such as dry toast with black coffee and pulp-free juice, have been shown to clear within 4 hours.

Perioperative fasting protocols vary between institutions and between patients and may depend on comorbidities that influence gastric emptying and how urgently surgery is needed. For example, some institutions and anesthesiologists wait only 2 hours when performing surgery on babies fed breast milk. Patients with diabetes mellitus, particularly those with autonomic neuropathy, are at risk for gastroparesis (more than 50% of patients with long-term diabetes); therefore, these patients may have a prolonged gastric emptying time. Pregnant patients have a higher-than-normal risk of aspiration. Patients with known gastroesophageal reflux disease and those with peptic ulcer disease may also have an increased risk of aspiration.

Note that a pediatric patient who fasts for 10–12 hours preoperatively may become hypotensive as a result of dehydration. The use of clear liquids orally up to 2 hours before surgery does not lead to a higher incidence of aspiration or other gastrointestinal complications in the setting of general or local anesthesia and is encouraged for the pediatric population.

Oral administration of an H_2 blocker such as ranitidine or famotidine 2–4 hours before surgery reduces the percentage of patients with low gastric pH or high gastric volume. Metoclopramide promotes intestinal motility and decreases reflux, which may be especially useful in a nonfasting patient who requires urgent surgery, but it is associated with a higher risk for extrapyramidal adverse effects.

Latex Allergy

According to the US Centers for Disease Control and Prevention, the prevalence of latex allergy in the general population is 1%–6% and is 8%–12% among health care workers. Health care workers and hospital employees can experience progressive sensitization to latex because of repeated occupational exposure. This sensitivity is accentuated in those with a history of atopy.

Certain medical populations are also at significant risk for this allergy, for example, patients with myelodysplasia or spina bifida and those who have undergone repeated urinary catheterization or frequent surgical procedures. A cross-reactivity with bananas, avocados, mangoes, and chestnuts has been demonstrated, and allergies to these foods and others have been associated with latex allergy. A history of reactivity to balloons also suggests a latex allergy.

Patients suspected of having latex allergy should be clearly identified, and the operating room environment made latex free. Latex is an aeroallergen and can be present in the operating room air for at least 1 hour after the use of latex gloves. Thus, whenever possible, an allergic patient should be the first case of the day. Alternatively, surgery may be performed in a latex-free surgical facility.

Sussman GL, Gold M. Guidelines for the management of latex allergies and safe latex use in health care facilities. ResearchGate website. www.researchgate.net/publication/242182348_Guidelines_for_the_Management_of_Latex_Allergies_and_Safe_Latex_Use_in_Health_Care_Facilities. Accessed September 10, 2021.

Universal Protocol

The definition of *wrong-site surgery* includes operating on the wrong site, performing the wrong procedure, or performing a procedure on the wrong person. In ophthalmology, the definition includes operating on the wrong eye or performing the wrong procedure, including implantation of a lens whose style and/or power differs from that chosen during preoperative surgical planning. For example, inserting a monofocal lens during cataract surgery, when the plan was to implant a premium intraocular lens, is considered the wrong procedure.

In 2004, the Joint Commission enacted the Universal Protocol (www.jointcommission.org/standards/universal-protocol), which was developed to eliminate wrong-site surgery in the United States. The Universal Protocol includes several key elements:

- agreeing on and documenting the procedure to be performed (typically done on the surgical consent form)

- marking the surgical site in the preoperative period (done by a designated member of the team, typically the surgeon)
- pausing before the beginning of surgery (performing a time-out) to verify that all members of the surgical team agree that this is the correct patient and correct procedure; that the necessary equipment is present, including implants; that the patient is correctly positioned; that the medical information on the patient, including x-rays, is for the correct patient; and that appropriate preoperative antibiotics, if indicated, have been given.

To reduce potential errors, including performing surgery on the wrong patient, 2 unique patient identifiers are required to be confirmed by the surgical team before the initiation of surgery. These identifiers, used during the time-out, include name, date of birth, and medical record number. For the time-out to be effective, it is important that members of the surgical team feel empowered to speak up and invoke a hard stop if they do not agree that all elements of the Universal Protocol have been satisfied. Wrong-site surgery is considered a sentinel event and, in many states, must be reported to the state board of medicine.

The AAO has a wrong-site-wrong-IOL checklist that surgeons may find very useful and can be used to ensure that the necessary steps are adhered to in every patient before cataract surgery to eliminate the risk of wrong-site surgery or wrong-IOL implantation. This type of checklist can be adapted/modified to any other type of surgery.

AAO Wrong-Site Task Force, Hoskins Center for Quality Eye Care. Patient Safety Statements. *Recommendations of American Academy of Ophthalmology Wrong-Site Task Force—2014.* San Francisco: American Academy of Ophthalmology; 2014. www.aao.org/patient-safety-statement/recommendations-of-american-academy-ophthalmology-. Accessed September 10, 2021.

Intraoperative Considerations

Systemic Anesthetic Agents

The use of balanced general anesthesia, in which small amounts of several different types of medications are titrated to avoid the adverse effects of a large dose of any one type, has been effective in reducing prolonged anesthesia and prolonged recovery time. The use of neuromuscular blocking agents of short duration (12 minutes for mivacurium and 30 minutes for atracurium and vecuronium) administered with an infusion pump allow the anesthesiologist to fine-tune the degree of neuromuscular blockade during balanced anesthesia.

The shorter-acting narcotics such as sufentanil have potencies up to 1000 times those of morphine. These agents help provide short-term stability of hemodynamics during intensive stimulation without prolonged excessive postoperative sedation, as seen with fentanyl. Using such agents immediately before intubation as part of an anesthetic induction has become nearly universal.

Management of postoperative nausea and vomiting after general anesthesia has become easier with the use of more powerful antinausea medications such as ondansetron. Postoperative pain can be prophylactically treated during the procedure with IV ketorolac in a 30-mg to 60-mg dose or with small titrated doses of IV fentanyl in the range of 50–100 μg. Because of its pain-reducing qualities, there is evidence that IV ketorolac can also reduce the amount of postoperative nausea and vomiting in patients who have undergone strabismus surgery or other procedures requiring general anesthesia. There is no evidence that this particular nonsteroidal anti-inflammatory drug increases postoperative bleeding after ophthalmic surgery. However, because of the reported gastrointestinal complications of higher doses of ketorolac, patients older than 60 years should receive a total of no more than 30 mg of IV ketorolac.

Sedation is an important part of comfortable regional or general anesthesia in a patient undergoing elective surgery. Anxiolytics such as midazolam can be given intramuscularly (1–4 mg) 30–60 minutes before the procedure or intravenously (0.5–2.0 mg) 2–3 minutes before the stimulus of the anesthetic block. Midazolam is a more appropriate sedative than diazepam for outpatient surgery because its elimination half-life is 2–4 hours whereas diazepam's half-life is 20–40 hours. The effects of midazolam can also be reversed with flumazenil. Careful IV titration of sedatives and narcotics is important in older patients to avoid oversedation or respiratory depression.

Alfentanil can be given intravenously in titrated doses with appropriate anesthesia monitoring. Its peak effect occurs in 1–2 minutes and lasts 10–20 minutes. Fentanyl citrate, which has a peak effect in 3–5 minutes and lasts approximately 30 minutes, is also given in titrated doses during regional or topical anesthesia. These agents are used for sedation as well as for their analgesic properties. The effects of narcotics can be reversed with the antagonist naloxone, given intravenously.

Thiopental sodium, a barbiturate used for rapid sequence induction, is no longer available in the United States. Propofol is the drug of choice for most patients due to its rapid hypnotic effect, antiemetic effects, rapid clearance, and fast recovery. It must be given through a large-bore vein or administered after a lidocaine flush of the IV line to avoid significant burning on administration. Propofol is a lipid-based medication that supports rapid bacterial growth at room temperature. Extrinsically contaminated propofol has been associated with postoperative infections, including endogenous endophthalmitis. It is therefore imperative that hospital personnel involved in the preparation, handling, and administration of this drug adhere to strict aseptic technique during its use.

Local Anesthetic Agents

Local anesthetic injection into the retrobulbar space can lead to apnea, respiratory arrest, and cranial nerve palsies on the side being injected, or even on the opposite side. Anatomical studies of the position of the retrobulbar needle in relation to the optic nerve during injection show that it is possible to inject anesthetic into the subdural space with a standard Atkinson-type needle. Cases of cranial nerve palsies associated with respiratory difficulties represent actual brainstem anesthesia from injection of the anesthetic agent into the subdural space, with subsequent diffusion into the circulating cerebrospinal fluid.

Several suggestions have been made to avoid such complications, including changing the traditional positioning of the eye during the retrobulbar anesthetic injection so that the nerve is rotated away from the track of the needle (ie, having the patient look straight ahead, rather than up). Using less sharp, disposable retrobulbar needles that are less than 1¼ inches long also reduces the chance of perforating the optic nerve sheath. Although one case series implicated the concentration of anesthetic as the cause of respiratory arrest, it is more likely that a larger volume and, therefore, a larger total dose of anesthetic was delivered to the brainstem through an inadvertent subdural injection. If apnea, respiratory arrest, or cranial neuropathies occur after a retrobulbar injection, the patient's airway must be supported with mask ventilation. Intubation and mechanical ventilation may be necessary. Apnea seldom lasts more than 30–50 minutes, but it is important that experienced medical personnel stabilize the patient's condition during this time. The peribulbar technique was devised, in part, to avoid such complications.

Respiratory distress and dysphagia can result from the Nadbath facial nerve block, an injection into the stylomastoid foramen that is used to provide facial akinesia. These complications occur when the anesthetic agent is injected deeply into the area of the facial nerve as it exits the stylomastoid foramen, and the anesthetic bathes cranial nerves IX, X, and XI as they exit the jugular foramen, leading to paralysis of these nerves. The patient becomes dysphagic, begins to cough or has a hoarse voice, and may develop stridor or severe respiratory insufficiency. These complications tend to occur in thin persons, in whom it is easier to bury the needle deeply. Managing the respiratory distress requires suctioning the pharynx, positioning the patient on his or her side, and supplementing the patient's inspired gases with oxygen or even intubation. This complication can be avoided by use of a short hypodermic needle, advancing it only partway into the area to be injected, and injecting a small volume (<3 mL).

Anesthetic toxicity can occur when high concentrations of anesthetic agent are given. For example, if lidocaine 4% is used for a peribulbar injection, the total volume that can be safely given to a 154-lb (70-kg) patient is limited to 8 mL. A smaller patient would be able to tolerate no more than 5 mL of lidocaine 4% without risking complications of systemic toxicity, including confusion, cardiac arrhythmias, and respiratory depression.

Seizures have occurred from the intra-arterial injection of local anesthetic agent into the ophthalmic artery. Such seizures are nearly instantaneous with injection; supportive measures should include airway maintenance and blood pressure support. The seizures are of short duration.

Malignant Hyperthermia

Malignant hyperthermia (MH) susceptibility is a complex genetic disorder characterized by hypermetabolic activity leading to crisis following skeletal muscle exposure to a triggering agent. The triggering agent leads to a sharp increase in unbound intracellular calcium from the sarcoplasmic reticulum, stimulating sustained muscle contracture. When the oxygen supply to the muscle is depleted, anaerobic metabolism shift develops, resulting in lactic metabolic acidosis. Finally, after all energy stores are depleted, rhabdomyolysis occurs, resulting in hyperkalemia and myoglobinuria, the latter of which causes acute renal failure. Hyperthermia results from the increased metabolic state.

The earliest signs of MH include tachycardia and elevated end-tidal carbon dioxide level. Labile blood pressure, tachypnea, sweating, muscle rigidity, blotchy discoloration of skin, cyanosis, and dark urine all signal progression of the disorder. Elevation of temperature, which can reach extremely high levels, is a relatively late sign. Ultimately, respiratory and metabolic acidosis, hyperkalemia, hypercalcemia, elevated creatine kinase myoglobinuria, and renal failure can occur, as can disseminated intravascular coagulation and death.

Genetics, risk factors, and triggering agents

Approximately 50% of cases of MH susceptibility are autosomal dominant, and the others arise as de novo mutations. According to the Malignant Hyperthermia Association of the United States (MHAUS; www.mhaus.org), the prevalence is 1 in 2000 individuals, but because of variable expressivity and penetrance, the actual number of cases is far fewer than gene prevalence would indicate. The affected genes are those that code for proteins involving the calcium channel in the sarcoplasmic reticulum.

In addition to known familial susceptibility, diagnosis of certain muscle disorders raises suspicion for MH susceptibility, especially those disorders associated with ryanodine receptor mutations. Conditions previously associated with MH that are no longer felt to represent a greater risk include Noonan syndrome, osteogenesis imperfecta, myotonias, and neuroleptic malignant syndrome. The preoperative history can also help determine whether a patient is at risk for malignant hyperthermia. However, a negative history *does not* rule out MH susceptibility, because nearly 50% of patients who develop MH have had 1 or 2 prior uneventful exposures to a triggering agent. Patients with a history of unexpected exertional- or heat-induced rhabdomyolysis, as well as those with a history of severe statin-induced myopathy, are at increased risk for MH.

Triggering agents for MH include volatile halogenated inhalational anesthetics such as halothane, sevoflurane, isoflurane, desflurane, and enflurane as well as succinylcholine.

Susceptibility testing

Patients determined to be at high risk for MH may require a muscle biopsy for muscle contracture evaluation (caffeine halothane contracture test) or genetic testing. A negative contracture test essentially rules out MH susceptibility. However, the false-positive rate is 20%, and a positive contracture test should be followed by genetic analysis. However, even if no DNA variation or a DNA variation of undetermined significance is found, this does not mean that MH susceptibility is definitely ruled out. Treatment is indicated based on the preoperative clinical impression.

Prevention and treatment

Patients who are deemed susceptible for MH can be safely anesthetized using nontriggering agents. The anesthesia machine should be cleaned of any traces of volatile anesthetics. Safe, nontriggering agents include all intravenous anesthetics and sedative agents (eg, propofol, ketamine, and barbiturates), all local anesthetics (eg, lidocaine, bupivacaine, and ropivacaine), nondepolarizing muscular blockers, analgesics, and anxiolytics. Prophylactic dantrolene is not recommended.

When MH occurs, it is treated as a medical emergency (see Table 15-1 for the treatment protocol). Before dantrolene, mortality was as high as 70%–80%; now, the rate is less than 5%. MHAUS staffs a 24-hour hotline to advise medical personnel on the diagnosis and treatment of MH: 800-644-9737 (within the United States) or 00 + 1 209-417-3722.

Table 15-1 Malignant Hyperthermia Protocol

1. Stop the triggering agents immediately and conclude surgery as soon as possible. If surgery cannot be aborted, intravenous anesthetics or propofol may be used to complete the procedure.
2. Hyperventilate with 100% oxygen at high flow rates.
3. Administer:
    a. Dantrolene: 2.5 mg/kg initial bolus with increments up to 10 mg/kg total. Continue to administer dantrolene until symptoms are controlled. Occasionally, a dose greater than 10 mg/kg may be needed.
    b. Sodium bicarbonate: 1–2 mEq/kg increments guided by arterial pH and P_{CO_2}. Bicarbonate will combat hyperkalemia by driving potassium into cells.
4. Actively cool patient if core body temperature >39°C:
    a. If needed, administer IV iced saline (not lactated Ringer's) 15 mL/kg every 10 minutes × 3. Monitor closely.
    b. Lavage stomach, bladder, rectum, and peritoneal and thoracic cavities with iced saline.
    c. Surface cool with ice and hypothermia blanket.
5. Maintain urine output. If needed, administer mannitol 0.25 g/kg IV, furosemide 1 mg/kg IV (up to 4 doses each). Urine output greater than 2 mL/kg/h may help prevent subsequent renal failure.
6. Calcium channel blockers *should not* be given when dantrolene is administered, as hyperkalemia and myocardial depression may occur.
7. Insulin for hyperkalemia: Add 10 units of regular insulin to 50 mL of 50% glucose and titrate to control hyperkalemia. Monitor blood glucose and potassium levels.
8. Postoperatively: Continue dantrolene 1 mg/kg IV every 6 hours × 72 hours to prevent recurrence. Lethal recurrences of MH may occur. Observe in an intensive care unit for at least 24 hours.
9. Key indicators of stability include declining or normal end-tidal CO_2, stable heart rate with no signs of ominous dysrhythmia, resolution of hyperthermia, and, if present, resolution of generalized muscular rigidity.
10. For expert medical advice and further medical evaluation, call the MHAUS MH hotline at 800-644-9737 (outside the United States: 00 + 1 209-417-3722). For nonemergency professional or patient information, call 1-607-674-7901 or go to www.mhaus.org.

Hopkins PM, Rüffert H, Snoeck MM, et al; European Malignant Hyperthermia Group. European Malignant Hyperthermia Group guidelines for investigation of malignant hyperthermia susceptibility. *Br J Anaesth.* 2015;115(4):531–539.

Litman RS, Griggs SM, Dowling JJ, Riazi S. Malignant hyperthermia susceptibility and related diseases. *Anesthesiology.* 2018;128(1):159–167.

CHAPTER 16

Medical Emergencies and Ocular Adverse Effects of Systemic Medications

This chapter includes related videos, which can be accessed by scanning the QR codes provided in the text or going to www.aao.org/bcscvideo_section01.

Highlights

- In 2015, guidelines for cardiopulmonary resuscitation changed; the emphasis switched to chest compressions and the immediate use of an automated external defibrillator.
- The availability of portable defibrillators in public places increases the probability of survival for patients with out-of-hospital ventricular fibrillation.
- Persons with suspected ischemic stroke should be transported to a facility capable of initiating fibrinolytic therapy within 1 hour of arrival and within 3 hours of onset of symptoms.

Introduction

Though only occasionally called on to manage a medical emergency, the ophthalmologist must be aware of the diagnostic and therapeutic steps necessary for proper care of a patient in acute distress. Infrequent use of these life-support techniques makes periodic review particularly important. Also, it is advisable for a member of the office staff to be trained in basic life support. Both the American Red Cross and the American Heart Association offer courses in basic life support (BLS), advanced cardiac life support (ACLS), and pediatric advanced life support (PALS). In addition to a review of life-support techniques, it is appropriate to periodically review office procedures, medications, and the equipment needed for each category of medical emergency.

Cardiopulmonary Arrest

Cardiopulmonary resuscitation (CPR) is intended to rescue patients with acute circulatory failure, respiratory failure, or both. The most important determinant of short-term and long-term neurologically intact survival is the interval from onset of the arrest to restoration of effective spontaneous circulatory and respiratory function. Numerous studies have shown that early defibrillation is the most important factor influencing survival and the minimization of sequelae. The sequences included here have been developed to optimize treatment. They are useful guidelines for most patients but do not preclude other measures that may be indicated for individual patients. The most crucial aspects of treatment are contained in the mnemonic *CAB*—chest compressions, airway maintenance, and breathing. The most recent published CPR protocols are the 2020 American Heart Association Guidelines for cardiopulmonary resuscitation and emergency cardiovascular care; these basic CPR steps for adults, children, and infants can be found online at https://cpr.heart.org/en/resuscitation-science/cpr-and-ecc-guidelines, along with extensive resources, including text, graphics, and video demonstrations of CPR techniques.

The following are steps for CPR using CAB; they are performed with an unconscious patient (Table 16-1, Video 16-1):

1. Determine the level of responsiveness. Attempt to arouse the patient by tapping on his or her shoulder and shouting, "Are you all right?" Do not shake the head or neck until this area has been evaluated for trauma. Quickly note if breathing is absent or abnormal (eg, gasping).
2. Activate the Emergency Medical Services (EMS) system if there is no patient response (in the United States, call 911 where available). Rescuers should "phone first" for unresponsive adults and give the location and nature of the emergency.
3. Retrieve an automated external defibrillator (AED) or send someone for the AED.
4. Position the victim supine on a firm, flat surface.
5. In an unresponsive patient without respirations, initiate chest compressions. (Determination of a pulse is no longer indicated.) Place the heel of 1 hand at the midsternal region, with the bottom of the hand 1–2 finger-breadths above the xiphoid process.
6. "Push hard and push fast." The recommended cardiac compression rate is at least 100 compressions per minute (100–120/min). The depth of chest compression is critical; optimal compression depths are 1.5 inches in infants (⅓ of body depth), 2.0 inches in children (⅓ of body depth), and at least 2.0 inches in adults. The chest must be allowed to fully recoil between compressions; therefore, leaning on the chest between compressions should be avoided.
7. Deliver 30 chest compressions.
8. As soon as the AED is available, the unit should be connected to the patient and instructions followed for assessing the heart rhythm. Interruptions to chest compressions should be minimized by having a second rescuer (eg, the person

Table 16-1 Quick Reference Chart: 2015 CAB Guidelines

	Adults over 8 years of age	Children aged 1 to 8 years	Infants aged 0 to 1 year
Recognition	No breathing or abnormal breathing (ie, only gasping)	Unresponsive	Unresponsive
Pulse	No pulse palpated within 10 seconds		
CPR sequence	C-A-B (chest compressions, airway maintenance, breathing)		
Compression rate	At least 100 per minute		
Compression depth	At least 2 inches	At least ⅓ body depth (about 2 inches)	At least ⅓ body depth (about 1 ½ inches)
Chest wall recoil	Allow complete chest recoil between compressions. Health care providers should rotate compressions every 2 minutes.		
Compression interruptions	Minimize interruptions in chest compressions. Attempt to limit interruption lengths to less than 10 seconds.		
Airway	Head-tilt, chin-lift maneuver (if neck injury is suspected, use modified jaw thrust without head extension)		
Compression-to-ventilation ratio (until advanced airway is placed)	30:2, with 1 or 2 rescuers	30:2, with 1 rescuer 15:2, with 2 rescuers	
Defibrillation	Attach and use AED as soon as available. Minimize interruptions and chest compressions before and after shock; resume CPR beginning with compressions immediately after each shock. If pediatric pads are not available, adult pads may be used on children and infants (put 1 pad on back and 1 pad on chest).		

Adult: Get help first

Child and infant: If alone, perform 5 cycles of 30 compressions and 2 breaths before leaving child to call 911

Rescue Breathing

(For victims with pulse present, but *no* breathing)

Infants aged 0 to 1 year	Child aged 1 to 8 years	Adult over the age of 8 years
1 breath every 3 seconds	1 breath every 3 seconds	1 breath every 5 seconds

AED = automated external defibrillator; CPR = cardiopulmonary resuscitation.

who retrieved the AED) charge and apply the AED. Resume chest compressions immediately after the shock and continue until 30 compressions are given.

9. Open the airway. Rescue breathing (see step 10 for technique) should be performed at a rate of 10–12 ventilations per minute. Use the head-tilt, chin-lift maneuver to provide a good airway. This is done by applying firm pressure to the forehead while placing the fingers of the other hand under the chin, supporting the mandible. If a neck injury is suspected, the modified jaw thrust without head extension should be used.

10. Pinch the nose closed. Cover the patient's mouth with yours, making a tight seal, and ventilate twice with full breaths (1 second each). A 2-second pause should be observed between breaths. Visible chest rise should be seen with each breath. Resume chest compressions immediately. The "Help" button on the AED can be pressed for guidance with both compression and rescue breathing frequency.
11. For 1- and 2-rescuer CPR: When the victim's airway is unprotected, 30 compressions should be performed before the victim is ventilated twice. About 4 seconds should be taken for 2 ventilations, including the pause between ventilations.
12. If 2 rescuers are present, chest compression duties should be switched every 2 minutes or 5 compression/ventilation cycles.
13. Continue with compression/ventilation cycles until EMS arrives.

VIDEO 16-1 CPR and use of AED in an office setting.
Courtesy of A. Luisa Di Lorenzo, MD.
Access all Section 1 videos at www.aao.org/bcscvideo_section01.

CPR is most effective when started immediately after cardiac arrest. If cardiac arrest has persisted for more than 10 minutes, CPR is unlikely to restore the patient's central nervous system (CNS) to prearrest status. If there is any question about the exact duration of cardiac arrest, the patient should be given the benefit of the doubt and resuscitation should be started.

The risk of disease transmission through mouth-to-mouth ventilation is very low, but a variety of face shields and masks are available for the health care professional. Masks are more effective than face shields in delivering adequate ventilation. Alternative airway devices (eg, a laryngeal mask airway or a esophageal/tracheal dual lumen airway device) may also be acceptable for rescuers trained in their use.

Patients with suspected stroke should be rapidly transported to a hospital capable of initiating fibrinolytic therapy within 1 hour of arrival and within 3 hours of the onset of symptoms. These patients merit the same priorities for dispatch as patients with acute myocardial infarction or major trauma. See Chapter 6 in this volume for further discussion of stroke.

The following adjuncts are helpful in CPR and are suggested components for a medical emergency tray or crash cart:

- oxygen, to enhance tissue oxygenation and to prevent or ameliorate a hypoxic state
- airways, adult and child, oral and nasal, to be used on unconscious or sedated patients
- a barrier device, such as a face shield or mask-to-mouth unit, to prevent disease transmission. Both can be used with supplemental oxygen and are especially useful if the rescuer is inexperienced in using a standard bag-valve device, which should also be included as standard equipment to help secure the airway.
- Intravenous (IV) drugs (for use by those with ACLS training)
- IV solutions: dextrose 5% and water, D5 Ringer's lactate, normal saline
- syringes (1, 5, and 10 mL), hypodermic needles (20, 22, and 25 gauge), and venous catheters
- a suction apparatus, tourniquet, taped tongue blade, and tape
- laryngoscope and endotracheal tubes (adult and child)

If there is no 911 community emergency phone system, it is essential to have the phone number of the local paramedic emergency squad posted near all office telephones.

BLS also outlines methods for aiding persons who are choking. These methods include the Heimlich maneuver and appropriate manual techniques for removing foreign bodies from the oral pharynx. Epigastric thrusts should be attempted; up to 10–12 thrusts may be necessary. If these techniques fail to restore effective respiratory function, ventilation should be attempted. Using a finger sweep to clear a foreign body from the oral pharynx is recommended by the American Medical Association but is not indicated in many modern protocols. Transtracheal ventilation by means of cricothyrotomy may be necessary if other techniques fail to clear the airway.

The American Heart Association has established guidelines and procedures for ACLS. ACLS includes intubations, defibrillation, cardioversion, pacemaker placement, administration of drugs and fluids, and communication with ambulance and hospital systems. Because of the comprehensive and changing nature of ACLS algorithms, these procedures are beyond the scope of this chapter.

Competency in pediatric emergency care may be enhanced with training in pediatric life support (PLS) and PALS. In addition, ophthalmologists should be familiar with the ophthalmic manifestations of child abuse and abusive head trauma (shaken baby syndrome). These are discussed in BCSC Section 6, *Pediatric Ophthalmology and Strabismus.*

Neumar RW, Shuster M, Callaway CW, et al. Part 1: Executive summary: 2015 American Heart Association Guidelines Update for cardiopulmonary resuscitation and emergency cardiovascular care. *Circulation.* 2015:132(18 Suppl 2):S315–367.

Syncope

Vasovagal episodes (syncope) are common, usually benign, events. These reactions are centered around the "fight or flight" response, such as when a person experiences a perceived or actual danger or threat. Common scenarios that can trigger a vasovagal attack in an ophthalmology office include dilation, applanation tonometry, contact lens insertion, and foreign body removal. Often, the patient has premonitory signs and symptoms before the episode; these include lightheadedness, nausea, the sensation of changes in temperature, or tinnitus. Physiologically, during an episode the vagus nerve is stimulated, causing peripheral blood vessels to dilate, which lowers blood pressure and slows the heart rate. Cerebral hypoperfusion and subsequent loss of consciousness can occur. Fortunately, these episodes are short-lived; the patient typically recovers within seconds. If these episodes occur in older persons, cardiac abnormalities should be considered. Patients with a history of cardiac problems who experience a syncopal episode have a higher risk of morbidity and mortality and should be evaluated thoroughly. A person experiencing a syncopal episode should be placed supine—preferably in a cool, quiet place—and the legs should be elevated.

Video 16-2 depicts the management of a vasovagal episode in the office setting.

VIDEO 16-2 Management of a vasovagal episode.
Courtesy of A. Luisa Di Lorenzo, MD.

Hypoglycemia

Ophthalmologists treat patients with diabetes mellitus daily and therefore should be familiar with the management of a hypoglycemic episode. There are 2 types of hypoglycemia: postprandial hypoglycemia and fasting hypoglycemia. Causes of hypoglycemia are varied but include diabetes mellitus treated with insulin or insulin secretagogues; adrenal insufficiency; the presence of pheochromocytoma; hyperthyroidism; substance abuse, including alcohol, cocaine, and salicylate toxicity; nutritional deficiency; eating disorders; liver disease such as cirrhosis; and medications such as insulin, insulin secretagogues, methadone, and tramadol. Symptoms include perspiration, tremor, tachycardia, anxiety, hunger, dizziness, changes in vision, confusion, convulsions, and syncope. Management of these episodes depends on the severity of the hypoglycemia. It is important to recognize the signs of hypoglycemia; if possible, blood glucose should be tested, but treatment should not be delayed. Mild to moderate hypoglycemia can be treated orally with glucose gel or tablets, fruit juice, regular soda, milk, honey or corn syrup, and crackers. Unconscious patients with severe hypoglycemia should be treated with intravenous dextrose and intramuscular glucagon.

Shock

Shock is a state of tissue hypoperfusion that leads to impaired cellular metabolism and—if uncorrected—progresses to multiple organ failure and death.

Classification

Shock is classified according to the 4 primary pathophysiologic mechanisms involved:

- oligemic, or hypovolemic (eg, hemorrhage, diabetic ketoacidosis, burns, or sequestration)
- cardiogenic (eg, myocardial infarction or arrhythmia)
- obstructive (eg, pericardial tamponade, pulmonary embolus, or tension pneumothorax)
- distributive, characterized by maldistribution of the vascular volume secondary to altered vasomotor tone (eg, sepsis, anaphylaxis, spinal cord insult, beriberi, or arteriovenous fistula)

The type of shock can often be determined by the history, physical examination, and appropriate diagnostic tests. Regardless of the event that precipitated the state of shock, microcirculatory failure is the common factor that eventually leads to death in individuals in advanced shock. Ventilatory failure appears to be the most significant factor in the morbidity and mortality of shock, with subsequent hypoxemia and metabolic acidosis leading to many complications.

If vasovagal syncope is ruled out (due to its short duration and because of familiarity with the situations that produce this condition), the basic life-support measures for the initial emergency care of the unconscious patient are similar to the measures used when treating patients with shock. The most important aspects of treatment are the CABs, the same principles used in CPR (see the section Cardiopulmonary Arrest earlier in this chapter).

Failure of respiratory gas exchange is the most frequent single cause of death in patients with shock; thus, respiratory obstruction must be ruled out first. Oxygen is then given by mask; if respiratory movements are shallow, mechanical ventilation is necessary. Respiratory obstruction can be assumed if there is stridor with respiratory movements or if cyanosis persists even when adequate ventilatory techniques have been applied. A conscious patient in distress who cannot speak and who is developing cyanosis may be choking on food or a foreign body.

Assessment

The patient's vital signs must be monitored. The clinical syndrome is usually characterized by an altered sensorium, relative hypotension, tachycardia, tachypnea, oliguria, metabolic acidosis, weak or absent pulse, pallor, diaphoresis, and cool skin (however, in cases of septic shock the skin may be warm). Decreased pulse pressure is often an early sign of shock, and systolic blood pressures of less than 90 mm Hg are often associated with vital organ hypoperfusion. Blood pressure is not always a reliable indicator of tissue perfusion, however.

Treatment

Specific guidelines for the treatment of shock, which is often quite complex, are beyond the scope of this text. General guidelines are as follows:

- The EMS system should be activated, or the patient should be transferred to an emergency department.
- The patient should be positioned supine, with the legs elevated.
- Supplemental oxygen should be administered to enhance tissue oxygenation. Mechanical ventilation may be necessary to maintain the Po_2 at normal levels and to prevent respiratory acidosis.
- Fluid resuscitation with IV infusion of a crystalloid solution (ie, normal saline or Ringer's lactate) should be administered rapidly.
- Vasopressor drugs (norepinephrine first) may be necessary for augmentation of systemic vascular tone and/or cardiac output to help perfuse vital organs after an adequate circulating volume is established. Vasopressin, or antidiuretic hormone (ADH), has been suggested for septic shock because of its potent vasoconstrictor effect but it should only be reserved for salvage therapy. In December 2017, the US Food and Drug Administration approved synthetic human angiotensin II (Giapreza) for adults with septic or other distributive shock.
- If sepsis is suspected, blood cultures should be drawn and antibiotic therapy initiated promptly.
- Sodium bicarbonate, given intravenously, is indicated for correction of severe metabolic acidosis.

Experimental drugs used in the treatment of septic shock include polyclonal IV immunoglobulin, because it can bind endotoxin, but no existing studies substantiate its use.

Genga KR, Russell JA. Update of sepsis in the intensive care unit. *J Innate Immun.* 2017;9(5):441–455.

Jones AE, Puskarich MA. The Surviving Sepsis Campaign guidelines 2012: update for emergency physicians. *Ann Emerg Med.* 2014;63(1):35–47.
Rhodes A, Evans LE, Alhazzani W, et al. Surviving Sepsis Campaign: international guidelines for management of sepsis and septic shock: 2016. *Intensive Care Med.* 2017;43(3):304–377.

Anaphylaxis

Anaphylaxis is an acute allergic reaction following antigen exposure in a previously sensitized person; it requires immediate and specific therapy. It is usually mediated by immunoglobulin E antibodies and involves release of chemical mediators from mast cells and basophils. *Anaphylactoid reactions,* which are more common and less severe, are triggered by nonantigenic agents and are the result of direct release of these chemical mediators. Anaphylaxis or anaphylactoid reactions may occur after exposure to pollen, drugs, foreign serum, insect stings, diagnostic agents such as iodinated contrast materials or fluorescein, vaccines, local anesthetics, and food products. The most important parameter for predicting such an attack is a history of a previous allergic reaction to any other drug or possible antigen. Unfortunately, a history of known sensitivity may not always be elicited. Studies indicate that the prevalence of anaphylaxis has been increasing steadily since 2008.

Anaphylaxis is particularly important to the ophthalmologist, in view of the increasing number of surgical procedures and fluorescein angiograms performed in the office setting. It is estimated that allergic reactions to fluorescein (including urticaria) occur in up to 1% of all angiograms. In 1 survey, the overall risk of a severe reaction was 1 in 1900 patients, including a risk of respiratory compromise in 1 in 3800 subjects. If diaphoresis, apprehension, pallor, a rapid and weak pulse, or any combination thereof develops in a patient after administration of a drug, the patient should be considered to have an allergic reaction until proven otherwise. The diagnosis is confirmed if the patient experiences associated generalized itching, urticaria, angioedema of the skin, dyspnea, wheezing, or arrhythmia. Anaphylaxis may rapidly lead to loss of consciousness, shock, cardiac arrest, coma, or death.

Once an acute allergic reaction is suspected, prompt treatment is indicated:

- Oxygen should be administered to patients in respiratory distress.
- Epinephrine (0.3 mL of a 1:1000 solution) injected intramuscularly in a limb opposite to the antigenic agent exposure site is usually effective for the maintenance of circulation and blood pressure.
- IV volume expansion may be necessary to restore and maintain tissue perfusion. Methylprednisolone should be administered for serious or prolonged reactions. When given early, corticosteroids help control possible long-term sequelae.
- Antihistamines are helpful in slowing or halting the ongoing allergic response but are of limited value in acute anaphylaxis.
- Tracheotomy or cricothyrotomy is indicated when laryngeal edema is unresponsive to the previous methods or when oral intubation cannot be performed.
- All patients with anaphylaxis or anaphylactoid reactions should be kept under observation for at least 6 hours.

In cases of mild allergic reactions, the physician can administer 25–50 mg of diphenhydramine hydrochloride orally or intramuscularly and observe the patient closely to determine whether further treatment is necessary. Pretreating high-risk patients with an antihistamine, corticosteroids, or both prior to fluorescein angiography may reduce the risk of an allergic reaction. In all cases of anaphylaxis, supportive treatment should be maintained until the emergency medical team arrives.

For patients with a known history of anaphylaxis, personal emergency kits containing epinephrine are available and can be used until medical help arrives. The kits are designed to allow self-treatment by the patient or administration by a family member or an informed bystander. One commercially available allergy kit contains a syringe and needle preloaded with 0.6 mL of 1:1000 epinephrine. The physician who prescribes this kit must give detailed instructions concerning the use of the device. Epinephrine auto-injectors are also available. Each contains a spring-loaded automatic injector, which does not permit graduated doses to be given but automatically injects 0.3 mg of epinephrine (0.15 mg in the pediatric version) when the device is triggered by pressure on the thigh. The epinephrine ampules contained in these self-treatment kits have a limited shelf life and should be replaced when the expiration date is reached or if the solution becomes discolored. Any person given epinephrine requires 4–6 hours of observation to ensure that there is no rebound effect. In recent years, there has been renewed interest in treatment of allergic reactions with sublingual immunotherapy, in which the patient is exposed to the offending antigen via the gastrointestinal system to improve tolerance.

Seizures and Status Epilepticus

A *seizure* is a paroxysmal episode of abnormal electrical activity in the brain, resulting in involuntary transient neurologic, motor activity, behavioral, or autonomic dysfunction. Typically, seizures are divided into 2 major categories, partial and generalized. Although seizures can present with many different clinical manifestations, most fit into the subcategories of simple partial, complex partial, or generalized tonic–clonic. See Chapter 11 for detailed discussion of these categories.

Status epilepticus is defined as a prolonged seizure (30 minutes or longer) or as multiple seizures without intervening periods of normal consciousness. Like seizures, status epilepticus may have a local onset with secondary generalization or may be generalized from onset. This condition often occurs concomitantly with hyperthermia, acidosis, hypoxia, tachycardia, hypercapnia, and mydriasis and, if persistent, may be associated with irreversible brain injury. Status epilepticus that is completely stopped within 2 hours usually has relatively minor morbidity compared with episodes lasting longer than 2 hours.

Major causes of seizures and status epilepticus include

- drug withdrawal, such as from anticonvulsants, benzodiazepines, barbiturates, or alcohol
- metabolic abnormalities, such as hypoglycemia, hyponatremia, hypocalcemia, or hypomagnesemia
- conditions that affect the CNS, such as infection, trauma, stroke, hypoxia, ischemia, or sleep deprivation
- toxic levels of various drugs

Emergency *medical* management of seizures is best left to physicians who perform this routinely. However, the clinician should be aware of some general considerations in the treatment of seizures. The first priority is now the maintenance of circulation as opposed to airway maintenance. Maintenance of circulation becomes particularly important if the seizure progresses to status epilepticus.

During seizure management, it is important not only to stop the seizure activity but also to identify and treat the underlying cause when possible. Additional steps include noting the time of seizure onset, monitoring and maintaining an airway, and monitoring vital signs. Activation of the emergency response (911) team is indicated in all cases of acute seizure onset. In the setting of an ophthalmology office, it may be appropriate to check blood glucose levels, because many seizure patients have diabetes mellitus.

Refractory cases of status epilepticus have responded successfully to repeated electroconvulsive therapy sessions, IV sedatives such as ketamine or propofol, surgical ablation and stimulation procedures, and topiramate and levetiracetam.

Riviello JJ Jr, Claassen J, LaRoche SM, et al; Neurocritical Care Society Status Epilepticus Guideline Writing Committee. Treatment of status epilepticus: an international survey of experts. *Neurocrit Care.* 2013;18(2):193–200.

Toxic Reactions to Local Anesthetic Agents and Other Drugs

Toxic overdose can cause acute distress and unconsciousness. Clinicians should be prepared to respond to this emergency whenever a patient is undergoing a procedure that requires local anesthesia. Table 16-2 lists commonly used local anesthetics and their maximum safe dose.

Reactions following administration of local anesthetics are almost always toxic and only rarely allergic. A high blood level of local anesthetic can be produced by the following: too large a dose, unusually rapid absorption (including inadvertent administration directly into a vein), and unusually slow detoxification or elimination (especially in individuals with liver disease). Though rare, hypersensitivity (ie, decreased patient tolerance) and idiosyncratic reactions to local anesthetic agents may occur, as with any drug. True allergic or anaphylactic reactions are also uncommon but may occur, particularly with agents belonging to the amino ester class (eg, tetracaine).

Toxic reactions cause overstimulation of the CNS, which may lead to excitability, restlessness, apprehension, disorientation, tremors, and convulsions (cerebral cortex effects), as well as nausea and vomiting (medulla effects). Cardiac effects initially include tachycardia and hypertension. Ultimately, depression of the CNS and the cardiovascular system occurs, which may result in drowsiness or coma (cerebral cortex effects), as well as in irregular respirations, sighing, dyspnea, and respiratory arrest (medulla effects). Cardiac effects of CNS depression are bradycardia and hypotension.

Injected local anesthetic can have a direct toxic effect on muscle tissue. In peribulbar or retrobulbar injections, this can result in muscle weakness, which in some patients is followed by muscle contracture. Extraocular motility can be affected, resulting in diplopia (usually hypertropia) that may require surgical revision. Hyaluronidase may be partially protective by allowing more rapid diffusion of the anesthetic agent following injection.

Table 16-2 Maximum Recommended Local Anesthetic Doses

Agent	Commercially Available Concentrations (%) 1% = 10 mg/mL	Plain Solutions, mg	Epinephrine-Containing Solutions, mg
Chloroprocaine	1.0, 2.0, 3.0	800	1000
Lidocaine	0.5, 1.0, 1.5, 2.0, 4.0, 5.0	300	500
Mepivacaine	1.0, 1.5, 2.0	300	225
Bupivacaine	0.25, 0.5, 0.75	175	225
Tetracaine	1.0	100	100

Increased metabolic activity of the CNS and poor ventilation can lead to cerebral hypoxia. Treatment consists of oxygenation, supportive airway care, and titrated IV administration of midazolam, which is used to suppress cortical stimulation.

Other emergency procedures that must be applied in cases of toxic overdose include suctioning if vomiting occurs and using a taped tongue blade if convulsions develop. If shock develops, the appropriate drugs can be administered by IV infusion.

The addition of *epinephrine* to the local anesthetic can also cause adverse reactions. Reactions to epinephrine can produce symptoms similar to those of early CNS overstimulation by local anesthetic, such as anxiety, restlessness, tremor, hypertension, and tachycardia. Unlike local anesthetic toxicity, however, epinephrine overdose does not produce convulsions or bradycardia as the toxic reaction progresses. Oxygen is useful in the treatment of epinephrine overdoses.

Although rare, death can occur as a result of retrobulbar or peribulbar local anesthetic; for example, the administration of retrobulbar *bupivacaine* has been associated with respiratory arrest. This reaction may be caused by intra-arterial injection of the local anesthetic, with retrograde flow to the cerebral circulation. It can also result from puncture of the dural sheath of the optic nerve during retrobulbar block, with diffusion of the local anesthetic along the subdural space in the midbrain. Initial symptoms are a gradual or sudden change in consciousness, such as coma with tonic-clonic seizures; apnea; and blood pressure lability. A large prospective study that compared retrobulbar injection of 0.75% bupivacaine plus 2.0% lidocaine to 0.75% bupivacaine plus 4.0% lidocaine found that the patients receiving 4.0% lidocaine mixed with bupivacaine had an almost 9 times greater risk of respiratory arrest than patients receiving 2.0% lidocaine mixed with bupivacaine. Ophthalmologists should be prepared for these possible adverse effects by having the proper resuscitative equipment at hand and training office staff in CPR.

The use of IV *edrophonium chloride* in the diagnosis of myasthenia gravis can have toxic adverse effects. The signs and symptoms result from cholinergic stimulation and may include nausea, vomiting, diarrhea, sweating, increased bronchial and salivary secretions, muscle fasciculations and weakness, and bradycardia. Some of these signs may be transient and self-limited because of the very short half-life of IV edrophonium. However, whenever the test is to be performed, a syringe containing 0.5 mg of atropine sulfate must be immediately available. (Some physicians routinely pretreat with atropine all patients undergoing such testing.)

As noted, if signs of excess cholinergic stimulation occur, 0.5 mg of atropine sulfate should be administered intravenously. This dose may be repeated every 3–10 minutes if necessary. The total dose of atropine necessary to counteract the toxic effects is seldom more than 2 mg. If toxic signs progress, the treatment described earlier for toxic overdose may be necessary.

Guo S, Wagner R, Gewirtz M, et al. Diplopia and strabismus following ocular surgeries. *Surv Ophthalmol.* 2010;55(4):335–358.

Kumar CM, Eke T, Dodds C, et al. Local anaesthesia for ophthalmic surgery—new guidelines from the Royal College of Anaesthetists and the Royal College of Ophthalmologists. *Eye (Lond).* 2012;26(6):987–898.

Moorthy SS, Zaffer R, Rodriguez S, Ksiazek S, Yee RD. Apnea and seizures following retrobulbar local anesthetic injection. *J Clin Anesth.* 2003;15(4):267–270.

Palte HD. Ophthalmic regional blocks: management, challenges, and solutions. *Local Reg Anesth.* 2015;8:57–70.

The Opioid Crisis

The opioid crisis is a national socioeconomic and public health issue with which every ophthalmologist should be familiar. Opioid abuse includes misuse and addiction to prescription pain relievers, heroin, and synthetic opioids such as fentanyl. In the United States, 115 individuals die of opioid overdose daily. The US Centers for Disease Control and Prevention estimates the economic burden of this crisis at $78.5 billion a year. This figure includes the cost of health care for the addicted individuals, productivity loss, addiction treatment, and the ultimate involvement of the criminal justice system in many of these cases.

The cause of this epidemic is multifactorial; its origins can be traced back to the late 1990s when pharmaceutical companies assured the medical community that patients would not become addicted to prescription opioid pain relievers. Prescription of these medications to patients led to their widespread use and subsequent misuse, and it soon became clear that these drugs were indeed highly addictive. Opioid overdose rates began to increase; in 2015 alone, more than 33,000 individuals in the United States died as a result of overdose from prescription pain killers, heroin, and illegally manufactured synthetic fentanyl. Also in 2015, it was determined that approximately 2 million people were abusing pain medications, and over half a million people were suffering from heroin addiction, which unfortunately occurred in conjunction with prior opioid pain medication use in some cases.

Roughly 21%–29% of patients prescribed opioid-based chronic-pain medications ultimately abuse them. Of these, 8%–12% develop an opioid use disorder. Unfortunately, 4%–6% of those who abuse prescription opioids transition to heroin. In fact, 80.5% of individuals addicted to heroin once misused prescription pain medicine. In addition to the devastating public health issue created by this crisis, there is an increase in neonatal abstinence syndrome due to the misuse of opioids during pregnancy. Increased injection drug use has also led to increased incidence of blood-borne infections such as HIV and hepatitis C, resulting from the use of contaminated injection drug equipment.

The US Department of Health and Human Services and the National Institutes of Health (NIH) have aggressive strategies to manage this devastating problem by improving access to treatment and recovery programs, promoting the use of overdose-reversing drugs, advocating for better public health surveillance, improving research on pain and addiction, and, finally, improving prescribing patterns in the medical community for patients experiencing pain. The NIH is also exploring formal partnerships with pharmaceutical companies and academic centers to develop safe, effective nonaddictive approaches to managing long-term pain, to develop new medications and technologies to treat opioid-use disorders, and to improve prevention and reversal interventions to save lives and support recovery.

Collins F, Schuchat A, Ostroff S, Gingrich N, Kennedy P. Plenary Address: Rewriting the Prescription for Treating Opioid Addiction. Presented at: National Rx Drug Abuse & Heroin Summit; April 19, 2017; Atlanta, GA.

Volkow ND, Collins FS. The role of science in addressing the opioid crisis. *N Engl J Med.* 2017;377(4):391–394.

Ocular Adverse Effects of Systemic Medications

Because of the advancement of medical specialties and the proliferation of specific therapeutic agents, patients frequently have multiple simultaneous drug regimens. Often, no single physician is aware of all the drugs the patient is taking. The clinical problem is compounded by several factors. In addition, the physician may not be familiar with the types of drugs or the properties of drugs used outside his or her specialty. The patient may also have a drug interaction that affects a bodily system not usually monitored by the specialist. Finally, the patient might not associate a symptom with a particular drug if that symptom is not related to the system for which the drug was given. The growing use of electronic medical records has helped physicians become more aware of the multiple drug regimens, but it has not eliminated the problem.

The effects of some systemic drugs are widely known. For example, the commonly prescribed erectile dysfunction agent sildenafil has been noted to block photoreceptor signals, causing electroretinographic changes, visual disturbances (including changes in color perception), and increased light sensitivity. The spectrum of systemic side effects of commonly used ophthalmic drugs is covered extensively elsewhere in this series (see BCSC Section 9, *Uveitis and Ocular Inflammation,* and Section 10, *Glaucoma*). The ocular adverse effects of several commonly prescribed systemic medications are presented in Table 16-3. Drug interactions are always a concern in patients who use multiple topical and systemic medications.

The ophthalmologist can minimize adverse effects from multiple-drug therapy by doing the following:

- Maintain a high level of suspicion for drug interactions.
- Question the patient closely about other drug therapy and general symptoms.
- Encourage all patients to carry a card listing the drugs they use.
- Keep in close communication with the patient's primary care physician.
- Consult with a clinical pharmacologist or internist whenever a question of drug interaction arises.
- Utilize the resources provided through electronic medical records. For example, some electronic medical record systems link to pharmacy records.

Table 16-3 Potential Ocular Adverse Effects of Popular Drugs

Drug	Adverse Effects
Antibiotics	
Cefaclor	Mild inflammation of ocular surface (rare); eyelid problems; nystagmus; visual hallucinations
Cefuroxime axetil	Mild inflammation of ocular surface (rare)
Ciprofloxacin	Eyelid problems; exacerbation of myasthenia gravis; visual sensations; retinal detachment
Moxifloxacin (oral)	Iris transillumination; sphincter paralysis; retinal detachment
Rifampin	Conjunctival hyperemia; exudative conjunctivitis; increased lacrimation
Tetracycline, doxycycline, minocycline	Papilledema secondary to IIH; transient myopia; blue-gray, dark blue, or brownish pigmentation of the sclera; hyperpigmentation of eyelids or conjunctiva; diplopia
Antidepressants/anxiolytics	
Alprazolam	Diplopia; decreased or blurred vision; decreased accommodation; abnormal extraocular muscle movements; allergic conjunctivitis
Fluoxetine	Blurred vision; photophobia; mydriasis; dry eye; conjunctivitis; diplopia
Imipramine	Decreased vision; decreased accommodation; slight mydriasis; photosensitivity
Antiepileptics	
Topiramate	Conjunctivitis; abnormal accommodation; photophobia; strabismus; mydriasis; anterior uveitis; acute myopia; anterior chamber shallowing; secondary angle-closure glaucoma (bilateral); visual field defects; suprachoroidal effusions
Analgesics, anti-inflammatory drugs	
Aspirin	Transient blurred vision; transient myopia; hypersensitivity reactions
Ibuprofen	Blurred vision; decreased vision; diplopia; photosensitivity; dry eyes; decrease in color vision; optic or retrobulbar neuritis
Hydroxychloroquine	Retinopathy (bull's-eye maculopathy), with decreased vision and color perception
Naproxen	Decreased vision; changes in color vision; optic or retrobulbar neuritis; papilledema secondary to IIH; photosensitivity; corneal opacities
Disease-modifying agents	
Bisphosphonates	Anterior uveitis; conjunctivitis; scleritis; blurred vision
Interferon	Cotton-wool spots
Isotretinoin	Corneal opacities; night blindness; decreased color vision; sicca syndrome; papilledema
Asthma, allergy drugs	
Antihistamines	Decreased vision; may induce or aggravate dry eye; pupillary changes; decreased accommodation; blurred vision; decreased mucoid or lacrimal secretions; diplopia
Corticosteroids	Decreased vision; posterior subcapsular cataracts; increased intraocular pressure

Table 16-3 *(continued)*

Drug	Adverse Effects
Cardiovascular drugs	
Amiodarone	Photophobia; blurred vision; corneal deposits; anterior subcapsular lens opacities; optic neuropathy
β-Blockers	Decreased vision; dry eye syndrome; visual hallucinations; decreased intraocular pressure; decreased lacrimation
Selective α_{1a} antagonists	Intraoperative floppy iris syndrome, with a sluggish hypotonic iris, miosis, iris prolapse
Calcium channel blockers	Decreased or blurred vision; periorbital edema; ocular irritation (general)
Captopril, enalapril	Angioedema of the eye and orbit; conjunctivitis; decreased vision
Digitalis glycosides	Decreased vision; color vision defects; glare phenomenon; flickering vision
Diuretics (thiazide-type)	Decreased vision; myopia; color vision abnormalities; retinal edema
Flecainide	Blurred vision; decreased vision; decreased accommodation; abnormal visual sensations; decreased depth perception; nystagmus
Warfarin	Retinal hemorrhages in susceptible persons; hyphema; allergic reactions; conjunctivitis; lacrimation; decreased vision
Drugs used in the treatment of impotence	
Sildenafil Tadalafil	Possible retinal vascular occlusions; decreased color perception; conjunctivitis; photophobia
Hormones, hormone-related drugs	
Clomiphene	Visual sensations; decreased vision; mydriasis; visual field constriction; photophobia; diplopia
Danazol	Decreased vision; diplopia; papilledema secondary to IIH; visual field defects
Estradiol	Decreased vision; retinal vascular disorders; papilledema secondary to IIH; fluctuations of corneal curvature and corneal steepening; color vision abnormalities
Leuprolide	Blurred vision; papilledema secondary to IIH; retinal hemorrhage and branch vein occlusion; eye pain; eyelid edema
Oral contraceptives	Decreased vision; retinal vascular disorders; papilledema secondary to IIH; color vision abnormalities
Tamoxifen	Decreased vision; corneal deposits; retinal edema or hemorrhage; papilledema; retinopathy; decreased color vision; optic neuritis or neuropathy

IIH = idiopathic intracranial hypertension.

Unrecognized adverse effects of topical or systemic medications should be reported to the National Registry of Drug-Induced Ocular Side Effects, either via their website at www.eyedrugregistry.com, or in correspondence with the registry's director, Frederick T. Fraunfelder, MD, at eyedrug@OHSU.edu.

Fraunfelder FT, Fraunfelder FW, Chambers WA. *Drug-induced ocular side effects: clinical ocular toxicology*. 7th ed. Philadelphia, PA: Elsevier/Saunders; 2015.

CHAPTER 17

Social Determinants of Health

Highlights

- Social determinants of health (SDOH) are major drivers of health disparities.
- Addressing SDOH will "create social, physical, and economic environments that promote attaining the full potential for health and well-being for all" (Healthy People 2030).
- Minority ethnicity, lower educational attainment, lower income, and lack of insurance are all associated with greater visual impairment in the United States.
- Ophthalmologists should assess the impact of SDOH as part of every patient encounter and should address SDOH in their treatment of patients.

Introduction

Health is not the absence of disease but the presence of wellness. As illustrated in Figure 17-1, health is the result of the complex interplay of individual factors (eg, genetics, lifestyle), population factors (eg, ethnicity, gender, sexual orientation), and social determinants. *Social determinants of health (SDOH)* are conditions in the environment in which people grow, live, learn, work, and age that affect health outcomes. Over the past few decades, increasing evidence has suggested that complex social, physical, and economic conditions have a greater impact than medical care on health outcomes and life expectancy. In a 2008 report, the World Health Organization stated that "social justice is a matter of life and death. It affects the way people live, their consequent chance of illness, and their risk of premature death." The report calls for organized global action to address SDOH in order to achieve health equity. *Health inequities* are avoidable, systematic differences in health status between different population groups. SDOH are a major cause of *health disparities.* The pursuit of health equity requires a concerted, societal effort to remove barriers such as discrimination and poverty and their many consequences.

Categories of Social Determinants of Health

Recognizing the social, economic, and physical conditions that different populations experience because of their environments is fundamental to understanding and addressing SDOH, which can be grouped into 5 domains:

- health care access and quality (eg, insurance, physician availability, communication)
- economic stability (eg, employment, income, housing and food security)

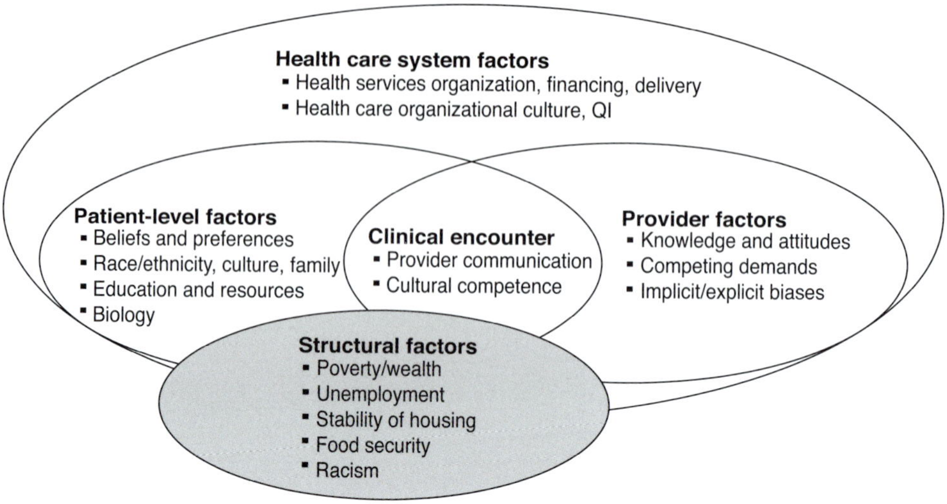

Figure 17-1 Key potential determinants of health and health care disparities. QI = quality improvement. *(From Bryant A. Racial and ethnic disparities in obstetric and gynecologic care and role of implicit biases. In:* UpToDate*. October 29, 2020. Used with permission from Kilbourne AM, Switzer G, Hyman K, Crowley-Matoka M, Fine MJ. Advancing health disparities research within the health care system: a conceptual framework.* Am J Public Health. *2006;96(12):2116. Copyright © 2006 American Public Health Association.)*

- education access and quality (eg, education, literacy, language skills)
- neighborhood and built environment (eg, transportation, safety, geography, parks)
- social and community context (eg, community engagement, social cohesion, incarceration rates)

Health Care Access and Quality

There are several barriers to accessing health care and receiving high-quality care. First, although the rates of uninsured Americans have decreased under the Affordable Care Act, approximately 10% of people in the United States remain uninsured. Vulnerable population groups, such as minority groups, account for over half of the uninsured population. Second, inadequate health insurance coverage resulting in high out-of-pocket costs continues to be one of the largest barriers to health care access. Other barriers include poor access to transportation, limited health care resources and provider availability in underserved areas, and poor provider-patient communication. Poor communication can be due to several factors, including patient fear or lack of trust, lack of time, cultural and language barriers, and lower literacy levels. These social complexity factors have been associated with poorer outcomes with respect to preventive health care and management of chronic disease.

Ophthalmic considerations Compared with White patients, Black and Latino patients and other ethnic minority groups have higher rates of diabetic retinopathy, impaired vision due to cataract, and primary open-angle glaucoma (POAG). But despite being at higher risk for visual impairment and blindness, Black and Latino patients are less likely than White patients to be seen by an ophthalmologist or to receive a dilated examination.

A study by Elam and colleagues found that Medicaid patients with a new diagnosis of POAG receive substantially less glaucoma testing in the 15 months following initial diagnosis compared with patients with commercial health insurance. This disparity is most striking in Black patients with Medicaid insurance, who had 291% increased odds of not undergoing glaucoma testing, compared with Black patients with commercial health insurance. Further, Black patients are more likely than White patients to go blind from POAG, highlighting the importance of efforts to improve the quality of glaucoma care for Medicaid recipients and ethnic minority groups.

Elam AR, Andrews C, Musch DC, Lee PP, Stein JD. Large disparities in receipt of glaucoma care between enrollees in Medicaid and those with commercial health insurance. *Ophthalmology.* 2017;124(10):1442–1448.

Priorities for addressing this domain should include the following:

- expanding access to appropriate insurance coverage and to primary care and health professionals, both in person and remotely
- focusing on preventive health care
- improving health communication between physicians and patients through cultural competency training and by ensuring availability of patient education material in various languages and at the appropriate education level
- offering telehealth to improve services and expand access
- providing vision services in community health centers and vision outreach in underserved areas
- optimizing the electronic health record for screening and patient communication

Economic Stability

A substantial body of research has demonstrated the detrimental effects of low socioeconomic status and poverty on health outcomes. Economic stability is one of the most important SDOH, as it affects all other domains. Without stable employment, one may not be able to access health insurance and may also experience food insecurity, housing instability, and poor work environments, all of which have complex effects on many aspects of health. One overarching goal of Healthy People 2030, an initiative by the US Department of Health and Human Services, relates specifically to SDOH: "Create social, physical, and economic environments that promote attaining the full potential for health and well-being for all." The program focuses on helping more people achieve economic stability through employment programs, career counseling, and provision of high-quality child care options, as well as through policies to help individuals secure quality food and stable housing and access health care and education.

Education Access and Quality

Higher education is strongly associated with improved health outcomes, positive health behaviors, and increased life expectancy. Early childhood education and primary and secondary education are key determinants of future health; therefore, addressing disparities in education access and quality as early as possible in life is critical.

Poor health literacy is associated with poor medical adherence, decreased utilization of preventive services, and increased mortality. When educational material is given to patients, it is necessary to understand the health literacy level of the target population and tailor this material accordingly.

Neighborhood and Built Environment

The neighborhood and built environment in which individuals live, learn, work, and play have a direct impact on health and well-being. High rates of crime and violence; unsafe air or water; poor walkability; and limited access to healthful food options, parks, playgrounds, healthy work environments, or transportation are some of the numerous factors that can negatively affect health outcomes. The Area Deprivation Index (ADI) is a metric derived from 17 US census variables—including education, employment, income, household characteristics, and housing—to assess the level of socioeconomic disadvantage by neighborhood.

Ophthalmic considerations In underserved urban communities, patients with a high school education or less are significantly less likely to have had a recent eye examination compared with those with greater than a high school education. They are also more likely to report difficulties with insurance and transportation and lack of knowledge as barriers to eye care.

A recent study by Yusuf and colleagues found that living in more disadvantaged neighborhoods, as measured by the ADI, is associated with nonadherence to first-time ophthalmology referrals for diabetic retinopathy screenings.

Yusuf R, Chen EM, Nwanyanwu K, Richards B. Neighborhood deprivation and adherence to initial diabetic retinopathy screening. *Ophthalmol Retina.* 2020;4(5):550–552.

Social and Community Context

Social, family, and community networks serve as important support systems for individuals and thus can significantly affect health outcomes. Factors such as civic participation, social cohesion, and community engagement can have positive health effects by reducing stress. Community engagement by health care providers may improve patient-provider relationships and build trust among patients. Research indicates that when patients and physicians are of the same ethnicity, patients report greater satisfaction with their treatment and improved communication. Although recent US census data show that underrepresented minority groups make up 30.7% of the US population, only 6% of practicing ophthalmologists are from these groups. Increasing the diversity of the ophthalmologic workforce may help improve patient outcomes for underserved populations.

Discrimination and Social Determinants of Health

Discrimination is a socially structured action resulting in the unfair treatment of individuals or groups based on their ethnicity, gender, sexual orientation, age, disability, religion, or other factors. This discrimination can significantly affect the health of different population groups, including ethnic minority groups; women; lesbian, gay, bisexual, transgender, and queer (LGBTQ+) individuals; older adults; and individuals with disabilities.

Ethnicity

Discrimination based on ethnicity, one definition of *racism,* is a major driver of SDOH and results in significant disparities in health outcomes for minority groups. In 2020, the American Medical Association adopted a policy that recognizes racism as a public health threat, and the organization committed to actively working to dismantle racist policies and practices across all of health care. Racism exists in different forms (eg, internalized, interpersonal, systemic), can manifest in various ways (eg, stereotypes, beliefs), and can be intentional or unintentional.

The effects of ethnicity and ethnic discrimination on SDOH are complex, multidimensional, and interrelated. For example, in the United States, ethnic minority groups are disproportionately affected by poverty (SDOH: economic stability). Individuals affected by poverty are more likely to have lower levels of education (SDOH: education). They are also more likely to live in neighborhoods with high rates of crime (SDOH: social and community context) and poor access to resources such as nutritious foods, safe outdoor spaces for exercise, and clean water (SDOH: neighborhood and built environment). All of these factors adversely affect health, quality of life, and health outcomes.

Gender

Gender is a social construct that refers to the roles and expectations attributed to men and women in society and evolves with time. The World Health Organization recognizes that gender is an important factor affecting SDOH, as gender inequality leads to health risks for women globally, and unbalanced power relations between men and women affect health-seeking behavior and health outcomes.

Sexual Orientation and Gender Identity

Research has demonstrated that LGBTQ+ individuals experience worse health outcomes than heterosexual individuals, and they have high rates of mental illness and substance abuse, beginning in adolescence. Factors such as societal stigma and harassment, lack of cultural competency among health care providers, and low rates of insurance coverage together contribute to the overall health burden in this population. LGBTQ+ individuals who are members of ethnic minority groups face even greater health disparities.

Age and Disability

Older adults and individuals with disabilities are particularly vulnerable to discrimination and its consequences. Older adults are more susceptible to illness and chronic disease with aging, but many face considerable barriers such as limited income and physical and cognitive limitations, in addition to discrimination. Adults with disabilities are more likely than those without disabilities to report their health to be fair or poor and to report higher rates of obesity, lack of physical activity, and smoking.

Approaches to Address Social Determinants of Health

Ophthalmologists can play an important role in addressing SDOH in vulnerable patient populations. Various strategies can be used:

- *Assess the impact of SDOH in patients' lives as part of every patient encounter.* Similar to the way that the history of the present illness, medical/ocular history, and other patient information are obtained, ophthalmologists and their health care teams can assess the role of SDOH in the lives of their patients, how SDOH might affect patient health, and how health care can more effectively be provided. A suggested screening tool, provided by the American Academy of Family Physicians, is available at https://www.aafp.org/dam/AAFP/documents/patient_care/everyone_project/hops19-physician-guide-sdoh.pdf.
- *Address biases in your practice.* How are people of a lower socioeconomic status or lower education or literacy level viewed? By acknowledging potential bias, ophthalmologists can work to mitigate the effects it may have on patient care. Consider taking an Implicit Association Test (implicit.harvard.edu) to illuminate your own unconscious bias.
- *Provide patient-centered care based on the principles of empathy, curiosity, and respect.* Consider the patient's culture and the possible roles of communication styles; mistrust and prejudice; family dynamics and decision making; traditions, customs, and spirituality; and sexual orientation and gender issues.
- *Integrate patient social support structures into your practice.* Empower other members of your team to identify and address SDOH. Provide support such as parking or transportation vouchers.
- *Improve access to care and quality of care.* This includes strategies such as improving patient-physician communication and patient health literacy and reducing cultural and linguistic barriers (see the section Health Care Access and Quality). It may be helpful to do a quality assurance assessment of your practice to identify any disparities in the care being provided to patients.

Carrillo JE, Green AR, Betancourt JR. Cross-cultural primary care: a patient-based approach. *Ann Intern Med.* 1999;130(10):829–834.

Elam AR, Lee PP. High-risk populations for vision loss and eye care underutilization: a review of the literature and ideas on moving forward. *Surv Ophthalmol.* 2013;58(4):348–358.

Goyal A, Richards C, Patel V, et al. The Vision Detroit project: visual burden, barriers, and access to eye care in an urban setting. *Ophthalmic Epidemiol.* 2021 Feb 12:1–12.

Healthy People 2030. US Department of Health and Human Services, Office of Disease Prevention and Health Promotion. Accessed May 19, 2021. https://health.gov/healthypeople/objectives-and-data/social-determinants-health

O'Reilly KB. AMA: Racism is a threat to public health. American Medical Association. November 16, 2020. Accessed May 19, 2021. https://www.ama-assn.org/delivering-care/health-equity/ama-racism-threat-public-health

Uhr JH, Chawla H, Williams BK Jr, Cavuoto KM, Sridhar J. Racial and socioeconomic disparities in visual impairment in the United States. *Ophthalmology.* 2021;128(7):1102–1104.

World Health Organization. Commission on Social Determinants of Health. *Closing the Gap in a Generation: Health Equity Through Action on the Social Determinants of Health. Final Report.* World Health Organization; 2008.

Basic Texts

General Medicine

Access Medicine [database online]. New York, NY. McGraw-Hill Medical; 2019. https://accessmedicine.mhmedical.com. Accessed September 10, 2021.

Advanced Cardiovascular Life Support Provider Manual. Dallas: American Heart Association; 2011.

Bhat P, Dretler A, Gdowski M, Ramgopal R, Williams D, eds. *The Washington Manual of Medical Therapeutics.* 35th ed. Philadelphia: Wolters Kluwer; 2016.

Blaser MJ, Bennett JE, Dolin R, eds. *Mandell, Douglas, and Bennett's Principles and Practice of Infectious Diseases.* 8th ed. Philadelphia: Elsevier/Saunders; 2015.

Bonow RO, Libby P, Mann DL, Zipes DP, Tomaselli GF, eds. *Braunwald's Heart Disease: A Textbook of Cardiovascular Medicine.* 11th ed. Philadelphia: Elsevier; 2019.

Bope ET, Kellerman RD, eds. *Conn's Current Therapy 2018.* Philadelphia: Elsevier/Saunders; 2018.

DeVita VT Jr, Lawrence TS, Rosenberg SA, eds. *DeVita, Hellman, and Rosenberg's Cancer: Principles and Practice of Oncology.* 11th ed. Philadelphia: Lippincott Williams & Wilkins; 2018.

Firestein GS, Budd RC, Gabriel SE, McInnes IB, O'Dell JR, eds. *Kelley & Firestein's Textbook of Rheumatology.* 10th ed. Philadelphia: Elsevier/Saunders; 2017.

Goldman L, Schafer AI, eds. *Goldman's Cecil Medicine.* 25th ed. Philadelphia: Elsevier/Saunders; 2015.

Ham RJ, Sloane PD, Warshaw GA, Potter JF, Flaherty E, eds. *Ham's Primary Care Geriatrics.* 6th ed. Philadelphia: Elsevier/Saunders; 2014.

Hochberg MC, Gravallese EM, Silman AJ, Smolen JS, Weinblatt ME, Weisman MH, eds. *Rheumatology.* 7th ed. Philadelphia: Elsevier; 2019.

Longo DL, Fauci AS, Kasper DL, Hauser SL, Jameson JL, Loscalzo J, eds. *Harrison's Principles of Internal Medicine.* 20th ed. New York: McGraw-Hill; 2018.

Louis ED, Mayer SA, Rowland LP. *Merritt's Neurology.* 13th ed. Philadelphia: Wolters Kluwer; 2016.

McGill JB, Henderson KE, Clutter WE, Baranski TJ, eds. *The Washington Manual Endocrinology Subspecialty Consult.* 3rd ed. Philadelphia: Lippincott Williams & Wilkins; 2012.

Melmed S, Polonsky KS, Larsen PR, Kronenberg HM, eds. *Williams Textbook of Endocrinology.* 13th ed. Philadelphia: Elsevier/Saunders; 2016.

Miller RD, Cohen NH, Eriksson LI, Fleisher LA, Wiener-Kronish JP, Young WL, eds. *Miller's Anesthesia.* 8th ed. Philadelphia: Elsevier/Saunders; 2015.

Papadakis MA, McPhee SJ, Rabow MW, eds. *Current Medical Diagnosis and Treatment 2019.* 58th ed. New York: McGraw-Hill; 2019.

Plotkin SA, Orenstein WA, Offit PA, Edwards KM. *Plotkin's Vaccines.* 7th ed. Philadelphia: Elsevier; 2018.

Porter RS. *The Merck Manual of Diagnosis and Therapy.* 20th ed. Whitehouse Station, New Jersey: Merck Sharp & Dohme Corp; 2018.

PubMed [database online]. Bethesda, MD. National Center for Biotechnology Information, US National Library of Medicine, National Institutes of Health; 2021. https://pubmed.ncbi.nlm.nih.gov. Accessed September 10, 2021.

Ropper AH, Samuels MA, Klein JP, eds. *Adams and Victor's Principles of Neurology.* 10th ed. New York: McGraw-Hill; 2014.

Stern TA, Fava M, Wilens TE, Rosenbaum JF. *Massachusetts General Hospital Comprehensive Clinical Psychiatry.* 2nd ed. Philadelphia: Elsevier; 2016.

Stommel M, Dontje KJ. *Statistics for Advanced Practice Nurses and Health Professionals.* New York: Springer; 2014.

UpToDate [database online]. Waltham, MA. Wolters Kluwer; 2019. www.uptodate.com. Accessed February 27, 2019.

Volberding PA, Sande MA, Lange J, Greene WC, Gallant JE, eds. *Global HIV/AIDS Medicine.* Philadelphia: Elsevier/Saunders; 2008.

Related Academy Materials

The American Academy of Ophthalmology is dedicated to providing a wealth of high-quality clinical education resources for ophthalmologists.

Print Publications and Electronic Products

For a complete listing of Academy products related to topics covered in this BCSC Section, visit our online store at http://store.aao.org/clinical-education/topic/comprehensive-ophthalmology.html. Or call Customer Service at 866.561.8558 (toll free, US only) or +1 415.561.8540, Monday through Friday, between 8:00 AM and 5:00 PM (PST).

Online Resources

Visit the Ophthalmic News and Education (ONE®) Network at https://www.aao.org/comprehensive-ophthalmology to find relevant videos, online courses, journal articles, practice guidelines, self-assessment quizzes, images, and more. The ONE Network is a free Academy-member benefit.

Access free, trusted articles and content with the Academy's collaborative online encyclopedia, EyeWiki, at aao.org/eyewiki.

Get mobile access to the *Wills Eye Manual,* watch the latest 1-minute videos, and set up alerts for clinical updates relevant to you with the AAO Ophthalmic Education App. Download today: Search for "AAO Ophthalmic Education" in the Apple app store or in Google Play.

Requesting Continuing Medical Education Credit

The American Academy of Ophthalmology is accredited by the Accreditation Council for Continuing Medical Education (ACCME) to provide continuing medical education for physicians.

The American Academy of Ophthalmology designates this enduring material for a maximum of 10 *AMA PRA Category 1 Credits*™. Physicians should claim only the credit commensurate with the extent of their participation in the activity.

To claim *AMA PRA Category 1 Credits*™ upon completion of this activity, learners must demonstrate appropriate knowledge and participation in the activity by taking the posttest for Section 1 and achieving a score of 80% or higher.

This activity meets the Self-Assessment CME requirements defined by the American Board of Ophthalmology (ABO). Please be advised that the ABO is not an accrediting body for purposes of any CME program. ABO does not sponsor this or any outside activity, and ABO does not endorse any particular CME activity. Complete information regarding the ABO Self-Assessment CME Maintenance of Certification requirements is available at https://abop.org/maintain-certification/cme-self-assessment/.

To take the posttest and request CME credit online:

1. Go to www.aao.org/cme-central and log in.
2. Click on "Claim CME Credit and View My CME Transcript" and then "Report AAO Credits."
3. Select the appropriate media type and then the Academy activity. You will be directed to the posttest.
4. Once you have passed the test with a score of 80% or higher, you will be directed to your transcript. *If you are not an Academy member, you will be able to print out a certificate of participation once you have passed the test.*

CME expiration date: June 1, 2023. *AMA PRA Category 1 Credits*™ may be claimed only once between June 1, 2019, and the expiration date.

For assistance, contact the Academy's Customer Service department at 866-561-8558 (US only) or +1 415-561-8540 between 8:00 AM and 5:00 PM (PST), Monday through Friday, or send an e-mail to customer_service@aao.org.

Study Questions

Please note that these questions are not part of your CME reporting process. They are provided here for your own educational use and identification of any professional practice gaps. The required CME posttest is available online (see "Requesting CME Credit"). Following the questions are a blank answer sheet and answers with discussions. Although a concerted effort has been made to avoid ambiguity and redundancy in these questions, the authors recognize that differences of opinion may occur regarding the "best" answer. The discussions are provided to demonstrate the rationale used to derive the answer. They may also be helpful in confirming that your approach to the problem was correct or, if necessary, in fixing the principle in your memory. The Section 1 faculty thanks the Self-Assessment Committee for developing these self-assessment questions.

1. What type of study design offers the highest level of evidence?
   a. randomized controlled double-masked study
   b. meta-analysis
   c. case-control study
   d. cohort study

2. A theoretical intervention produces a 20% absolute risk reduction in cases of worsening multiple sclerosis. How many multiple sclerosis patients would have to receive this treatment in order to prevent the worsening of the disease in 1 patient?
   a. 20
   b. 10
   c. 5
   d. 2

3. What is the most frequent psychiatric disorder seen in the older population?
   a. depression
   b. schizophrenia
   c. bipolar disorder
   d. dementia

4. What class of medications commonly used in older patients has been associated with an increased incidence of inflammatory eye disease?
   a. bisphosphonates
   b. anticoagulants
   c. thiazide diuretics
   d. HMG CoA reductase inhibitors (ie, statins)

5. What is the lifetime risk of developing a major depressive disorder in women, as compared to men?
   a. The risk for women is 4 times the risk for men.
   b. The risk for women is about twice that for men.
   c. Women and men are at equal risk of developing a major depressive disorder.
   d. The risk for women is half the risk for men.

6. A former nurse presents with a white cornea, blurred vision, a central corneal abrasion and minimal to no pain. She has no evidence of vesicles or rash on her face, and there are no dendrites or pseudodendrites on her cornea. She denies experiencing any trauma, stating that these changes have developed slowly over time. She volunteers in a emergency department twice a month. After numerous examinations, the ophthalmologist determines that the patient has factitious disorder. What treatment is recommended for this somatization?
   a. antianxiety medication
   b. antipsychotic medication
   c. electroconvulsive therapy
   d. psychotherapy

7. What varicella-zoster vaccine may be safe for use in immunocompromised patients?
   a. Varivax
   b. Shingrix
   c. Zostavax
   d. ProQuad

8. Given the basic tenets of screening for prevention of disease, what scenario best exemplifies appropriate screening?
   a. A healthy 6-year-old child receives a vision test at school.
   b. A 70-year-old woman with normal results from an eye examination receives antibody testing for myasthenia gravis.
   c. A 15-year-old sexually inactive girl receives a rapid plasma reagin (RPR) test.
   d. A healthy 80-year-old man traveling to Saudi Arabia receives the meningococcus vaccine.

9. What virus has been associated with Burkitt lymphoma and nasopharyngeal carcinoma?
   a. herpes simplex virus
   b. Epstein-Barr virus
   c. cytomegalovirus
   d. hepatitis B virus

10. What agent, used in the treatment of neovascular age-related macular degeneration, works by serving as a decoy vascular endothelial growth factor (VEGF) receptor?
    a. bevacizumab
    b. aflibercept
    c. ranibizumab
    d. pegaptanib

11. A healthy 52-year-old former nuclear submarine engineer asks about whether his prior occupation exposed him to any health risks. What complication associated with radiation exposure is most likely to be observed on slit-lamp examination?
    a. nuclear sclerosis
    b. punctate epithelial erosions
    c. cotton-wool spots
    d. optic nerve head hemorrhage

12. What is a life-threatening complication of toxoplasmosis in immunocompromised patients?
    a. disease reactivation
    b. chorioretinitis
    c. lymphadenopathy
    d. encephalitis

13. What severe neurological sequelae can occur following varicella-zoster virus reactivation?
    a. Guillain-Barré syndrome
    b. unilateral vesicular eruption
    c. postherpetic neuralgia
    d. Stevens-Johnson syndrome

14. Hemorrhagic conjunctivitis is a presenting sign of what virus?
    a. herpes simplex virus
    b. varicella-zoster virus
    c. Ebola virus
    d. cytomegalovirus

15. What procedure described in the Universal Protocol of the Joint Commission is designed to eliminate wrong-site surgery?
    a. confirming 2 patient identifiers prior to the start of the case
    b. confirming at the end of the case that the procedure described on the consent form was the procedure actually performed
    c. identifying all of the people in the operating room and their roles prior to the start of the case
    d. stating the level of fire risk prior to the start of the case

16. What raises suspicion for susceptibility to malignant hyperthermia, a potentially lethal complication of anesthesia?
    a. diagnosis of Noonan syndrome, osteogenesis imperfecta, or neuroleptic malignant syndrome
    b. history of exertional or heat-induced rhabdomyolysis
    c. negative history of malignant hyperthermia with prior anesthesia
    d. muscle biopsy with negative muscle contracture evaluation

17. How should anticoagulants/antiplatelet agents be managed for most routine cataract surgeries performed via a clear corneal incision with topical anesthesia?
    a. Warfarin should be discontinued prior to surgery.
    b. Direct anticoagulants, such as apixaban or dabigatran, should be discontinued prior to surgery.
    c. Dual antiplatelet therapy (aspirin plus clopidogrel) prescribed after a drug-eluting stent placement should be discontinued prior to surgery.
    d. Anticoagulants and antiplatelet agents can be continued.

18. After the onset of symptoms of a suspected ischemic stroke, fibrinolytic therapy should be instituted within what time period?
    a. 1 hour
    b. 3 hours
    c. 6 hours
    d. 12 hours

19. What is 1 of the main products of the posterior pituitary?
    a. growth hormone–releasing hormone
    b. vasopressin
    c. dopamine
    d. thyrotropin-releasing hormone

20. Multiple endocrine neoplasia (MEN) syndromes are rare hereditary syndromes of benign and malignant neoplasms. What feature is commonly seen in cases of MEN 2A and 2B but is not commonly seen in MEN 1?
    a. hyperparathyroidism
    b. gastrinomas
    c. pituitary adenomas
    d. medullary thyroid cancer

21. Use of β-blockers should be avoided in patients with what condition?
    a. systolic heart failure
    b. reactive airway disease
    c. atrial fibrillation
    d. essential tremor

22. Certain signs of hypertensive retinopathy, independent of other risk factors, are associated with increased cardiovascular risk. What sign has a strong association with death from cardiovascular causes?
    a. focal arteriolar narrowing
    b. arteriovenous nicking
    c. copper wiring
    d. cotton-wool spot

23. What lipoprotein is protective against atherosclerosis?
    a. very-low-density lipoprotein (VLDL)
    b. low-density lipoprotein (LDL)
    c. intermediate-density lipoprotein (IDL)
    d. high-density lipoprotein (HDL)

24. What lipid profile is recommended to decrease the risk of cardiovascular disease?
    a. high LDL and low HDL levels
    b. low LDL and high HDL levels
    c. high LDL and high HDL levels
    d. low LDL and low HDL levels

25. An 80-year-old man who takes an oral anticoagulant to treat chronic atrial fibrillation needs emergency surgery. What agent is reversible with an antibody?
    a. apixaban
    b. dabigatran
    c. rivaroxaban
    d. warfarin

26. An 80-year-old woman with heart failure with a reduced ejection fraction (HFrEF) remains symptomatic despite taking diuretics, a β-blocker, and an angiotensin-converting enzyme (ACE) inhibitor. What drug could be added to her existing medications that acts by a mechanism other than decreasing afterload?
    a. amiodarone
    b. amlodipine
    c. digoxin
    d. hydralazine

27. What oral antithrombotic agent works by preventing factor Xa from cleaving prothrombin to thrombin?
    a. clopidogrel
    b. warfarin
    c. rivaroxaban
    d. aspirin

28. A 65-year-old man with diabetes and hypertension is brought to the emergency department 2 hours after the onset of weakness on the right side. What imaging study is the most important in guiding acute management?
    a. brain magnetic resonance imaging (MRI)
    b. cerebral angiography
    c. noncontrast head computed tomography (CT)
    d. transcranial Doppler ultrasonography

29. A 60-year-old woman presents with the sudden onset of left-sided eye pain accompanied by ipsilateral ptosis, impaired ocular motility–sparing abduction, and a fixed and dilated pupil. What are head imaging studies most likely to show?
    a. intracerebral hemorrhage
    b. intraventricular hemorrhage
    c. saccular aneurysm
    d. arteriovenous malformation

30. A 52-year-old man is brought to the emergency department with a 3-hour history of severe headache, accompanied by altered mental status and decreased vision in his right eye. His medical history includes chronic hypertension. Dilated fundus examination of the right eye reveals a vitreous hemorrhage obscuring the posterior pole. The peripheral retina is appears normal. What is the most important diagnostic tool?
    a. B-scan ultrasonography
    b. CT of the brain
    c. urine toxicology tests
    d. serum erythrocyte sedimentation rate (ESR) and C-reactive protein (CRP) tests

31. A 48-year-old woman presents with a history of total, painless loss of vision affecting her right eye and lasting approximately 10 minutes. The left eye was unaffected, and there were no prodromal symptoms. The episode occurred 6 hours prior to presentation. Her ocular examination is normal, and her visual acuity is 20/20 in both eyes. She recently had an annual physical examination that was unremarkable, and she takes no medications. What is the most appropriate management?
    a. observation only unless the symptoms recur
    b. urgent referral for cardiac and carotid imaging
    c. urgent referral for neuroimaging
    d. observation with repeat dilated examination in 4 weeks

32. A patient with a history of rheumatoid arthritis presents with severe dry eye. On review of systems, she reports a chronic, nonproductive cough and intermittent difficulty breathing. Pulmonary function tests reveal reduced total lung capacity. This constellation of symptoms is indicative of potential complications related to what medication?
    a. hydroxychloroquine
    b. methotrexate
    c. losartan
    d. prednisone

33. An obese patient reports the recent onset of extreme ocular discomfort and dryness upon awakening in the morning. What finding might elicit the etiology of the complaint?
    a. snoring
    b. dyspnea and walking up a flight of stairs
    c. swelling in the ankles
    d. abdominal bloating

34. A 43-year-old patient with a long history of asthma and multiple flare-ups presents with a progressive decrease in vision. The patient's visual acuity is 20/50, and dark defects are noted on retinoscopy. What long-term medication used in the treatment of this patient's asthma has most likely caused his ophthalmic findings?
    a. corticosteroids
    b. long-acting β_2-agonists
    c. leukotriene inhibitors
    d. anticholinergic agents

35. During a routine eye examination, multiple telangiectatic lesions are found on a patient's lips. Some lesions are also present on the palpebral conjunctiva. The patient reports that the lip lesions sometimes bleed spontaneously or with minimal trauma. What disorder is consistent with these findings?
    a. Rendu-Osler-Weber disease
    b. Ehlers-Danlos syndrome
    c. osteogenesis imperfecta
    d. pseudoxanthoma elasticum

36. A patient with sickle cell anemia comes in for an examination. On examination, the ophthalmologist finds no ophthalmic manifestations. How often should the patient be re-evaluated?
    a. monthly
    b. yearly
    c. every 5 years
    d. only when symptomatic

37. What is the most common ocular manifestation of systemic lupus erythematosus (SLE)?
    a. retinal vascular occlusion
    b. discoid eyelid skin lesions
    c. sixth cranial nerve palsy
    d. keratoconjunctivitis sicca

38. A 65-year-old White man reports blurry vision. He has a known diagnosis of polymyalgia rheumatica and has recently experienced pain when chewing and tenderness when combing his hair. An urgent workup for what disease is indicated?
    a. optic neuritis
    b. embolic occlusion of the ophthalmic artery
    c. giant cell arteritis
    d. cavernous sinus syndrome

39. What is the most common symptom of Behçet disease?
    a. oral ulcers
    b. skin disease
    c. genital ulcers
    d. central nervous system disease

Answer Sheet for Section 1
Study Questions

Question	Answer	Question	Answer
1	a b c d	21	a b c d
2	a b c d	22	a b c d
3	a b c d	23	a b c d
4	a b c d	24	a b c d
5	a b c d	25	a b c d
6	a b c d	26	a b c d
7	a b c d	27	a b c d
8	a b c d	28	a b c d
9	a b c d	29	a b c d
10	a b c d	30	a b c d
11	a b c d	31	a b c d
12	a b c d	32	a b c d
13	a b c d	33	a b c d
14	a b c d	34	a b c d
15	a b c d	35	a b c d
16	a b c d	36	a b c d
17	a b c d	37	a b c d
18	a b c d	38	a b c d
19	a b c d	39	a b c d
20	a b c d		

Answers

1. **b.** Meta-analyses offer the highest level of evidence because they provide a methodology to analyze the data of multiple clinical trials. Case-control and cohort studies are observational studies that are useful for describing the presentation and progression of a disease, generating hypotheses, or using existing data to test hypotheses. Prospective randomized controlled double-masked studies provide better evidence regarding the effects of an intervention.
2. **c.** The number needed to treat (NNT) is helpful when describing how likely a treatment or medication will improve an outcome for an individual patient. If the absolute risk reduction is 20%, the NNT is 5 (100/20). In other words, a clinician could describe to their patient that they would need to treat 5 patients with this theoretical treatment to prevent 1 patient from developing worsening multiple sclerosis.
3. **a.** Depression is the most frequent psychiatric problem in the older population. Approximately one-quarter of older patients seen in primary care settings are clinically depressed. The prevalence of depression in patients with macular degeneration is even higher, at 30%–40%. Although dementia is common in persons older than 80 years, dementia is not a normal part of the aging process. Schizophrenia usually begins when patients are young and continues to a greater or lesser extent throughout their lives. Bipolar disorder has an average age of onset of 25 years and is found in approximately 4% of people.
4. **a.** Bisphosphonates are often prescribed to postmenopausal women to inhibit bone resorption. These drugs have been associated with inflammatory disease of the eye, including conjunctivitis, uveitis, and episcleritis. Scleritis, which can be vision threatening, has also been reported.
5. **b.** The lifetime risk of developing a major depressive disorder for women is 17%, which is almost twice that of men, who have a 9% risk.
6. **d.** Somatic disorders (conversion disorder; illness anxiety disorders, including body dysmorphic disorder; factitious disorder) are classified in the *Diagnostic and Statistical Manual of Mental Disorders,* Fifth Edition (DSM–5), as somatic symptom and related disorders. This term describes a syndrome of symptoms suggesting physical illness or injury in the absence of objective findings or a known physiological mechanism, following appropriate investigation. The prevalence of somatic disorders in the general population is around 6%. Associated risk factors are female sex, lower socioeconomic level, and minority ethnic status. In this scenario, the patient has been diagnosed with factitious disorder (previously known as Munchausen syndrome), which is characterized by the willful production, feigning, or exaggeration of physical or psychological signs or symptoms in the absence of external causes. Topical anesthetic abuse should be treated accordingly, and the patient should be referred to a psychotherapist. Although no medications are indicated specifically for the disorder, coexisting mental health disorders (eg, depression or substance abuse) may require prescribed psychotropic agents.
7. **b.** Shingrix is an effective inactivated recombinant zoster vaccine that was approved by the United States Food and Drug Administration (FDA) in 2017 for adults aged 50 or older to reduce the incidence of varicella-zoster virus (VZV) infection. It does not contain live virus and therefore may be safe in immunocompromised patients. Varivax is a live, attenuated varicella-zoster vaccine that is recommended for immunocompetent pediatric

patients older than 12 months with no history of previous infection with VZV, or for health care workers not previously exposed to varicella. Zostavax is another live, attenuated zoster vaccine that was previously recommended to reduce the risk of VZV infection and postherpetic neuralgia in adults. However, Zostavax appears to be less effective than Shingrix, and it cannot be used in adults receiving high-level immunosuppressive therapy. Neither Shingrix nor Zostavax can be used in place of Varivax in younger persons. Zostavax is no longer available in the United States as of November 2020. ProQuad is a combination vaccine for measles, mumps, rubella, and chickenpox (also called MMRV). It contains the same live, attenuated vaccine as Varivax.

8. **a.** Screening for nonresearch purposes is useful if the disease in question is detectable with some measurable degree of reliability, is treatable or preventable, is significant because of its impact (prevalence or severity), is progressive, and is generally asymptomatic (or has symptoms a patient might deny or might not recognize). The scenario that fits these principles best is the 6-year-old child who receives a vision test at school. It fits the tenets of a good screening test because childhood refractive error is common and treatable. Screening can detect amblyopia, which may otherwise go undetected until development of strabismus or vision problems are noticed by a school teacher. In contrast, it is inappropriate for a 70-year-old woman with no ocular findings to receive antibody testing for myasthenia gravis, because it is a relatively rare disease; thus, testing for this condition should be performed only in patients with suspicious symptoms. Furthermore, the current tests are only 50% sensitive for ocular myasthenia gravis, although specificity raises its utility in a patient with signs of fatigable ptosis or incomitant strabismus. A 15-year-old sexually inactive girl does not need routine screening with a treponemal antibody syphilis test; syphilis is a sexually transmitted infection, and individuals who have not yet been sexually active are not at risk. Finally, the meningococcus vaccine is not a screening test; it is a preventive treatment for an acute and symptomatic disease and is required for persons applying for a visa for travel to Saudi Arabia.

9. **b.** Epstein-Barr virus, the causative agent in infectious mononucleosis, has been associated with Burkitt lymphoma and nasopharyngeal carcinoma. Herpes simplex virus has been associated with carcinoma of the lip and oropharynx, as well as cancer of the uterine cervix, vulva, kidneys, and nasopharynx. Cytomegalovirus has been associated with prostate cancer, Kaposi sarcoma, and carcinoma of the bladder and uterine cervix. Hepatitis B virus has been associated with hepatocellular carcinoma.

10. **b.** Aflibercept is a recombinant fusion protein that acts as a decoy receptor for vascular endothelial growth factor (VEGF). Aflibercept inactivates VEGF-A, VEGF-B, and placental growth factor and is effective in the treatment of neovascular age-related macular degeneration. Bevacizumab is a humanized monoclonal antibody directed against VEGF-A. Pegaptanib is an aptamer that specifically binds the human 165 isoform of VEGF. Ranibizumab is a recombinant humanized antibody fragment that binds all active isoforms of VEGF-A.

11. **a.** The lens is the most radiosensitive structure in the eye, followed by the cornea, the retina, and the optic nerve. Cataract formation is the most likely complication of radiation exposure that would be found in this patient. Low doses of radiation (as low as 2 Gy in 1 fraction) may cause cataract formation, and higher doses of radiation (7–8 Gy and higher) can cause progressive cataracts. The average latent period for the development of radiation-induced cataracts is 2 to 3 years.

    In severe cases, erosion of the corneal epithelium and secondary ulceration may result. Radiation retinopathy clinically resembles diabetic retinopathy; injury occurs first to the capillary vascular endothelium, then the capillary pericytes, and then the endothelium of larger vessels, resulting in ischemic changes. Cotton-wool spots develop first, followed by capillary nonperfusion, then ingrowth of telangiectatic vessels. Radiation optic neuropathy may present with optic nerve head pallor and splinter hemorrhages, but the exposure may also be clinically silent except for symptoms of unilateral headache and ocular pain.

12. **d.** The clinical picture and histopathology of toxoplasmosis are a reflection of the immune response. In immunocompromised patients, reactivation of latent disease can cause life-threatening encephalitis. Primary toxoplasmosis infection is usually subclinical, but in some patients cervical lymphadenopathy or ocular disease can be present. The ocular manifestations include uveitis and chorioretinitis with macular scarring.

13. **a.** Primary VZV infection usually occurs in childhood in the form of chickenpox (varicella), a generalized vesicular rash accompanied by mild constitutional symptoms. Reactivation may be heralded by pain in a sensory nerve distribution, followed by a unilateral vesicular eruption occurring over 1 to 3 dermatomic areas. New crops of lesions appear in the same area within 7 days. Severe neurologic sequelae following VZV reactivation include segmental myelitis, Guillain-Barré syndrome, and Ramsay Hunt syndrome. Postherpetic neuralgia may occur in up to 50% of patients older than 50 years. Stevens-Johnson syndrome is a rare, serious disorder of the skin and mucous membranes usually due to a reaction to a medication or an infection. Often, it begins with flulike symptoms, followed by a painful red or purplish rash that spreads and blisters.

14. **c.** The Ebola virus is contracted through contact with blood or bodily fluids or tissue of infected bats, nonhuman primates, or humans. Ophthalmologists working in endemic areas should suspect Ebola virus infection when patients present with hemorrhagic conjunctivitis. Later ocular findings include retinal scarring, cataracts, and optic neuropathy. The other viruses listed do not typically present with hemorrhagic conjunctivitis.

15. **a.** The Universal Protocol of the Joint Commission, which is designed to eliminate wrong-site surgery, includes performing a time-out before the initiation of surgery, during which the surgical team agree that the patient who is about to undergo a surgical procedure is the correct patient, that the procedure is correct for that patient, and that the correct site is identified. This requires the confirmation of 2 unique patient identifiers that include name, date of birth, and medical record number. In addition, the surgical team must agree on and document the procedure to be performed, and mark the surgical site in the preoperative period. Noting the level of fire risk, identifying the operating room staff, and confirming postoperatively that the planned procedure was completed are not part of the Universal Protocol of the Joint Commission.

16. **b.** Malignant hyperthermia is a genetic disorder in which skeletal muscle exposure to a triggering agent results in hypermetabolic activity and crisis. Factors that raise suspicion for malignant hyperthermia susceptibility include a positive family history, diagnosis of certain muscle disorders (in particular, those associated with ryanodine receptor mutations), or a history of unexpected exertional or heat-induced rhabdomyolysis, or severe statin-induced myopathy. Although Noonan syndrome, osteogenesis imperfecta, neuroleptic malignant syndrome, and myotonias were historically associated with malignant hyperthermia, they are no longer thought to impart a greater risk. A negative personal or family history of malignant hyperthermia does not raise suspicion for this disorder but neither does it rule out susceptibility. Individuals at greater risk for malignant hyperthermia may undergo muscle biopsy for muscle contracture evaluation (caffeine halothane

contracture test). A negative contracture test essentially rules out MH susceptibility. A positive contracture test should be followed by confirmatory genetic analysis.

17. **d.** The decision to maintain or discontinue anticoagulants/antiplatelet agents for ophthalmic surgery is contingent on the type of procedure, the bleeding risk, the effect of bleeding on postoperative outcome, and the risk of a serious or fatal thrombotic event after discontinuation. For uncomplicated cataract surgery via clear corneal incision under topical anesthesia, the benefit of discontinuing anticoagulants to prevent bleeding does not outweigh the potential risks. Studies found an increased risk of ophthalmic bleeding when warfarin was continued in patients undergoing cataract surgery, but the bleeding events were minor and did not impact vision. Continuation of aspirin or clopidogrel had similar findings. Direct-acting anticoagulants (eg, factor Xa inhibitors [apixaban, edoxaban, rivaroxaban] and a thrombin inhibitor [dabigatran]) have a 20% lower risk than warfarin of causing intraocular bleeding during surgery. In an emergent situation, the monoclonal antibody idarucizumab can reverse the effect of dabigatran within 15 minutes. In patients on dual antiplatelet therapy (aspirin plus clopidogrel) after cardiac stent placement, there is increased risk of thrombosis of the stented artery, with potentially fatal outcome if these agents are discontinued. Cataract surgery may be performed in these patients when cessation of anticoagulants is felt to be unnecessary.

18. **b.** The current recommendations are that fibrinolytic therapy should be initiated in a patient with suspected ischemic stroke within 3 hours of onset of symptoms and within 1 hour of arrival at the hospital.

19. **b.** The main products of the posterior pituitary are oxytocin and vasopressin. Growth hormone–releasing hormone, dopamine, and thyrotropin-releasing hormone are involved in anterior pituitary function.

20. **d.** Medullary thyroid cancer is seen in 90%–100% of patients with multiple endocrine neoplasia (MEN) syndrome types 2A and 2B. Hyperparathyroidism, gastrinomas, and pituitary adenomas are commonly seen in MEN 1.

21. **b.** β-Blockers can cause bronchospasm and should thus be avoided in patients with asthma and reactive airway disease. They also cause bradycardia and should be avoided in patients with second- and third-degree atrioventricular blocks. In patients with heart failure due to systolic dysfunction, the use of certain β-blockers reduces hospitalization for heart failure and improves survival rates. β-Blockers are beneficial in the treatment of atrial fibrillation and essential tremor.

22. **d.** In the simplified classification of hypertensive retinopathy, which was proposed in 2004, hypertensive retinopathy is categorized as mild, moderate, or malignant. The presence of retinal hemorrhage, microaneurysm, cotton-wool spot, hard exudates, or a combination of these signs indicates moderate hypertensive retinopathy, which has a strong association with stroke, cognitive decline, and death from cardiovascular causes. Moderate retinopathy plus optic nerve head edema indicates malignant hypertensive retinopathy, which is strongly associated with death. Mild hypertensive retinopathy has a modest association with risk of stroke, coronary disease, and death and is characterized by focal/generalized arteriolar narrowing, arteriovenous nicking, increased opacity of the arteriolar wall ("copper wiring"), or a combination of these signs.

23. **d.** High-density lipoprotein (HDL), or "good cholesterol," is protective against atherosclerosis. It has anti-inflammatory properties and transports cholesterol away from the blood vessel walls to the liver for disposal. Very-low-density lipoproteins (VLDLs) produced by

the liver carry most circulating triglycerides. Intermediate-density lipoproteins (IDLs) are less dense than low-density lipoprotein (LDL) molecules but denser than VLDL particles; some are cleared rapidly into the liver and some are degraded to LDLs. LDL, or "bad cholesterol," is a product of VLDL and IDL metabolism and is the primary carrier of cholesterol.

24. **b.** Current guidelines recommend a high HDL and low LDL concentration to decrease risk of cardiovascular disease. Lipoproteins, which transport cholesterol and triglycerides in the body, are classified based on the relative concentrations of their components. LDL is associated with atherogenesis; lowering LDL levels is associated with a reduction in risk for cardiovascular disease. In contrast, HDL has a protective effect against atherogenesis because it has anti-inflammatory properties and transports cholesterol from blood vessel walls to the liver for disposal.

25. **b.** The direct thrombin inhibitor dabigatran can be reversed with the monoclonal antibody idarucixumab. Warfarin has been a mainstay of anticoagulation treatment for patients with chronic atrial fibrillation, however, new classes of oral anticoagulants offer superior stroke prevention with comparable bleeding risks and without the need for regular international normalized ratio (INR) checks. Although warfarin can be reversed (historically with fresh frozen plasma and vitamin K), many of the new agents are not reversible at this time, including factor Xa inhibitors such as rivaroxaban and apixaban.

26. **c.** Reducing afterload by decreasing vascular resistance and lowering arterial blood pressure is a primary goal in the management of HFrEF. Digoxin is an inotropic agent that can be used to enhance left ventricle contractility in patients with HFrEF who are still symptomatic despite efforts to reduce afterload. Like β-blockers and angiotensin-converting enzyme (ACE) inhibitors, amlodipine and hydralazine both reduce afterload. Although intermittent arrhythmias can impair ventricular function in congestive heart failure (CHF), amiodarone was not effective in a clinical trial.

27. **c.** Rivaroxaban is a factor Xa inhibitor that prevents the cleaving of prothrombin to thrombin. Clopidogrel prevents the activation of glycoprotein IIb/IIIa and inhibits platelet aggregation. Warfarin is a vitamin K antagonist that reduces the synthesis of numerous clotting factors that require vitamin K. Aspirin blocks cyclo-oxygenase and inhibits platelet aggregation.

28. **c.** Multiple studies have shown that the administration of the fibrinolytic agent recombinant tissue plasminogen activator (rtPA) within a 3-hour window of symptom onset results in lower morbidity from ischemic strokes. Imaging with noncontrast head computed tomography (CT) is critical in evaluating for the presence of hemorrhage, which would be a contraindication to rtPA use. Magnetic resonance imaging (MRI) is more sensitive than CT in detecting evolving ischemia within hours of onset, particularly if diffusion-weighted MRI (DWI) with apparent diffusion coefficient (ADC) mapping is used. However, MRI is too time-intensive, considering the limited window during which rtPA can be administered. Cerebral angiography provides detailed information about vascular abnormalities, but it is not indicated in the acute setting and would not reveal either stroke or hemorrhage. Transcranial Doppler ultrasonography may reveal stenosis of the intracranial arteries but is not helpful in making decisions regarding initial management.

29. **c.** The possibility of an aneurysm at the origin of the posterior communicating artery from the internal carotid artery must be urgently evaluated in a patient presenting with a new-onset painful pupil-involving third cranial nerve palsy. Saccular ("berry") aneurysms are the most common cause of subarachnoid hemorrhage (SAH), and the origin

of the posterior communicating artery is a frequently involved site. Intracerebral hemorrhage, which is most commonly due to hypertension, can present with focal neurologic symptoms but a pupil-sparing third cranial nerve palsy would be atypical. Arteriovenous malformations (AVMs) can cause intracerebral hemorrhage as well as SAH. When associated with SAH, AVMs may manifest with focal seizures, progressive worsening of focal neurologic signs, and recurrent unilateral migraine-like headache. Intraventricular hemorrhage usually occurs as a secondary phenomenon in patients with an intracerebral or subarachnoid hemorrhage. It typically manifests with sudden-onset headache, nausea, vomiting, and varying degrees of impaired consciousness.

30. **b.** The presentation of acute-onset headache, altered mental status, and a vitreous hemorrhage is strongly suggestive of Terson syndrome (SAH that causes a subhyaloidal or vitreous hemorrhage). If left untreated, Terson syndrome has a high mortality rate, and the most important diagnostic test is thus neuroimaging with noncontrast CT of the brain. A lumbar puncture is indicated for cases in which the initial CT results are negative but suspicion remains high. Although B-scan ultrasonography may be useful to evaluate the posterior pole, neuroimaging is the most important imaging study for the initial consideration. Serum erythrocyte sedimentation rate (ESR) and C-reactive protein (CRP) tests are useful for the evaluation of suspected giant cell arteritis (GCA); however, this patient's presentation (as well as his younger age and history of hypertension) favor a diagnosis of SAH, not GCA. While urine toxicology tests may be warranted in patients with acute mental status changes, assessing for the presence of an intracranial hemorrhage is the primary consideration.

31. **b.** This patient has recent-onset transient monocular visual loss (TMVL). Patients presenting with new, recent (<48 hours) symptoms of TMVL should undergo urgent assessment for embolic etiology with cardiac and carotid imaging. Neuroimaging is unlikely to be diagnostic in cases of isolated TMVL. Observation without assessment of possible embolic disease is inappropriate because such patients may be at increased risk of stroke or myocardial infarction.

32. **b.** Methotrexate, a medication commonly used to treat rheumatoid arthritis (RA), can cause interstitial lung disease or pneumonitis, both of which reduce total lung capacity, indicating a restrictive lung disease process. Hydroxychloroquine and prednisone are also used to treat RA but have not been associated with restrictive lung disease. Losartan is an angiotensin II receptor blocker used to treat hypertension. It is also used as a second-line agent when patients develop a cough related to ACE inhibitors.

33. **a.** Dry eye syndrome has been reported to increase in patients with obstructive sleep apnea (OSA) syndrome and the use of a nasal continuous positive airway pressure (CPAP) mask. Dry eye syndrome is not associated with dyspnea, walking up stairs, ankle swelling, or abdominal bloating.

34. **a.** Corticosteroid use, especially long-term oral corticosteroid use, is known to potentiate the development of cataracts. Maintenance medications for the treatment of asthma include inhaled corticosteroids, chromones, leukotriene inhibitors, long acting β_2-agonists, anticholinergic agents, and oral corticosteroids. In this patient, the progressive decrease in vision and the dark defects on retinoscopy represent the development of cataracts resulting from long-term oral corticosteroid use.

35. **a.** A number of inherited and acquired disorders of blood vessels and their supporting connective tissues result in pathologic bleeding. Many of these disorders also have ocular

findings. Hereditary hemorrhagic telangiectasia (Rendu-Osler-Weber disease) is an autosomal dominant condition characterized by localized dilation of capillaries and venulae of the skin and mucous membranes. The telangiectasia are often located on the lips and tongue. These lesions increase in size and number over a period of decades. Ehlers-Danlos syndrome is characterized by hyperplastic fragile skin and hyperextensible joints. In patients with osteogenesis imperfecta, bone fractures and otosclerosis (leading to deafness) are common. Pseudoxanthoma elasticum is rare and is often complicated by gastrointestinal hemorrhage.

36. **b.** In sickle cell anemia, abnormal hemoglobin S damages the red blood cell (RBC) membrane and leads to sickling. This can lead to vascular occlusion, often precipitated by infection, dehydration, and/or hypoxia. Sickle cell disease is a systemic multiorgan disease that requires lifelong routine medical care, which includes regular updating of vaccinations, annual ophthalmologic examinations, and screening for hypertension, proteinuria, and pulmonary hypertension.

37. **d.** The most commonly associated ocular manifestation of systemic lupus erythematosus (SLE) is keratoconjunctivitis sicca from secondary Sjögren syndrome. Other ocular manifestations include retinal vascular occlusions, discoid skin lesions involving the eyelid, and cranial nerve palsies.

38. **c.** Approximately 10% of patients with polymyalgia rheumatica eventually develop the vasculitis underlying GCA. Symptoms include jaw claudication and scalp tenderness. Optic nerve insult may result from GCA, but it is an ischemic event rather than an inflammatory etiology, as with various causes of optic neuritis. GCA can be associated with retinal arterial occlusions, but an embolic workup is not indicated in this clinical scenario, because GCA-associated occlusion would result from local inflammatory damage to the vessel. Cavernous sinus syndrome would present with orbital apex impairment symptoms, including ophthalmoplegia and proptosis.

39. **a.** A multisystem vasculitis of unknown etiology, Behçet disease is most common in the Middle East and Asia. Oral ulcers occur in more than 95% of patients with Behçet disease, whereas genital ulcers and skin disease occur in about 75%, and central nervous system disease in about 20%.

Index

(*f* = figure; *t* = table)